Direct Microscopy in Gynecological Practice

Diagnostic Principles and Colposcopic Correlates

Giovanni Miniello

Direct Microscopy in Gynecological Practice

Diagnostic Principles and Colposcopic Correlates

edra

Publishing Manager: Costanza Smeraldi
Senior Editor: Arianna Ribichesu

Production Manager: Matteo Brambilla
Books Project Manager: Chiara Cucinella

Paper, Print and Binding Manager: Michele Ribatti

Cover: Paolo Ballerini

Illustrations: Giovanni Miniello

ISBN 978-88-2144-461-6
eISBN 978-88-2144-462-3

Knowledge and best practice in this field are constantly changing: As new research and experience broaden our knowledge, changes in practice, treatment, and drug therapy may become necessary or appropriate. Readers are advised to check the most current information provided (i) or procedures featured or (ii) by the manufacturer of each product to be administered, to verify the recommended dose or formula, the method and duration of administration, and contraindications. It is the responsibility of the practitioners, relying on their own experience and knowledge of the patient, to make diagnoses, to determine dosages and the best treatment for each individual patient, and to take all appropriate safety precautions. To the fullest extent of the law, neither the Publisher nor the Editors assume any liability for any injury and/or damage to persons or property arising out of or related to any use of the material contained in this book.

Edra S.p.A.
Via G. Spadolini 7, 20141 Milano
Tel. 02 881841
www.edizioniedra.it

Printed in Italy in April 2017 by LITOGRAFTODI srl, Todi (PG)

(*) Edra S.p.A. is part of LSWR GROUP

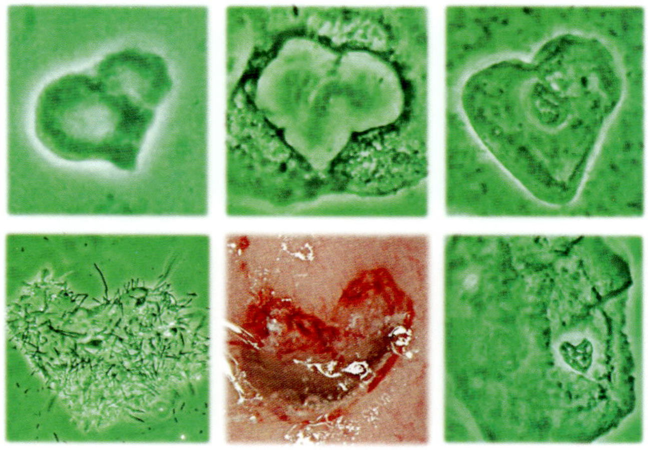

To my women
From the roots
to the buds

FOREWORD

It is a great pleasure for me to write a Foreword for this very interesting Atlas on Direct Microscopy.
The author and I have been involved in the cytology and colposcopy for over 25 years. We have contributed to introducing cytology in the diagnostic armamentarium of Gynecologists. We have witnessed the "revolution" caused by Pap smear, which decreased the incidence and mortality of invasive cervical cancer in some parts of the world.
We also learned to use the simple techniques like direct microscopy through phase contrast microscopy to rapidly identify hormonal disorders like amenorrhoea and infertility during a routine gynecological consultation. Other issues helped us understand that blood levels of circulating hormones or the presence of HPV virus are not the only elements reflected in the cellular pattern. Tissue receptors and their functionality, bioavailability of hormones and the diagnosis of cell metabolism and innate cell immunity all are key players. Finally, it is the end organ response which will need to be addressed and treated. Herein lies the innate value of cytology which alone indicates the end organ response to hormones or infective agents.
The author has dealt in details with all the patterns seen in health and disease. The text and diagrams are easy to follow and will certainly provide any clinician with an insight into the world of cellular response. Photographs are of exceptional quality, as usual.
Phase contrast microscopy is a new tool in the hands of clinicians. Without any laboratory support, staining, fixing, etc., this technique makes it possible to observe the floating cells and the organism and to formulate a diagnosis in 5 minutes. This atlas was written by a world renowned expert in phase contrast microscopy and will open up a new perspective for younger generations of clinicians who believe in evidence based medicine.
After Fritz Zernike, a Dutch physicist, developed phase contrast microscopy in 1935, this technique started to be employed by many European scientists. In 1953, post World War II, Zernike was awarded the Nobel Prize for this discovery. Since then, it has been gaining ground as a diagnostic tool for body fluids. It is mainly used by gynecologists and urologists.
This publication has great historic value. We must all congratulate the author Prof. Giovanni Miniello for undertaking and completing this atlas, as a gift to future generations.
And to all the readers, I wish them good luck and a pleasant reading. In this era of information technology, the whole world of vaginal cytology will be available to everyone all over the world at the click of a mouse. This is truly a miracle of the 21st century.
With warm personal regards and best wishes to all who made this publication a reality.

Dr. Usha Saraiya

Usha Saraiya

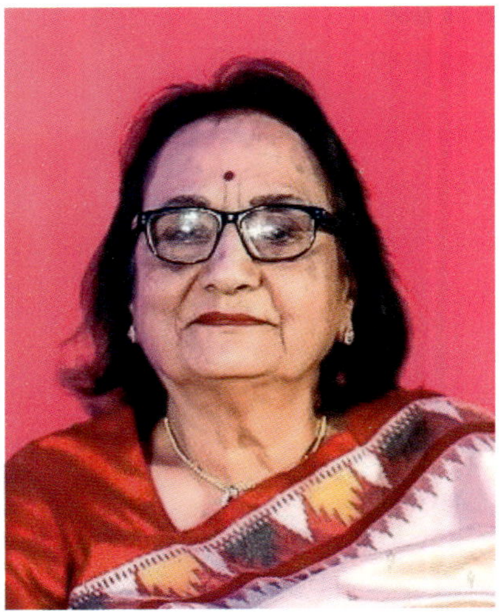

Dr. Usha Saraiya

- Founder Member & President 1984 – 86 Indian Academy of Cytologists.
- Colposcopy Recognition Award by American Society of Cervical Pathology & Colposcopy 1993
- President Mumbai Obst. & Gyn. Society 1997-1998.
- President, Federation of Obstetrics & Gynaecological Societies of India 2002.
- Chairman - Indian College of Obstetrics & Gynaecology – 2006-2009.
- Awarded Outstanding Woman Obstetrician Gynaecologist Award of FIGO in 2003.
- Dr. B N Purandare outstanding Services Award by MOGS in January 2015.
- Her current appointments include
  - Chairman – Ethics Committee for Clinical Research of the National Institute for Research Reproductive (ICMR)
  - Chairman, Board of Trustees – Mumbai Obstetric and Gynaecological Society (MOGS)
  - Vice President for Medical Women's International Association 2013-2016
- Hon. Member of Polish Obstetric & Gynaecological Society
- Hon. Member of Polish Society of Cervical Pathology & Colposcopy
- Editorial Board Member of Polish Journal of Obstetrician & Gynaecology

CONTENTS

INTRODUCTION

Conquer all the stars
for your trip
but save the last one
for your dreams
g.m.

Direct microscopy was developed in 1935 by a Dutch physicist named Fritz Zernike, on the grounds of Ernst Abbe's studies. Zernike was awarded the Nobel Prize in 1953 for his discovery of the phase contrast phenomenon. Direct microscopy was introduced into gynecological practice only in 1949 by Runge and Voge-Haselman.

This optical technique, which produces high-contrast images of unstained biological specimens, such as living cells and microorganisms, is also called phase contrast (Ph) microscopy or wet mount microscopy. Wet mounts cannot be stored over extended time periods, and for this reason are sometimes referred as "temporary mounts", to distinguish them from the "permanent mounts" which can be stored over longer times. One of the major advantages of direct microscopy is that living cells and microorganisms can be examined in their natural state without previously being killed, fixed, and stained.

In our current practice direct microscopy or phase contrast microscopy is usually performed as an extension of the routine gynecological check-up, in order to obtain more reliable information during patient examination.

Ideally, Ph microscopy should be used in every patient undergoing gynecological examination; this technically supported work-up may easily give very satisfactory results with a skilful application of such equipment. A rapid diagnosis by freshly mounted preparations was confirmed to be extremely useful in daily office practice, because it enables specific treatment to be prescribed during examination.

PHYSICS OF PHASE CONTRAST MYCROSCOPY

A microscope is a lens system producing an enlarged virtual image of a small object. It consists of two convergent lenses, each of a small focal length, called the objective lens (or objective) and the eyepiece (Figure 1).

In many medical and biological applications the majority of objects to be observed under microscope are represented by cellular microstructures in solution, with a refraction index slightly different from that of the surrounding medium.

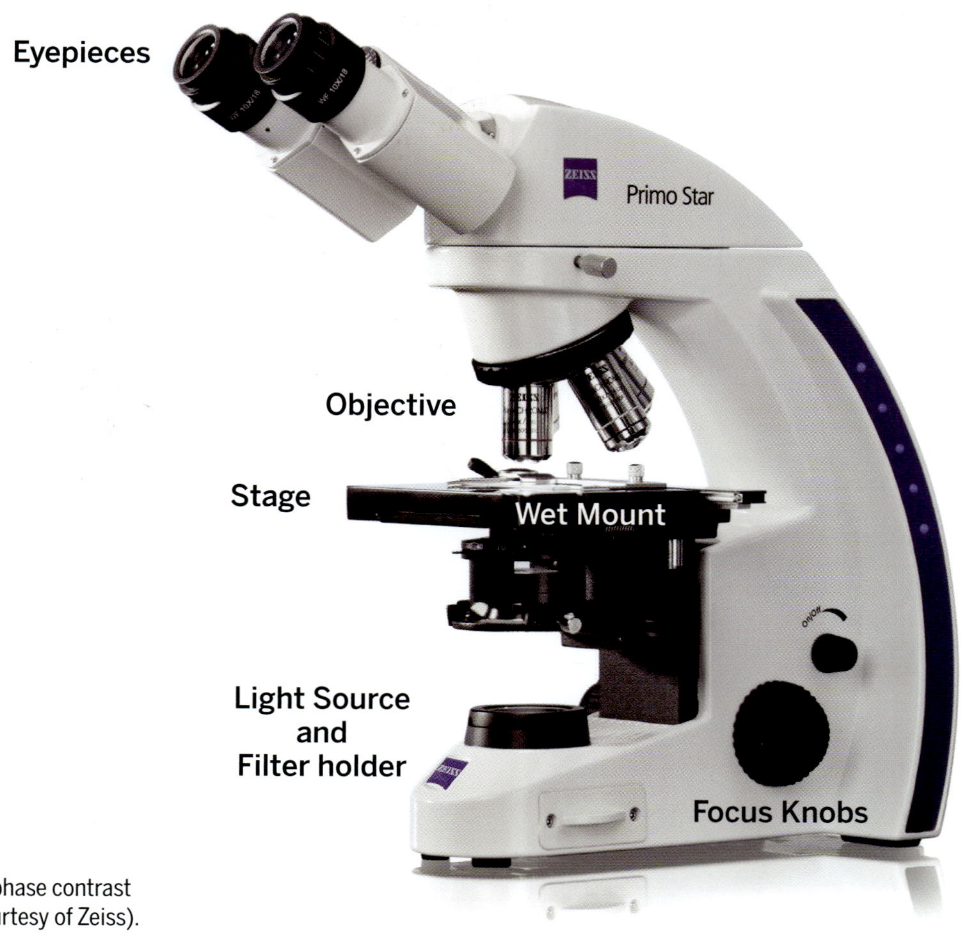

Figure 1 - Zeiss phase contrast microscope (Courtesy of Zeiss).

This weak contrast leads to ill defined and faded images when biological materials are observed by a bright-light microscope, without fixation and staining. On the other hand, these laboratory procedures alter the morphological characteristics of the object and modify the physicochemical properties of the matter.
When an unstained living object is observed under a normal microscope, the light coming from the object contains its "image", although it is hidden.
Phase contrast equipment makes these images discernible by the eye, so that tiny biological structures appear distinct, without any laboratory artefact due to fixation and staining.
In order to understand the physical features of the phase contrast technique, it must be noted that two types of objects can be encountered during microscope investigation: amplitude objects and phase objects (Figure 2).
Amplitude objects are visible because their components present differences in luminosity (depending on wave amplitude) and colours (depending on wavelength). These microscopic objects are so called because when the light beam passes through them, some of the waves are deflected by diffraction and reduce their amplitude. According to Abbe's theory, the image of this objects results from the interference between direct waves and diffracted ones. But the image becomes visible only if phase difference between the two types of waves amounts to about one half of a wavelength ($\lambda/2$).
On the other hand, the majority of biological materials belong to *phase objects*; their constituent parts have low density differences which do not modify light amplitude, but are able to delay wave phase of about one fourth of a wavelength ($\lambda/4$).
As mentioned above, this alone is not enough to make the object visible, since to accomplish that it is necessary to shift the phase of the direct waves of further $\lambda/4$ ($\lambda/4 + \lambda/4 = \lambda/2$).
The idea of Zernike (Figure 3) was to interfere in the path of direct waves by introducing an annular diaphragm (condenser annulus) in the condenser and an annular phase plate in the rear focal plane

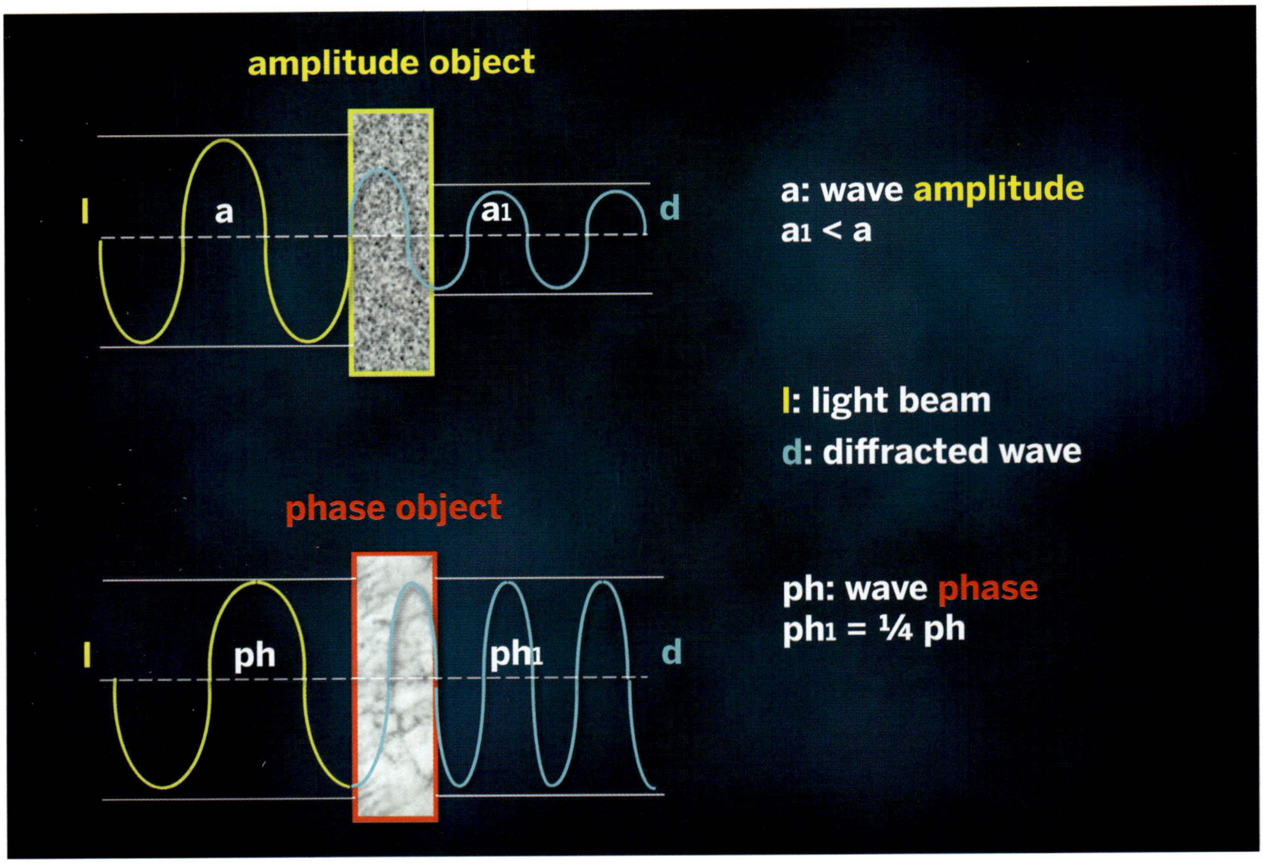

Figure 2 - Types of microscopic objects.

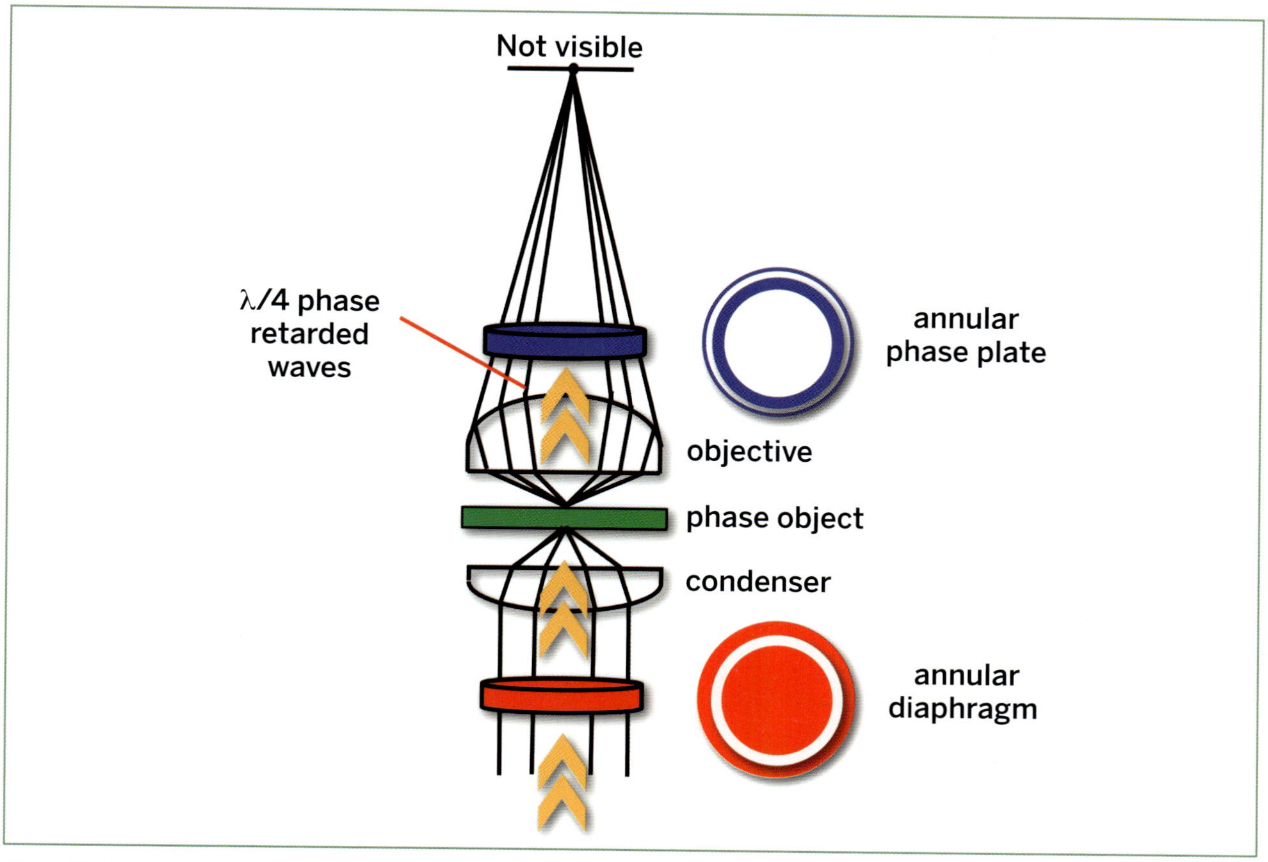

Figure 3 - Diagram of the phase contrast optical train: visible image.

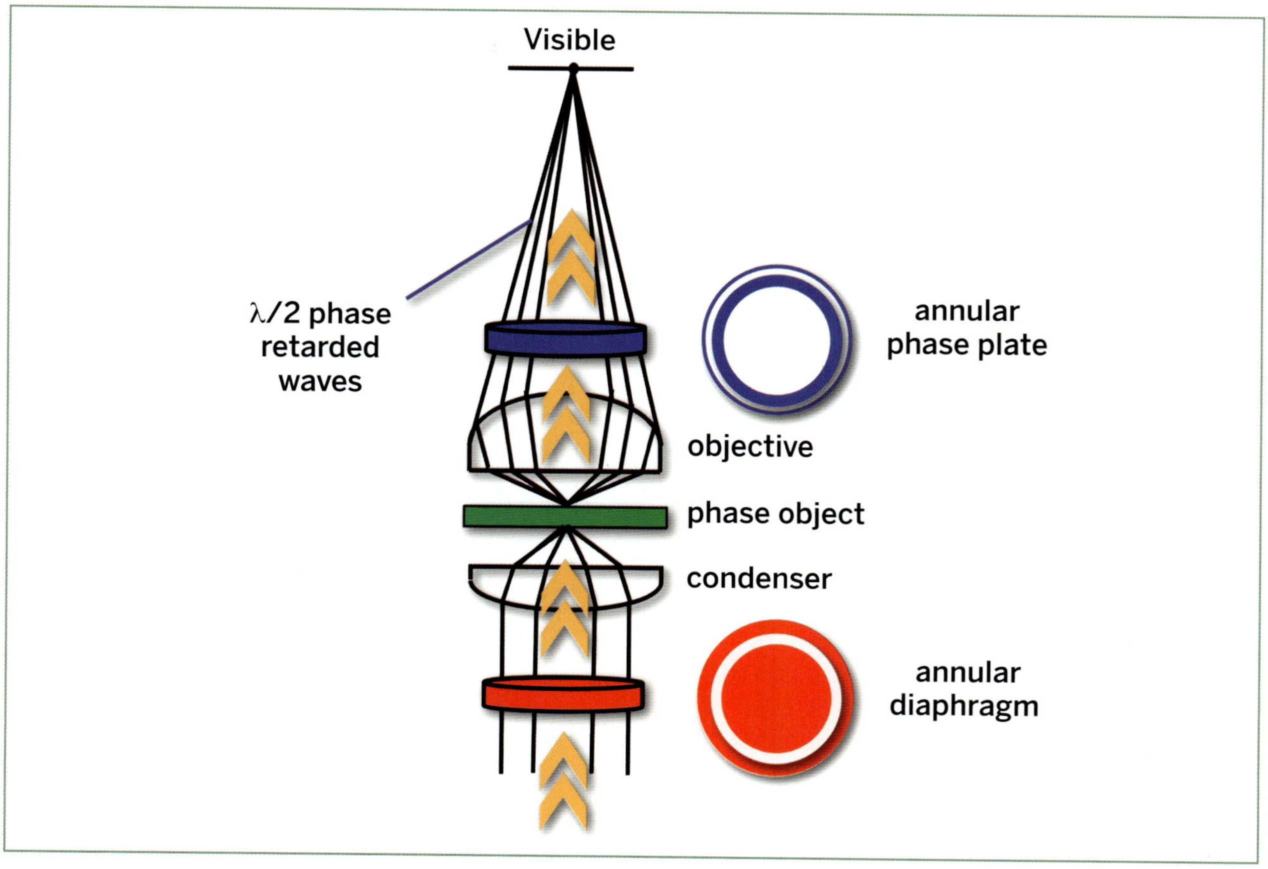

Figure 4 - Diagram of the phase contrast optical train: not visible image.

of the objective lens (specially labelled with *Ph* or *Phaco*).

The annular diaphragm turns the light beam into a light hollow cone and conveys it towards the annular phase plate of the objective lens, strictly aligned to the former.

The light waves passing through the specimen (phase object), both diffracted and non-diffracted, reach the annular phase plate of the objective lens with a phase difference of about $\lambda/4$.

Here (Figure 4) only direct waves are further retarded in phase of about $\lambda/4$, whereas diffracted waves pass through unaltered. In this way a final phase difference of $\lambda/2$ ($\lambda/4 + \lambda/4$) between direct and diffracted waves makes biological material visible, even being a phase object.

A green filter is placed on the filter holder (Figure 1) because, due to the physical peculiarity of phase contrast microscopy, optimum contrast is obtained with monochromatic light.

WET MOUNT PREPARATION

There are several types of wet mount, depending on the site of collection of the specimen:

- *cervico-vaginal* wet mount
- *urinary* wet mount or urocytogram
- *oral* wet mount
- *cutaneous* wet mount
- *rectal* wet mount.

Material

The following materials are needed to prepare a wet mount:

- *microscope glasses*
- *cover glasses* (coverslips)
- *sterile saline solution* (0,9% sodium chloride solution)
- 10% *potassium hydroxide solution*
- *dropper* for transferring saline solution onto the microscope slide
- *vaseline* or *clear nail polish.*

Cervico-vaginal wet mount technique

The patient should not have douched and used vaginal suppositories, creams, gels or foams for at least 48 hours prior to sampling.

With the patient lying down in gynaecological position, a non lubricated bivalve self retaining speculum is gently inserted into the vagina, so that vaginal walls, fornices and cervix can be thoroughly visualized.

A cotton swab or a spatula are used to collect discharge from the vaginal walls, the esocervix and the vaginal posterior fornix (Figure 5); a second cotton swab or an endocervical device can be rotated in the cervical canal.

The swabs, the spatula or the endocervical device are immediately and lightly dabbed (and not rubbed) in a drop of sterile normal saline, previously applied on a microscope slide (Figure 6a). Alternatively, 10% potassium hydroxide (KOH) solution is suggested when vaginal fungal infection is suspected. In fact, use of 10% KOH in wet preparations improves the visualization of yeasts and mycelia by disrupting cellular material that might obscure yeasts, pseudohyphae or hyphae.

Applying this type of solution between the slide and the coverslip is not recommended. In fact, despite the presence of a vaginal fungal infection and irritative symptoms, blastospores, hyphae and pseudohyphae may be not visible under direct microscopic examination and cultures give false negative results. In such cases, Candida uses protease to penetrate the vaginal epithelium, thus leaving a specific track on the cells, that the screener may easily detect. The use of KOH solution destroys the cells, thus hindering the recognition of the specific cytopathy induced by the fungal hyphae.

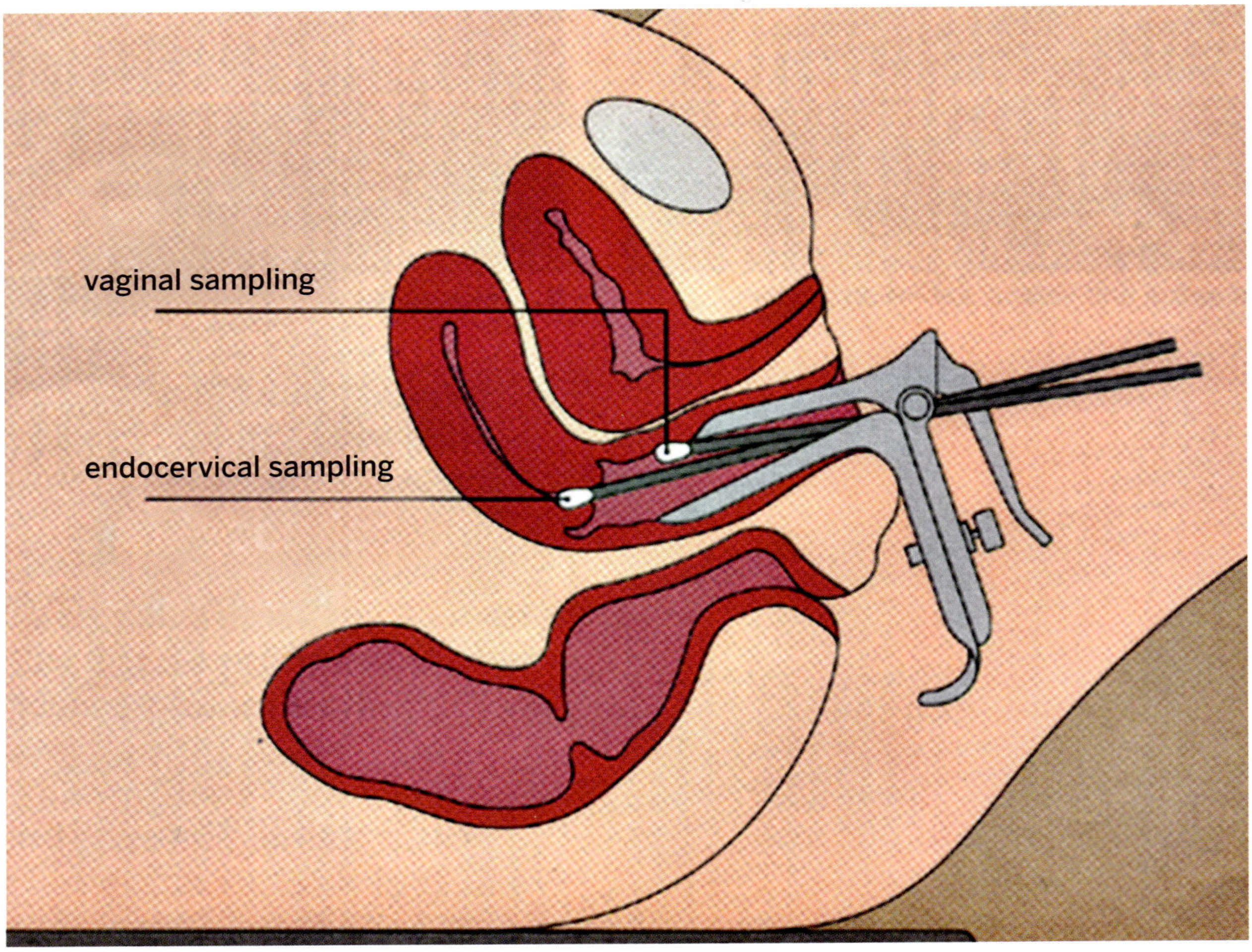

Figure 5 - Cervico-vaginal sampling.

The specimen is mounted with a cover glass (Figure 6b) immediately after. Be careful to lower the coverslip so that it forms an angle of 45 degrees with the microscope glass and one edge touches the slide. This precaution will prevent air bubbles from being entrapped under the coverslip, interfering with the viewing and hampering organisms' movements.
The sample is thus ready to be examined under the Ph microscope, without any artefact due to fixation and staining.
Each photomicrograph was taken through a Ph objective lens (x40) and an eyepiece (x10) connected with a camera, obtaining a 400x total magnification. Some images were magnified to highlight particular structures of cells or microorganisms.
The green shade of the pictures is due to the green filter placed on the filter holder.
When necessary, our microscopic findings had confirmatory cultures and the causative agents are indicated in brackets.

Advantages of a wet mount

- *No artefact*: direct microscopy makes living organisms and biological structures clearly and immediately visible, without artifacts due to dehydration, fixation and staining – used for processing permanent mounts – that may alter the morphological characteristics and modify the physicochemical properties of the matter.
- *Quick preparation.*
- *Observation of movements* of protozoas and cell organelles such as cilia in ciliated endocervical cells.

Disadvantages of a wet mount

- *Storage*: wet mounts cannot be stored over a long time because the specimen dries up. This problem may be easily solved by taking photos of the microscopic images using a digital camera system applied to the phase contrast microscope.

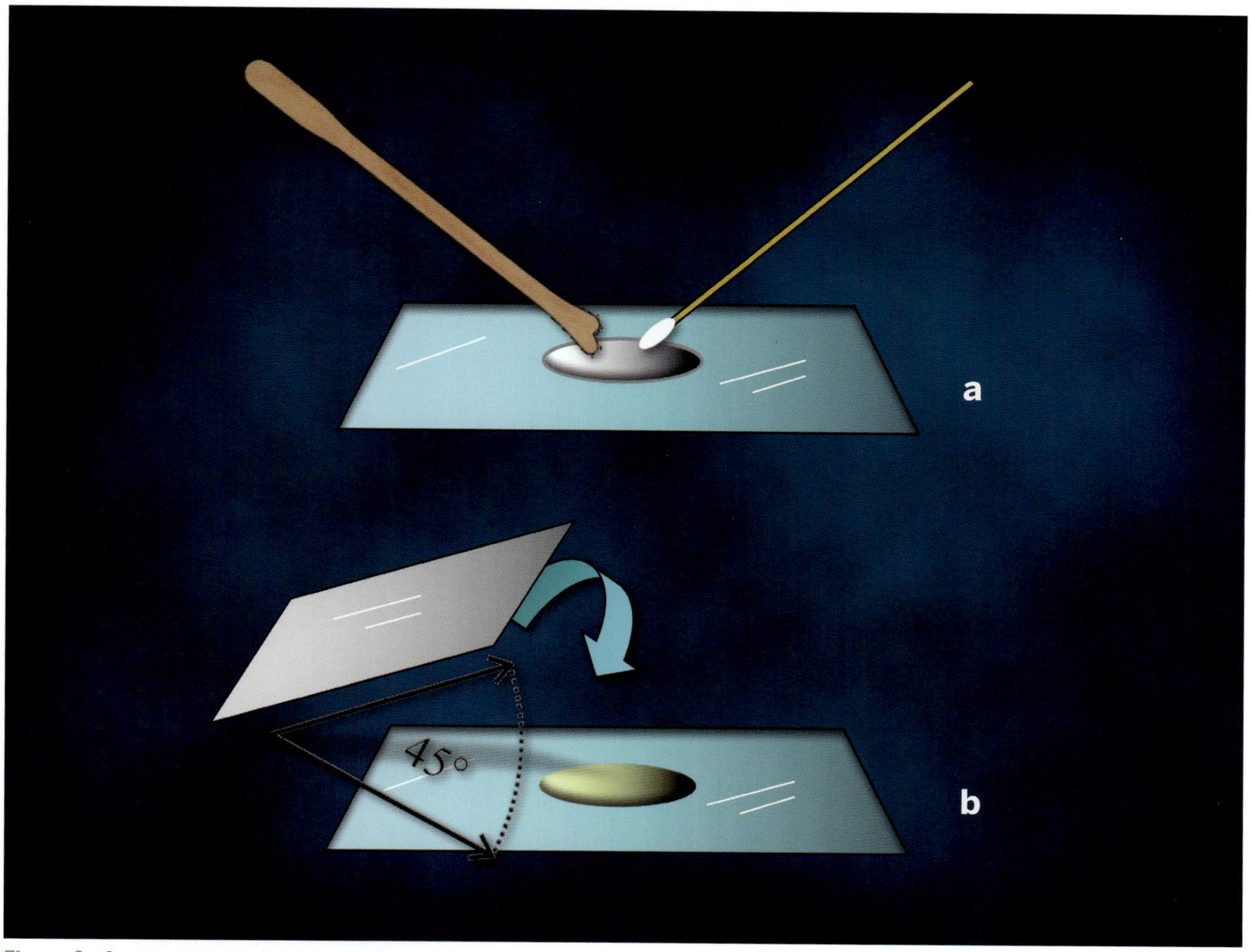

Figure 6 - Cervico-vaginal wet mount preparation.

- Difficulty in *taking pictures* due to the movement of protozoas or ciliated endocervical cells. However it is possible to film the moving organisms using the digital camera system or wait a few minutes for the movements to fade or disappear.

Technical tricks

- Your aim is to have sufficient water to fill up the space between coverslip and slide. The coverslip may float in case of excessive water. In such case, hold a paper towel close to one edge of the coverslip. This will draw out some water.
- If the wet mount is too dry, air bubbles may form and the specimen may be squeezed between the coverslip and the slide. This would interfere with the viewing and hamper the organisms' movements. In this case you can add a drop of water near the coverslip.
- Bringing the objective lens too near the edge of the slide will result in the saline smearing the objective; this may interfere with the viewing and can damage the lens.
- Touch the cover glass on the sides to avoid leaving fingerprints.
- Air-drying, a common artifact with wet mounts, causes artificial nuclear enlargement. When a longer observation of the wet mount is necessary, a vaseline chamber can be prepared to prevent that the specimen dries up due to the heat of the lamp. It is sufficient to gently rub the tip of a swab dibbed in vaseline on each edge of the coverslip, to form a thin and continuous vaseline ledge. The same result may be obtained by using a clear nail polish.

Urocytogram

With the patient's external genitalia exposed, the urethral meatus is thoroughly cleaned with sterile saline solution.

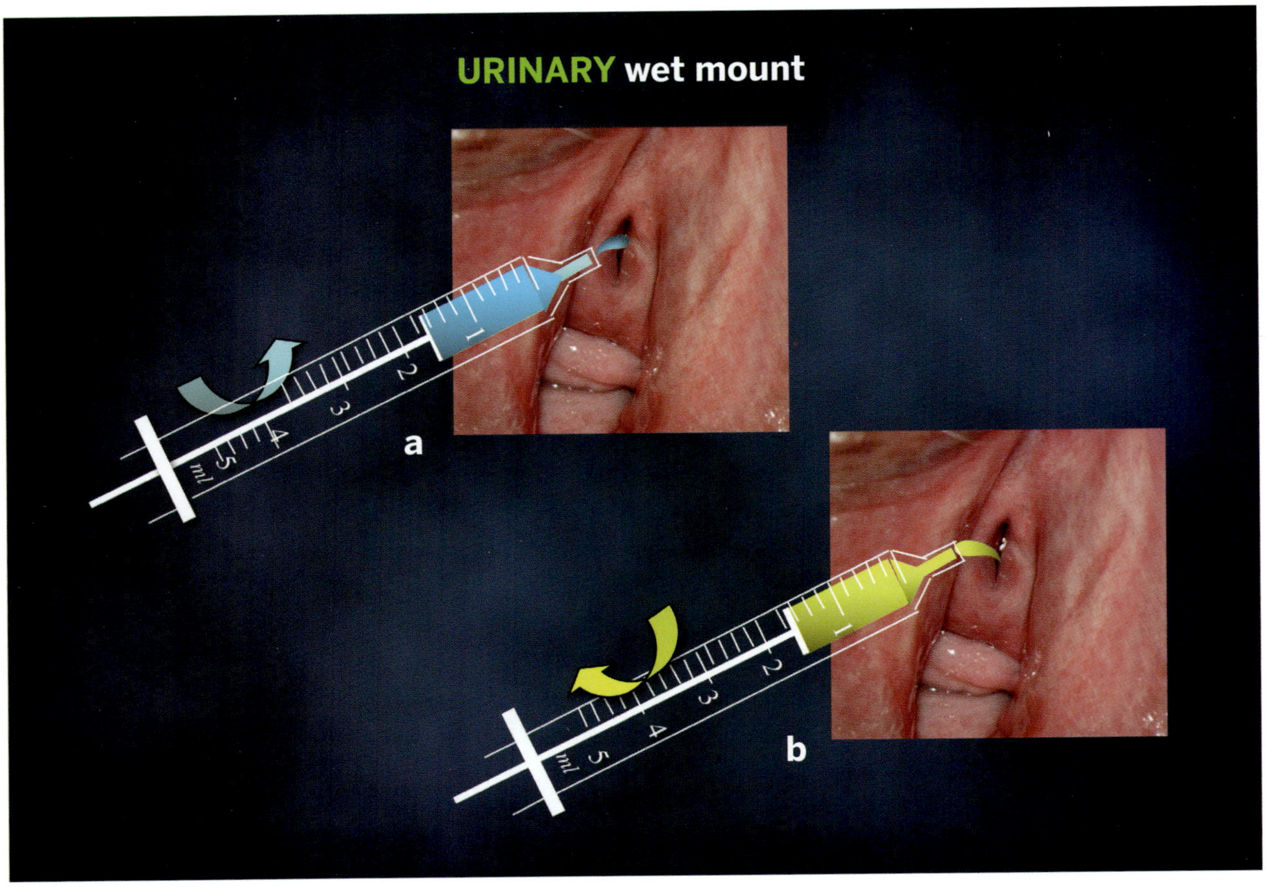

Figure 7 - Urinary wet mount sampling.

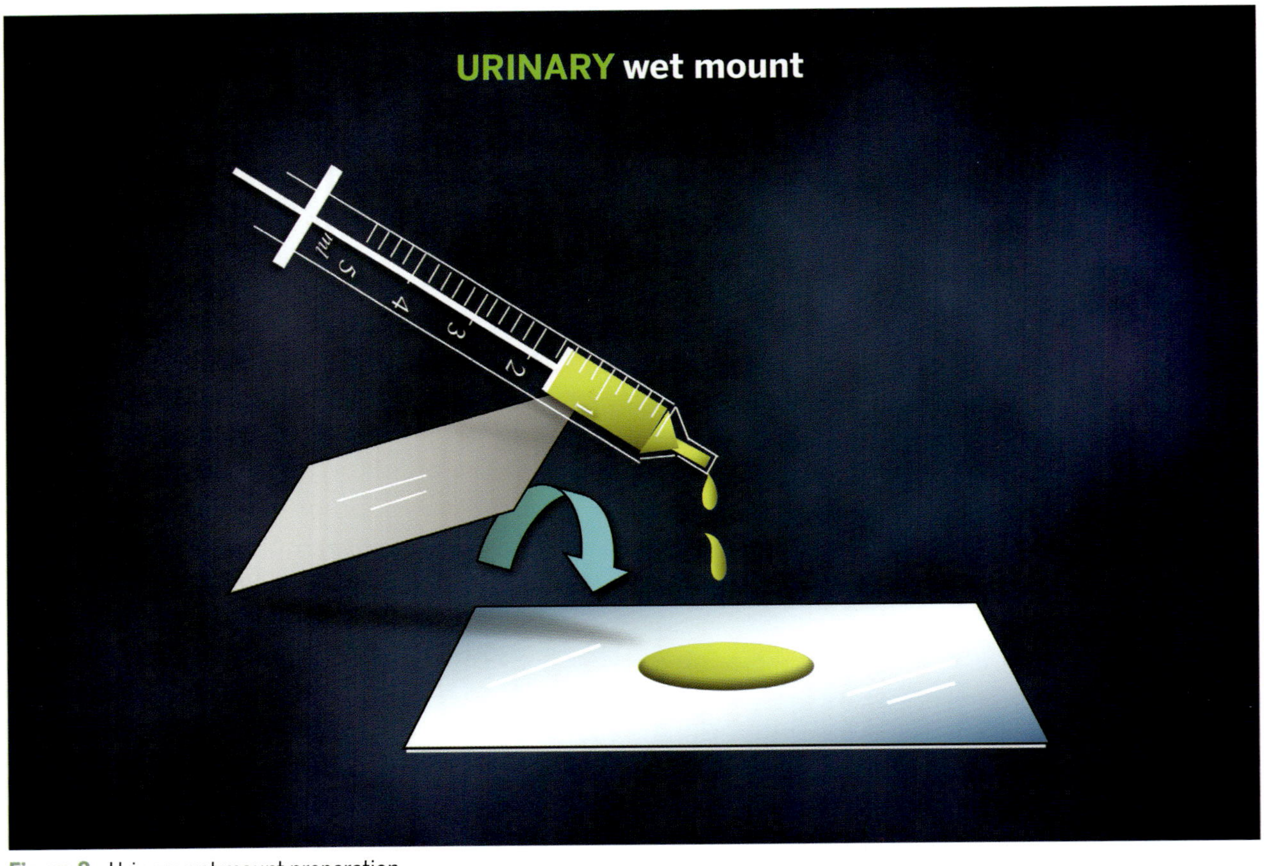

Figure 8 - Urinary wet mount preparation.

Using a disposable needless syringe, we introduce 5-10 ml of saline into the urethra and the bladder (Figure 7a).
Following this injection, a few drops of the urethral washing fluid are collected using the same syringe (Figure 7b). Soon after, one or two drops are poured onto the glass (Figure 8). The following procedures correspond to the ones used to process a cervico-vaginal wet mount.

Urinary epithelium

Two types of epithelia can be observed in the female urethra (Figure 9):

- transitional epithelium
- squamous epithelium.

All the cells of both epithelia show a pale nucleus with finely granular chromatin.
Transitional epithelium consists of multiple layers of epithelial cells able to contract and expand. It is called "transitional" because of this function in the transition from different degrees of distension.
This highly specialized and unique epithelium, known as urothelium, lines the proximal 2/3rds of the urethra.
Transitional epithelium also lines the renal pelvis, the ureters and the bladder.
Urothelium is composed of three types of cells, proceeding from the basement membrane towards the lumen (Figures 9, 10):

- basal cells
- club-shaped cells
- umbrella cells.

A basal layer of cuboidal cells rests on the basement membrane.
The intermediate layer is composed of club-shaped or columnar cells, whose expanded end lays in the concavity of umbrella cells which vary in

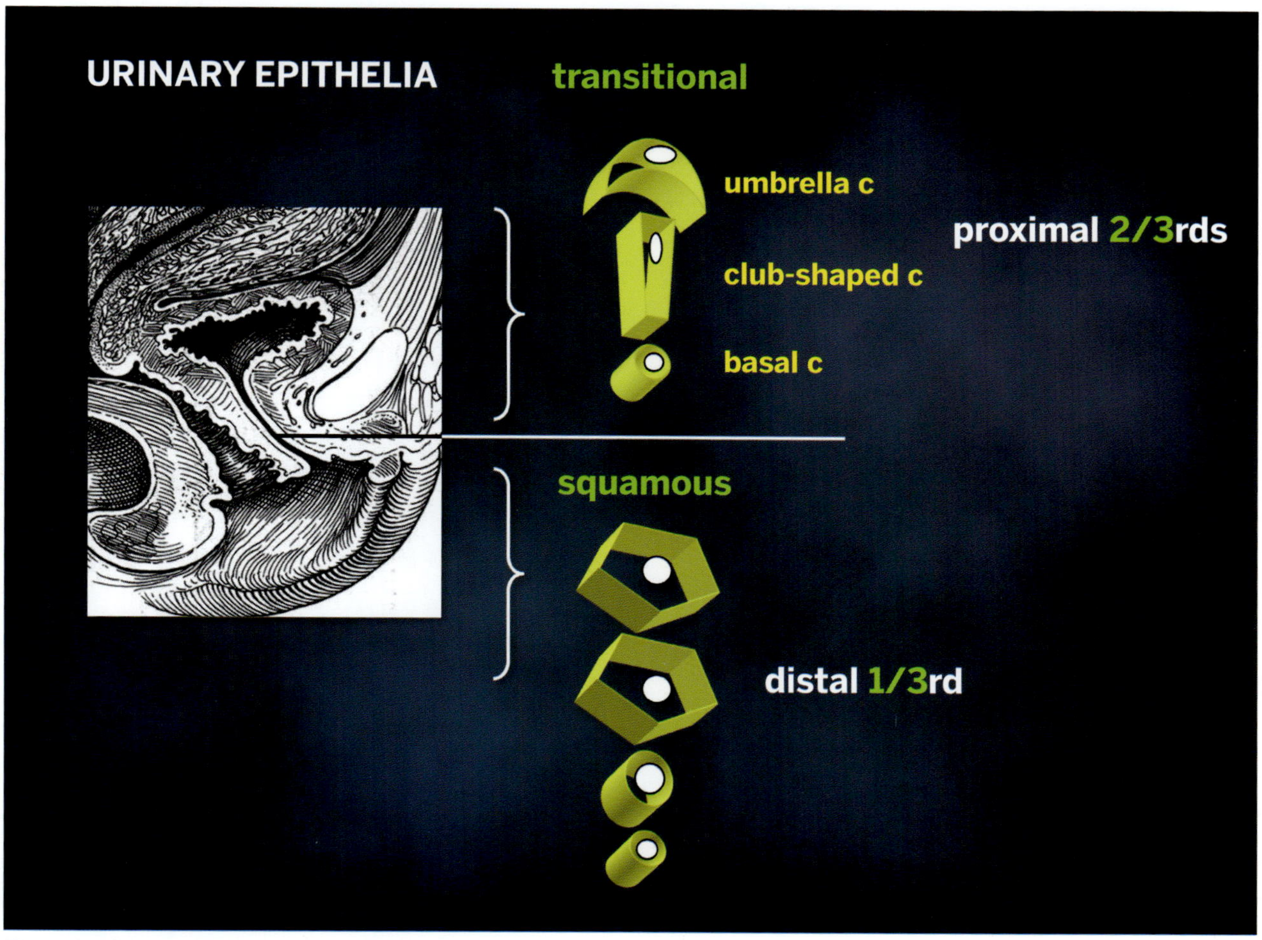

Figure 9 - Urinary epithelia.

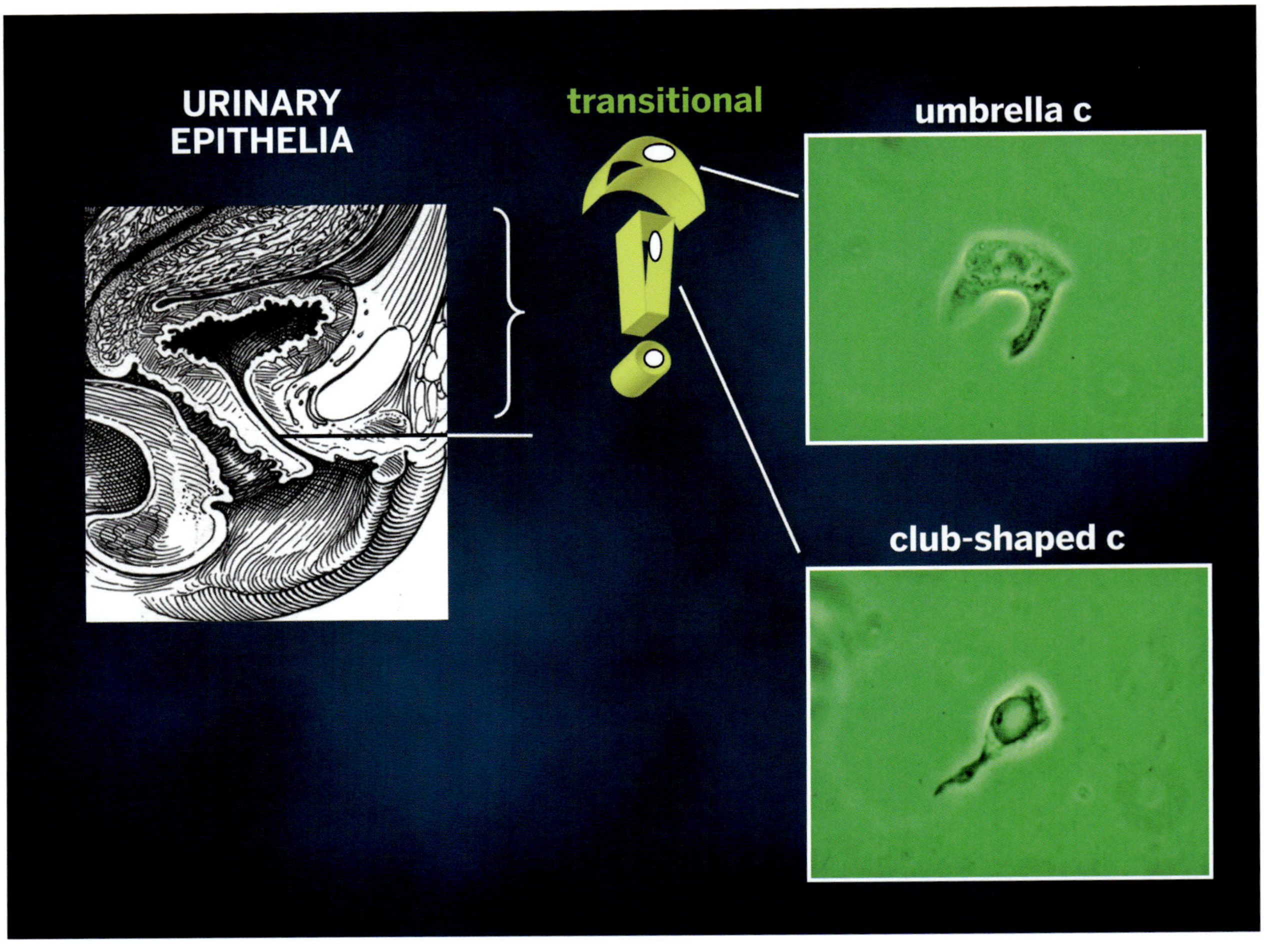

Figure 10 - Urinary transitional epithelium.

appearance, depending on the degree of distension. The superficial cells are referred to as umbrella cells with a domed apex when the organ or the tube in which they reside is not stretched. They are fairly large when released and may show multiple nuclei (Figure 11).
The distal 1/3rd of urethra is lined by a nonkeratinized stratified *squamous epithelium* (Figure 9). Urethral squamous cells differ from squamous cells lining the vagina only for the presence of pale nuclei (Figure 12). A gradual change from squamous to columnar epithelium can be observed with advancing age. More squamous epithelium is present at the distal end of the urethra. There are small mucus-secreting urethral glands, that help protect the epithelium from the corrosive urine.
The *urocytogram* is an essential diagnostic tool to observe bacterial adherence to urinary cells (Figures 13, 14), since it is not detectable by cultures and may cause recurrent urinary tract infections (UTIs). When urethral glands are interested by bacterial colonization or infection, bacteria can appear adhered to mucus filaments and the observation of clean filaments reveals the success of the pharmacological treatment (Figure 15).
Even in presence of negative urine culture and in absence of dysuric symptoms, the microscopic evidence of bacterial adherence enables to plan prophylactic antimicrobial regimens, such as (i) the use of long-term, low-dose prophylactic antimicrobials taken at bedtime; (ii) intermittent single-dose treatment with antimicrobials; (iii) post-coital prophylaxis for women whose episodes of infection are associated with sexual intercourse. These antimicrobial regimens have all been demonstrated to be effective in managing recurrent uncomplicated UTIs in women.
Furthermore, the screener can immediately recognize the same cell changes induced by pathogens, detectable in vaginal cells, like Candida cytopathy in urinary fungal infection (Figures 16, 17).

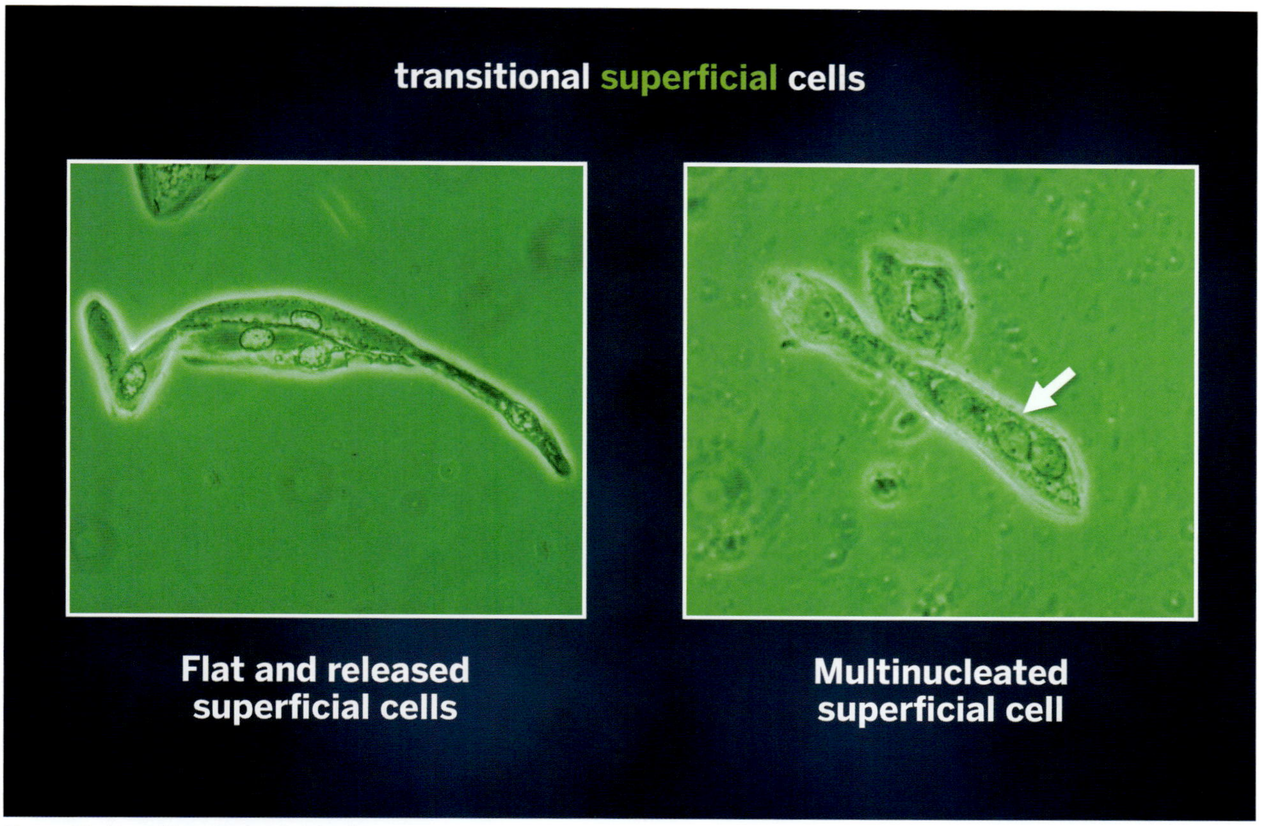

Figure 11 - Transitional superficial cells.

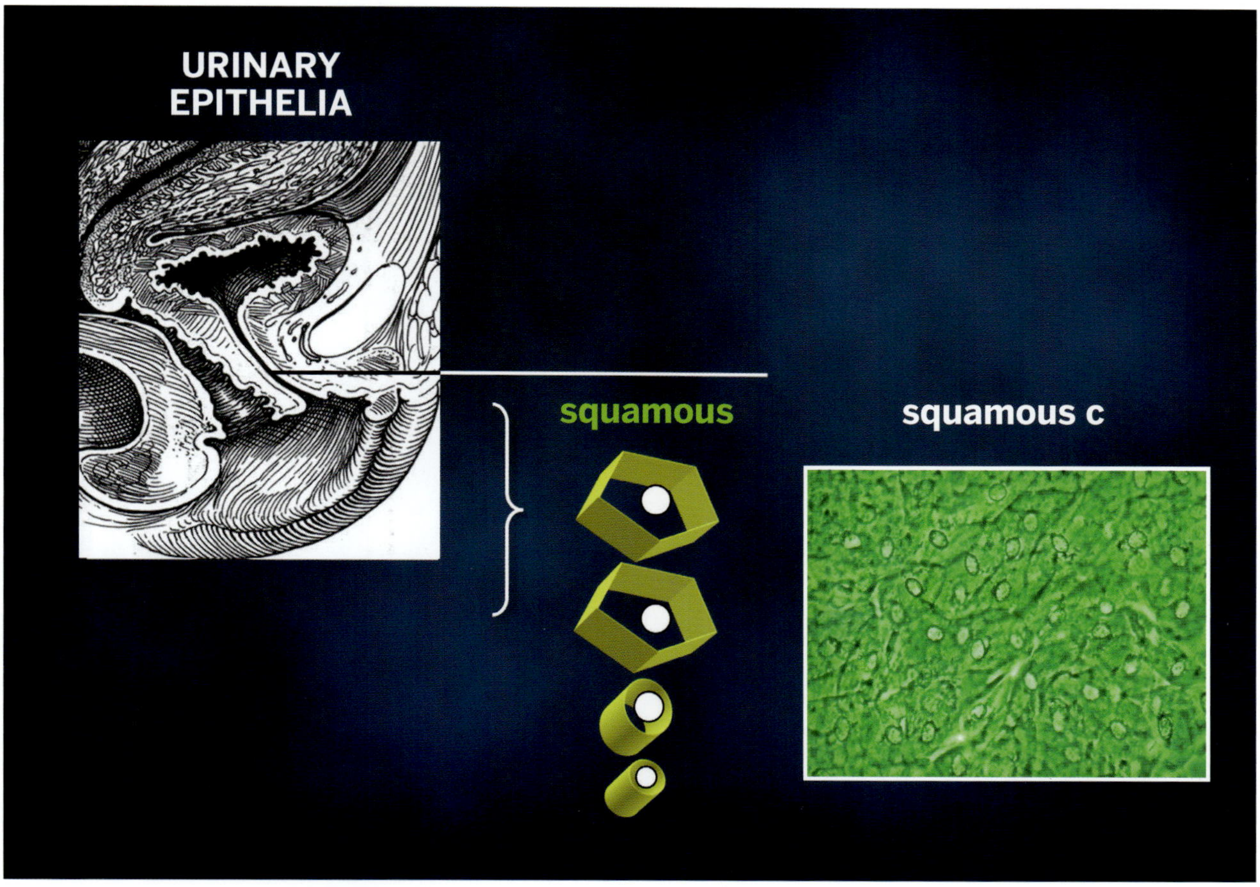

Figure 12 - Urinary squamous epithelium.

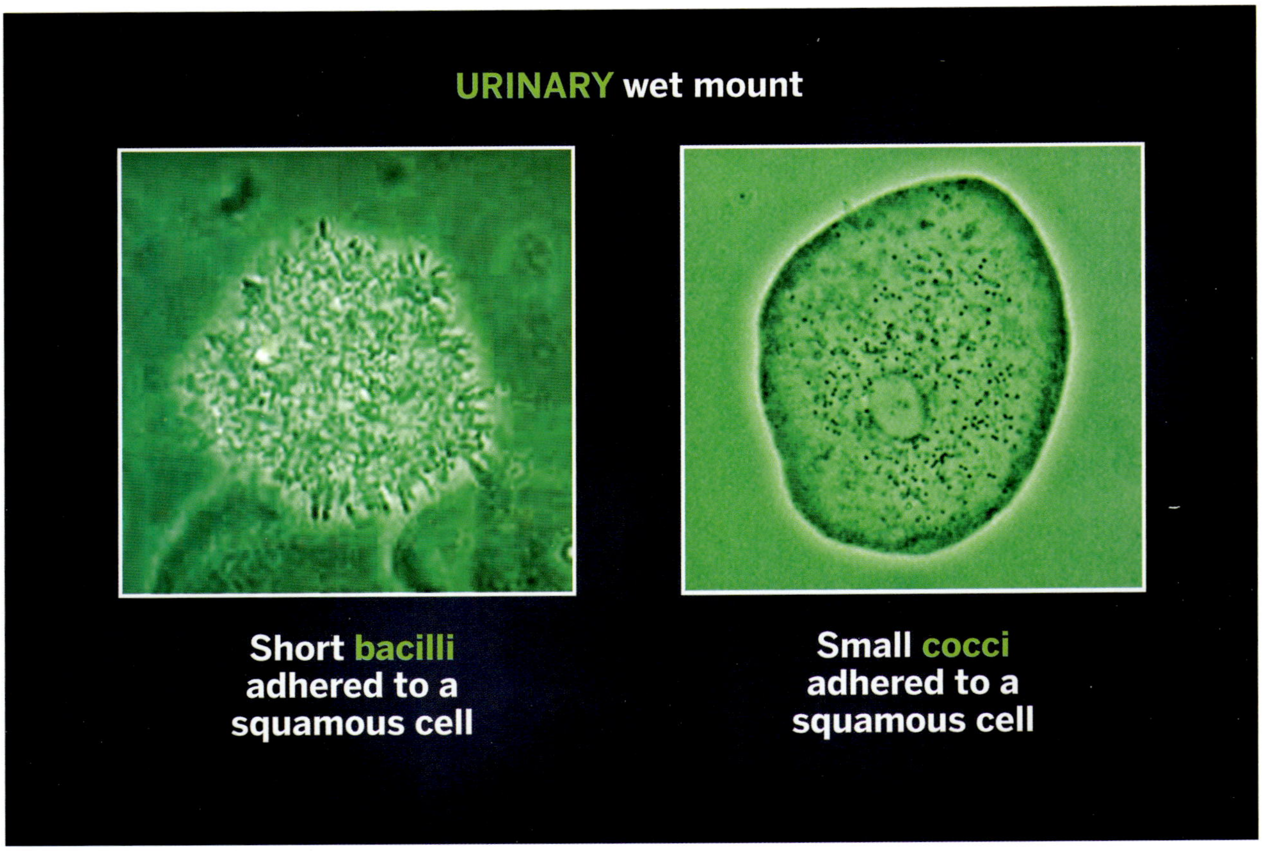

Figure 13 - Urinary wet mount: bacterial adhesion to squamous cells.

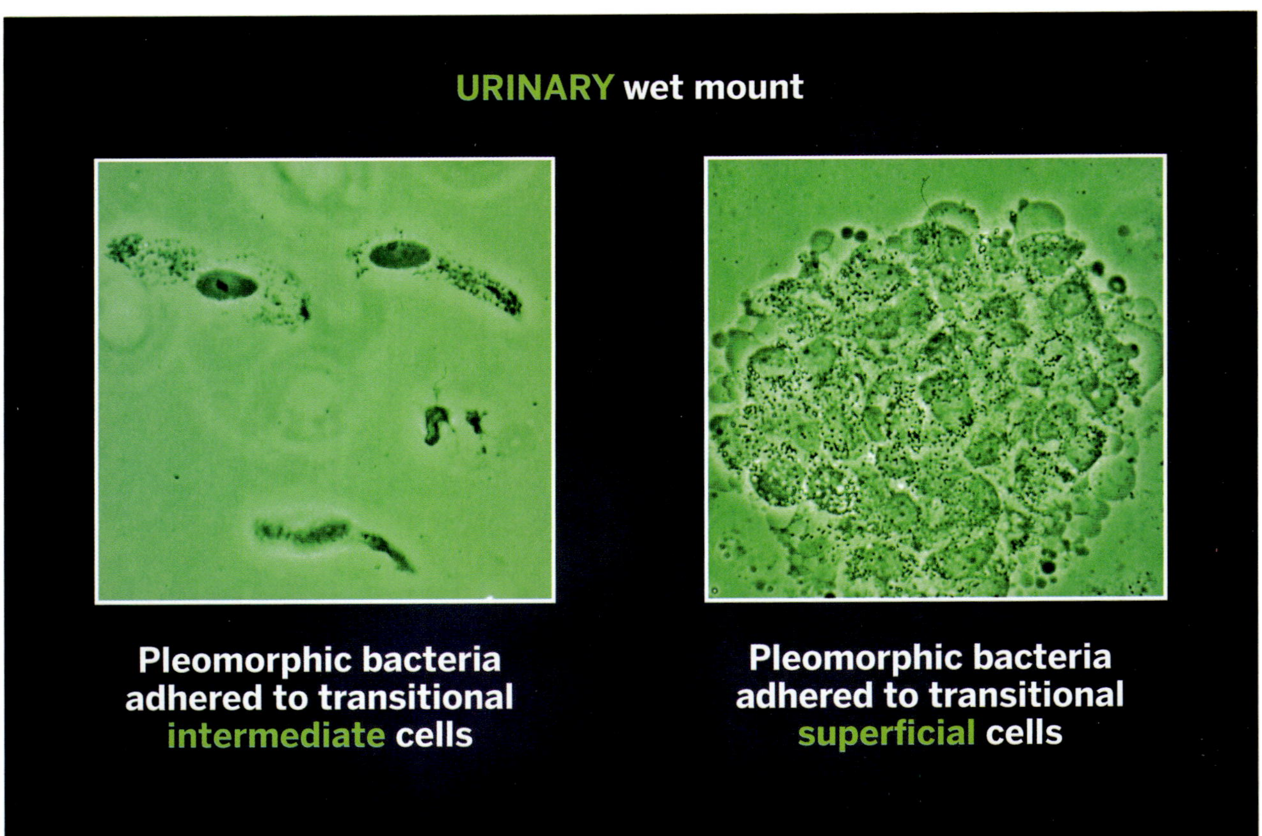

Figure 14 - Urinary wet mount: bacterial adhesion to transitional cells.

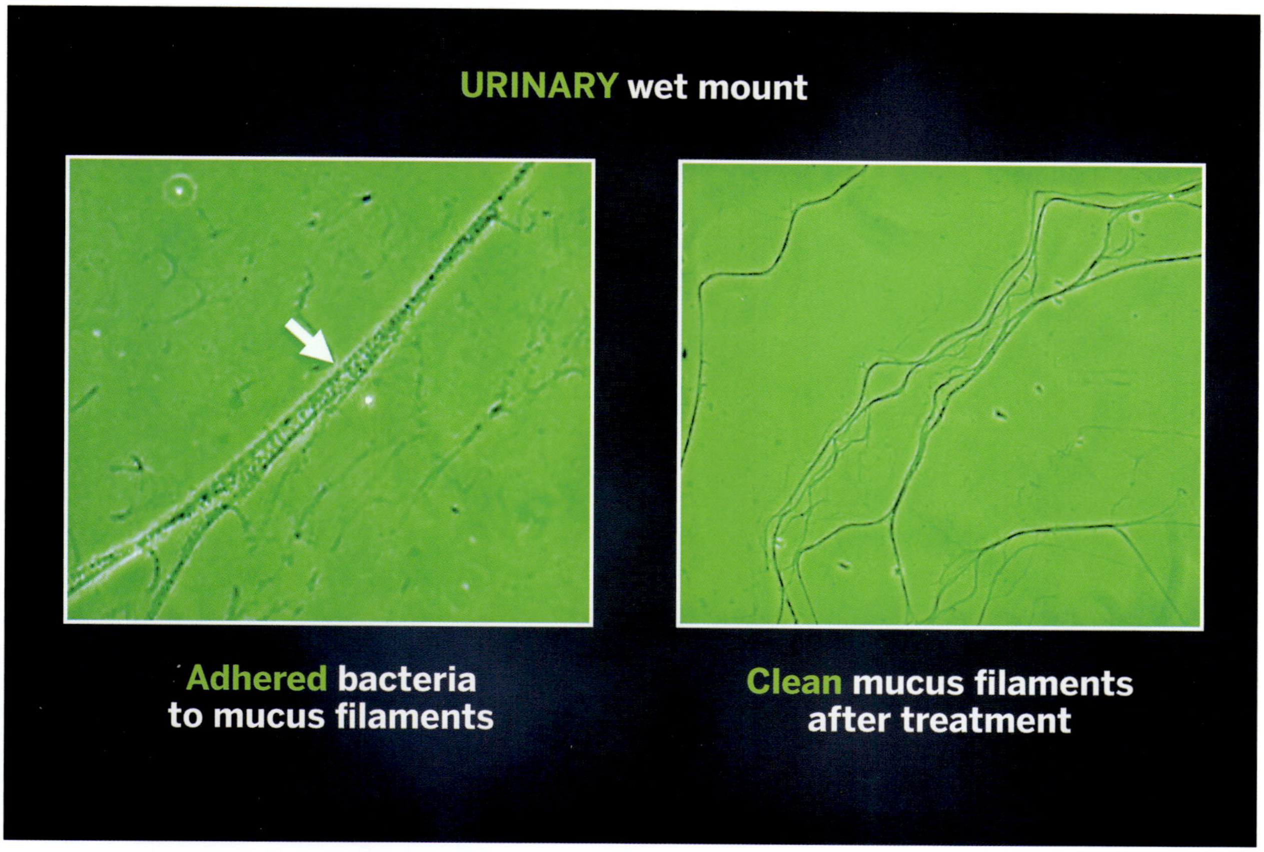

Figure 15 - Urinary wet mount: bacterial adhesion to mucus filaments.

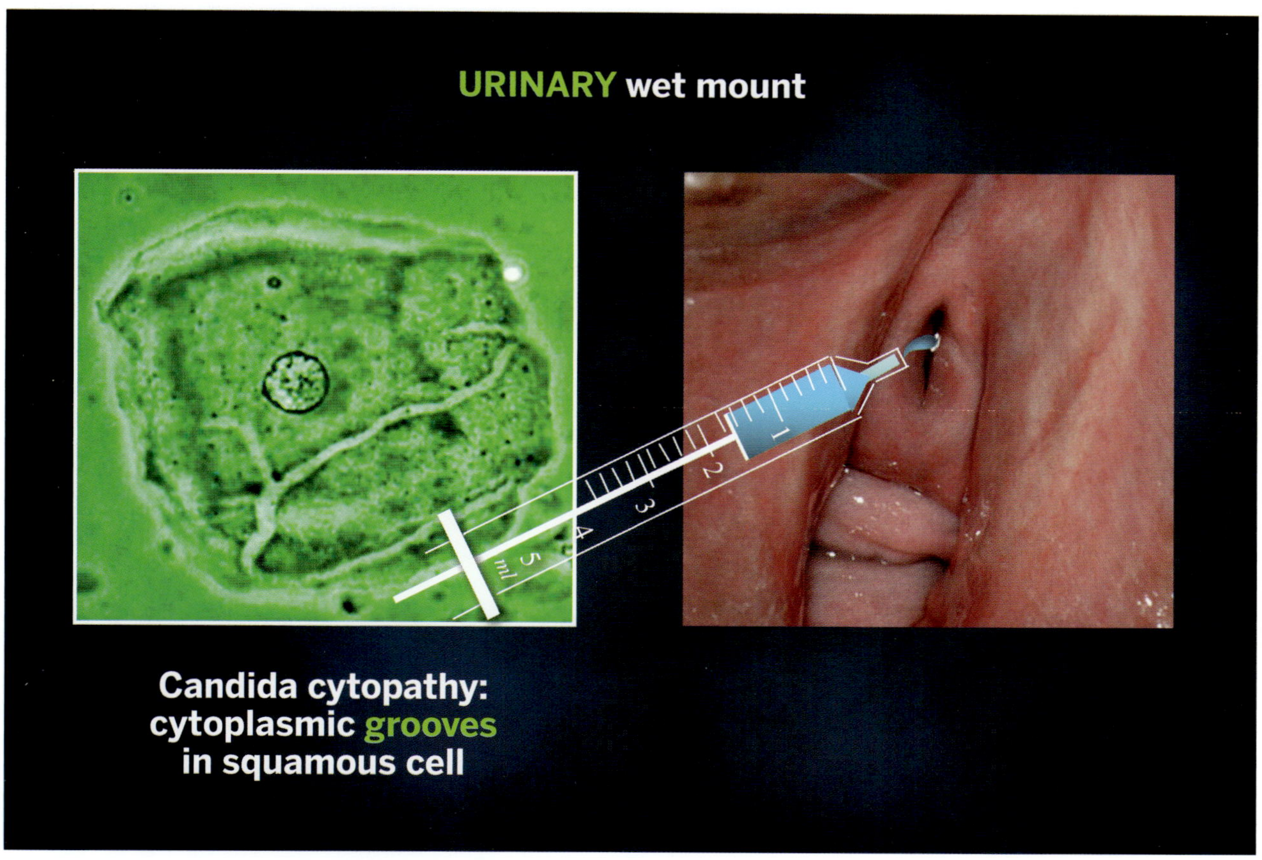

Figure 16 - Urinary wet mount: Candida cytopathy in a squamous cell.

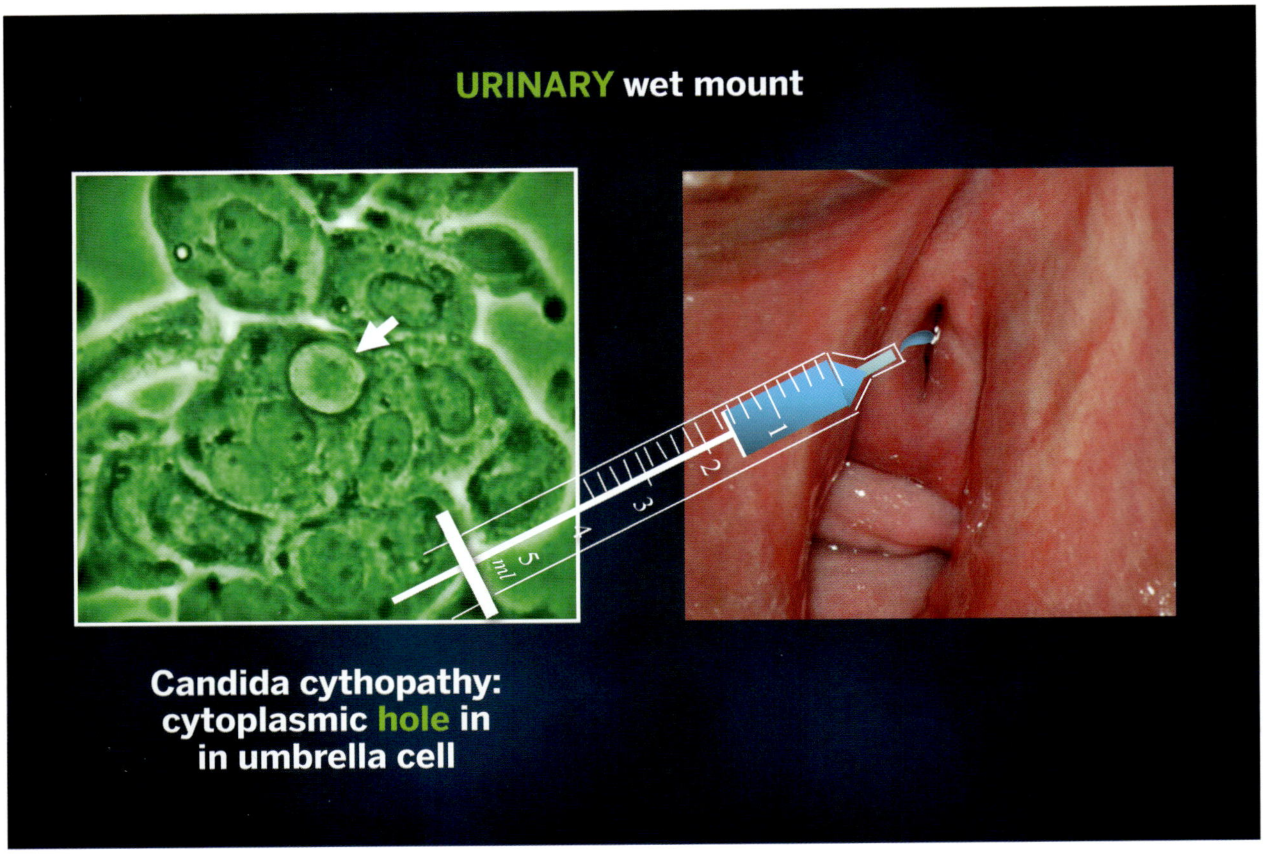

Figure 17 - Urinary wet mount: Candida cytopathy in a transitional cell.

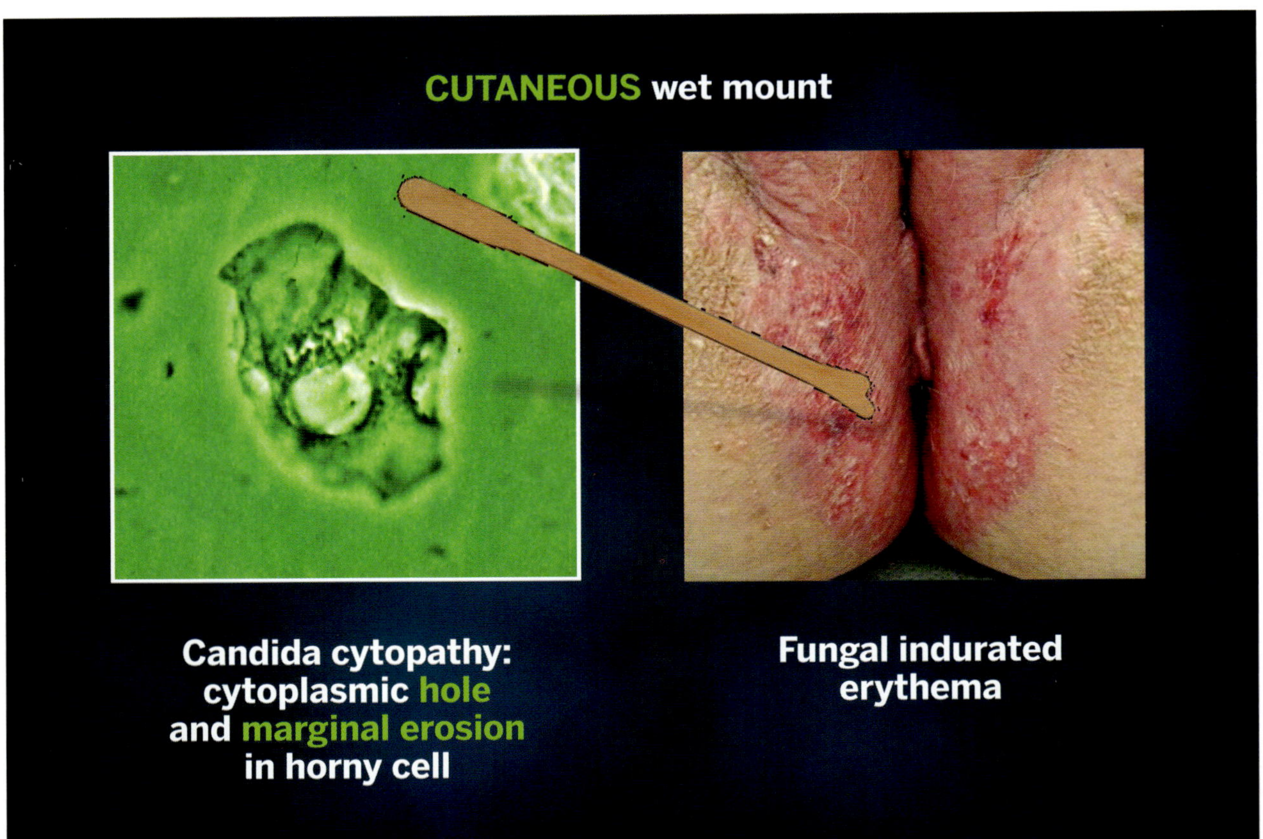

Figure 18 - Cutaneous wet mount: Candida cytopathy in a horny cell.

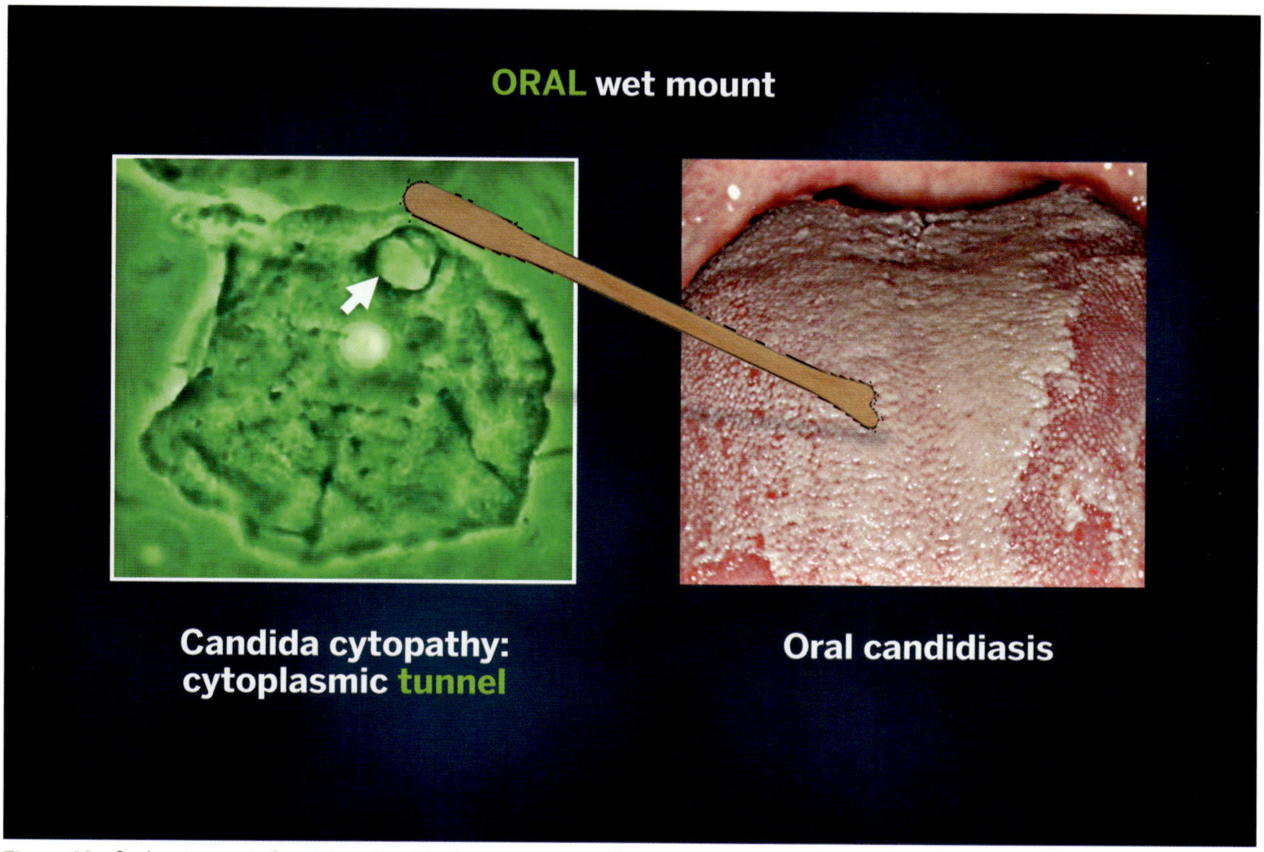

Figure 19 - Oral wet mount: Candida cytopathy in a squamous cell.

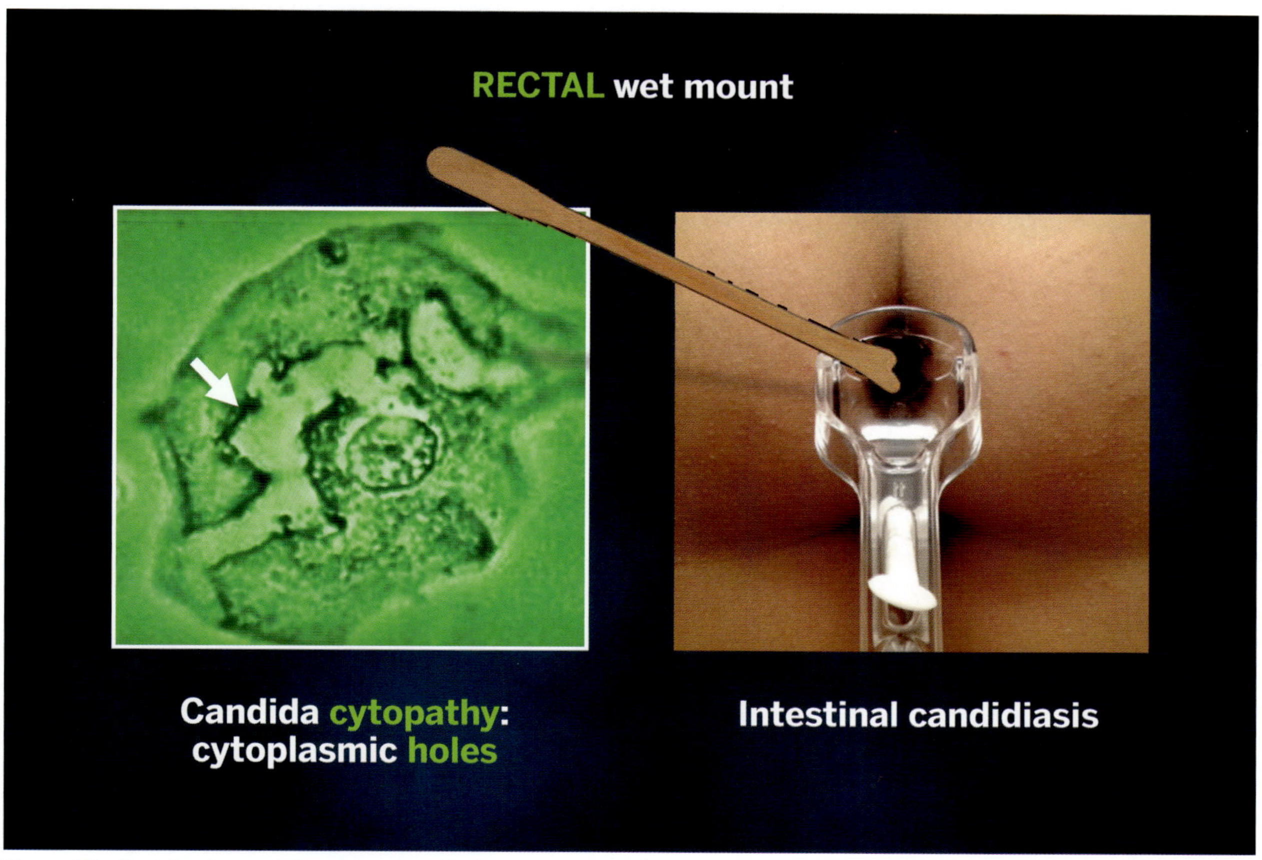

Figure 20 - Rectal wet mount: Candida cytopathy in a squamous cell.

When fungal infection is detected in the male sexual partner by urocytogram, it is advisable to treat him as well, in order to avoid recurrent vaginal candidiasis.

Different wet mounts

We use spatulas to collect the specimens for the preparation of cutaneous (Figure 18), oral (Figure 19) and rectal wet mounts (Figure 20). The following procedures correspond to the ones described to process a cervico-vaginal wet mount.

CLINICAL CORRELATES

A cervico-vaginal wet mount can provide immediate information about:

- *hormone status*
- *cervico-vaginal microbiology*
- *cell changes caused by pathogens*
- *stages of metaplastic process*
- *cell mediated immunity*
- *localization of occult bleeding and inflammation*
- *post coital sperm morphology and mobility*
- *presence of dyskaryotic or atypical cells.*

Hormone status

The observer may immediately gain precious information about the cell patterns in response to hormonal stimulation by means of Ph microscopy. It must be pointed out, in fact, that the peripheral effects caused by hormones on the vaginal mucosa express a reliable hormone status, whereas usual measurements of circulating hormones indicate a temporary determination of a variable quantity. In this respect, very often the cell pattern is not associated to hormone blood levels (blood-target dissociation).

The vaginal cytogram reflects not only estrogen activity but also the influence of other hormones, particularly progesterone and testosterone, so that patients with identical levels of circulating estrogens may show quite different vaginal cytograms.

The hormonal stimulation on the vaginal epithelium is responsible for the prevalence of different types of cells in the vaginal smear.

Vaginal and cervical epithelia are composed by four types of cells (Figure 21) proceeding from the basement membrane towards the surface:

- *basal* cells
- *parabasal* cells
- *intermediate* cells
- *superficial* cells.

With the maturation of the cells towards the surface, the cellular elements become progressively bigger, whereas the nuclei become smaller.

According to the peculiar cell predominance and aspect, we distinguish four cellular patterns (Figure 22):

- *atrophic* smear
- *progestinic* smear
- *cytolytic* smear
- *estrogenic* smear.

Basal and *parabasal* cells are the hallmark of atrophy. They have a round or oval shape and contain a large nucleus with finely granular chromatin. Nuclei generally show one or two nucleoli which appear dark for their density. Basal and parabasal cells have the same nucleus but can be distinguished for the amount of cytoplasm that is very scant in basal cells, appearing in the shape of a cytoplasmic ring. Wet mounts do not usually scrape off the entire

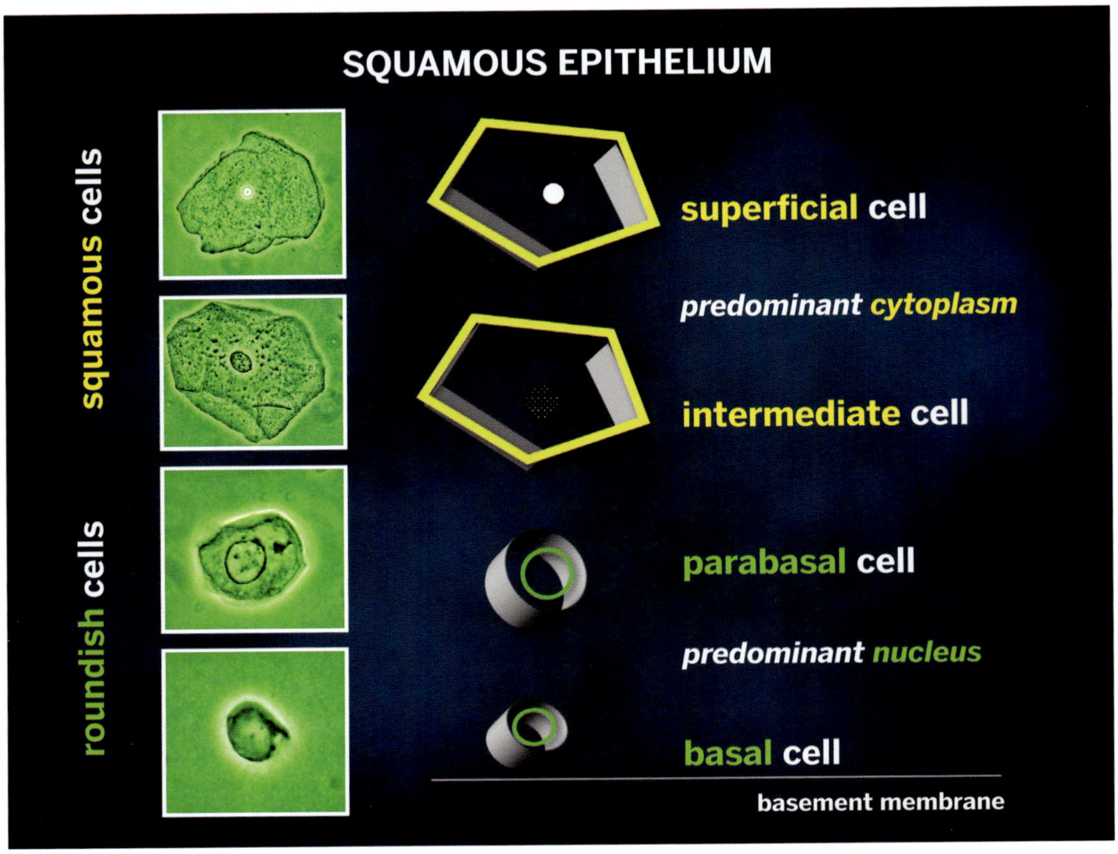

Figure 21 - Diagrammatic representation of the cervico-vaginal squamous epithelium.

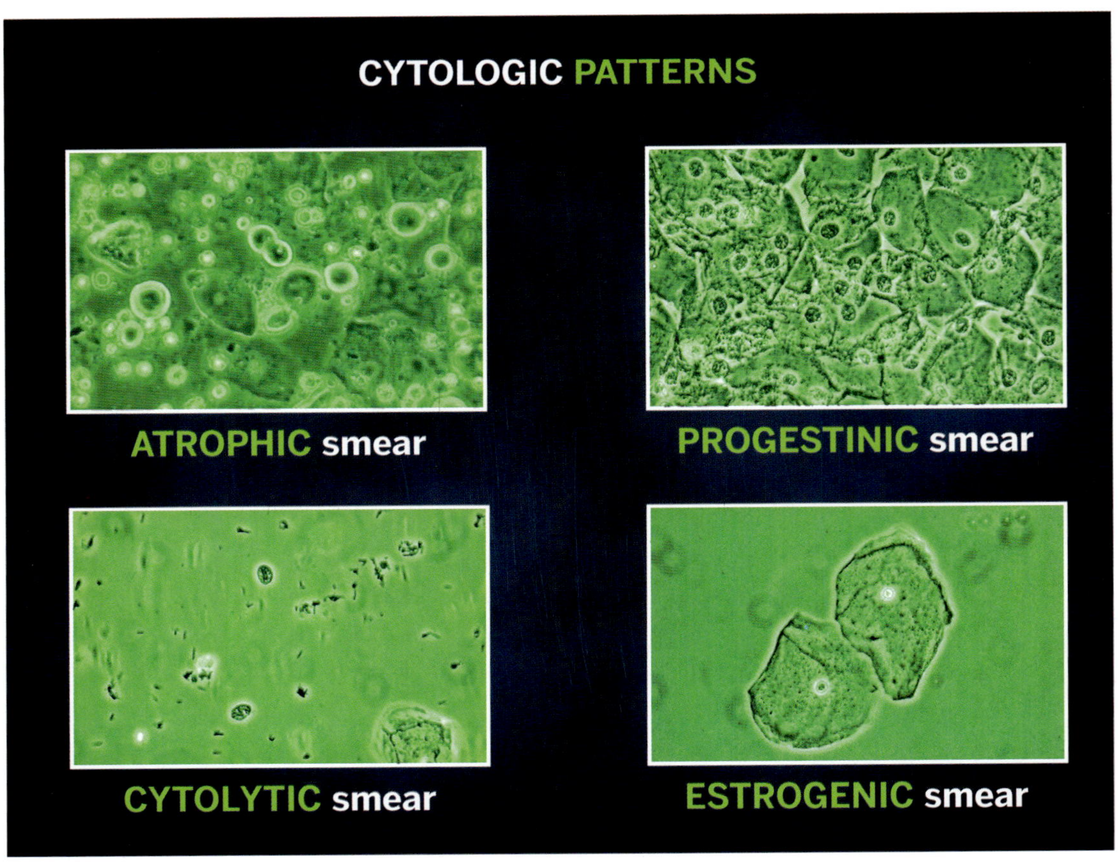

Figure 22 - Cytologic patterns.

thickness of the epithelium, but only the upper few layers, therefore immature basal cells near the base of a mature epithelium are not sampled.

If estrogen levels are low, the maturation level of the squamous epithelium is observable up to the layer of parabasal cells (Figure 23). The predominance of parabasal cells characterizes the *atrophic smear* (Figure 22).

Intermediate and *superficial* cells (Figure 21) are predominant in cytologic samples from women of reproductive age. They usually show the same polygonal shape and are flattened. For these reason, they are defined as squamous cells. Intermediate and superficial cells show the same cytoplasmic body, but can be distinguished for their different nuclear appearance: the nucleus of intermediate cells shows a gross chromatin texture, whereas the superficial cells contain a small nucleus which appears bright because it is densely pyknotic and chromatin characteristics cannot be discerned.

Progesterone stimulation on the epithelium leads the maturation level up to the intermediate cell layer (Figure 24) that predominates in the microscopical field, both in a discrete state or in cluster. This particular predominance is responsible for the *progestinic* pattern (Figure 22).

In presence of high levels of progesterone or androgens, cells undergo cytolysis (Figure 25). The microscopic field shows bare nuclei and cytoplasmic debris. This finding characterizes the *cytolytic* pattern (Figure 22).

When estrogens stimulate the epithelium, the *estrogenic* smear (Figure 22) shows the predominance of superficial cells, the most mature of the squamous epithelium (Figure 26).

A mechanical compression on cells may be responsible for the presence of the so called "fiber" cells (Figure 27) in the wet mount: they appear elongated and shaped as tape. Their aspect is probably due to a continuous friction on the epithelium, such as that caused by IUD strings or contraceptive vaginal rings. Some round, sharply edged and different in size inclusions may be found in cytoplasm. These evident inclusions are keratohyaline granules and precede the keratinization of the cytoplasm (Figure 28).

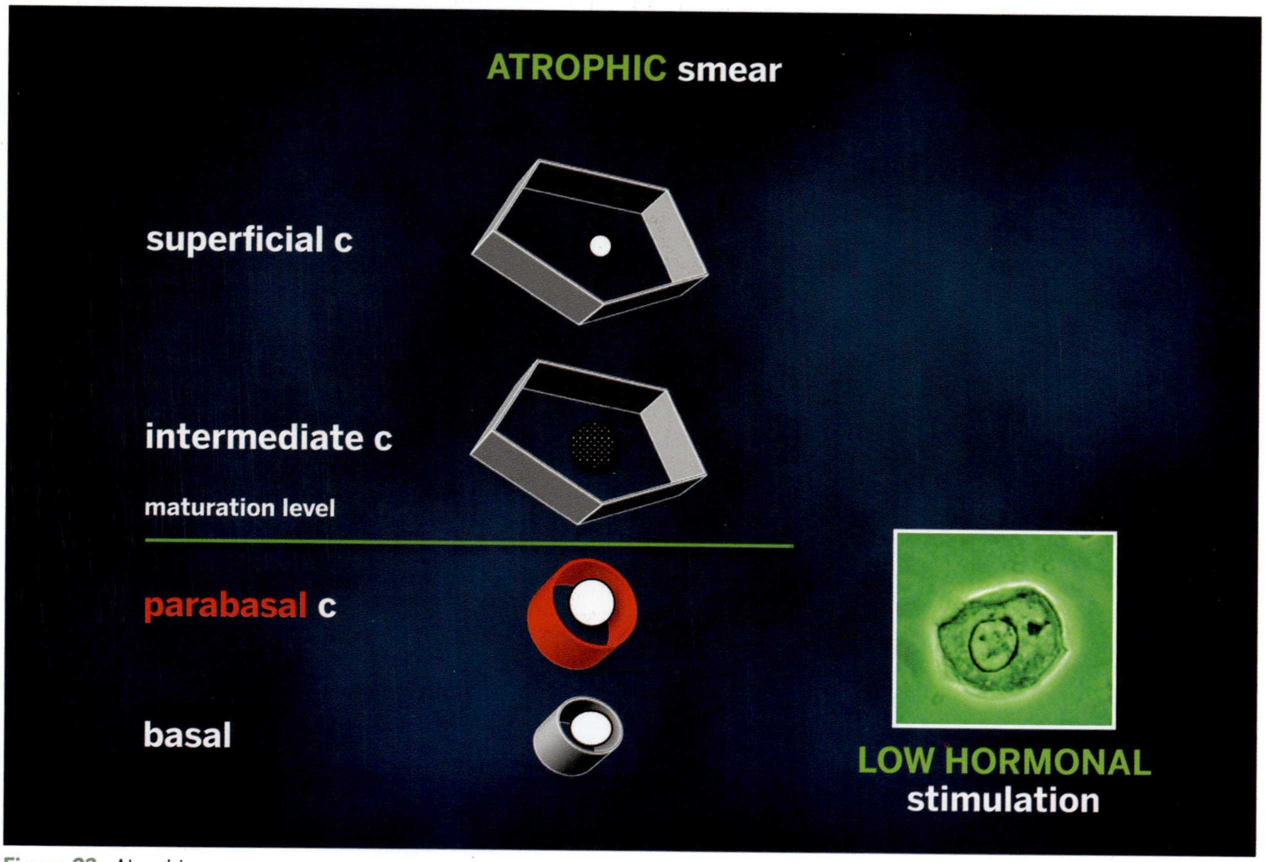

Figure 23 - Atrophic smear.

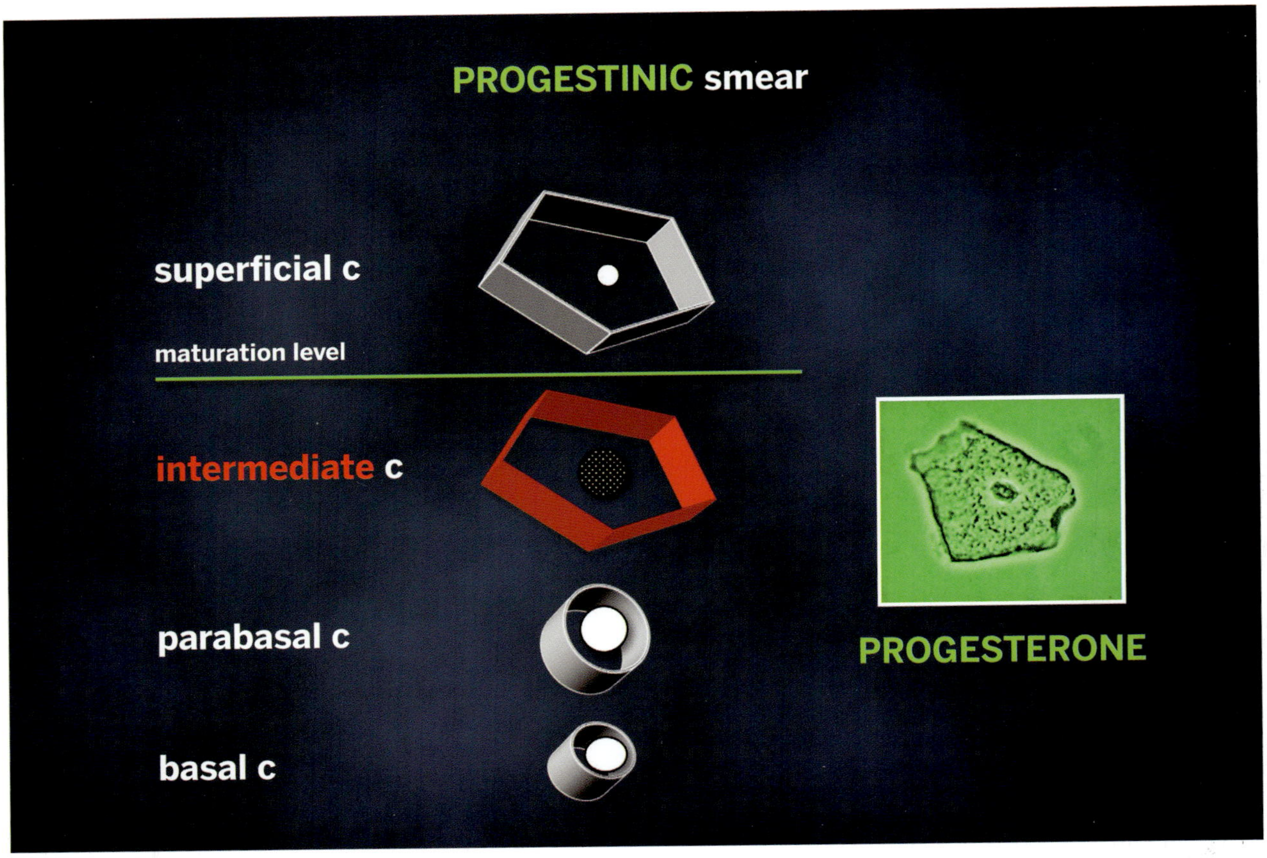

Figure 24 - Progestinic smear.

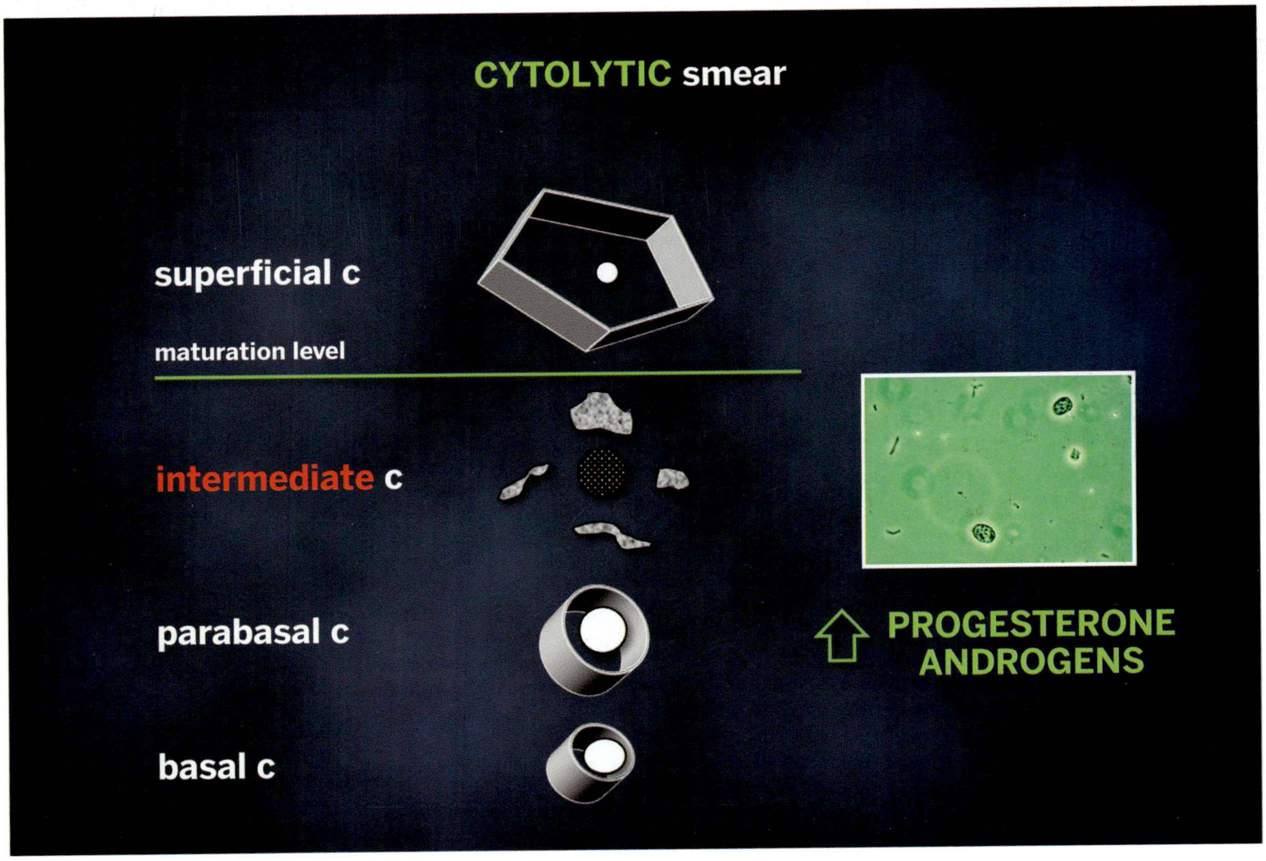

Figure 25 - Cytolytic smear.

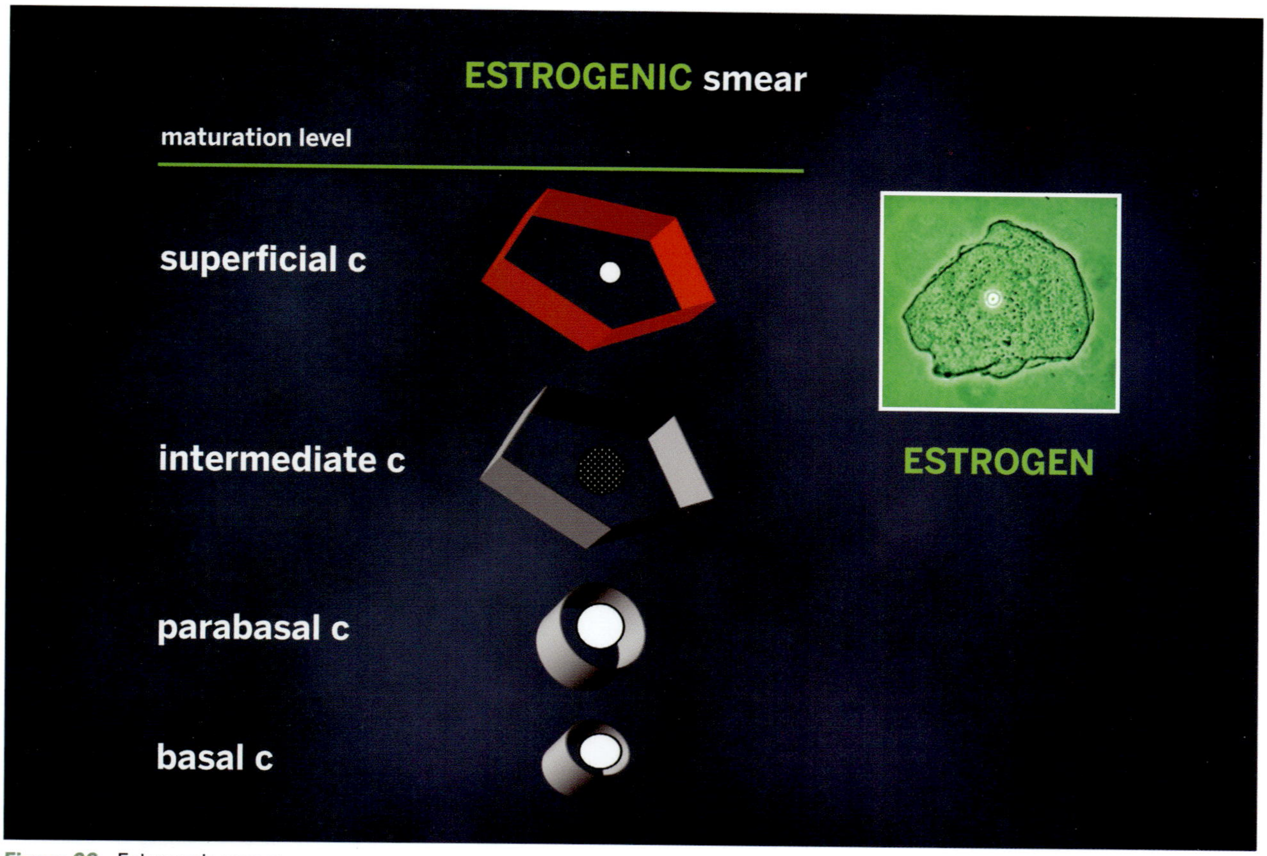

Figure 26 - Estrogenic smear.

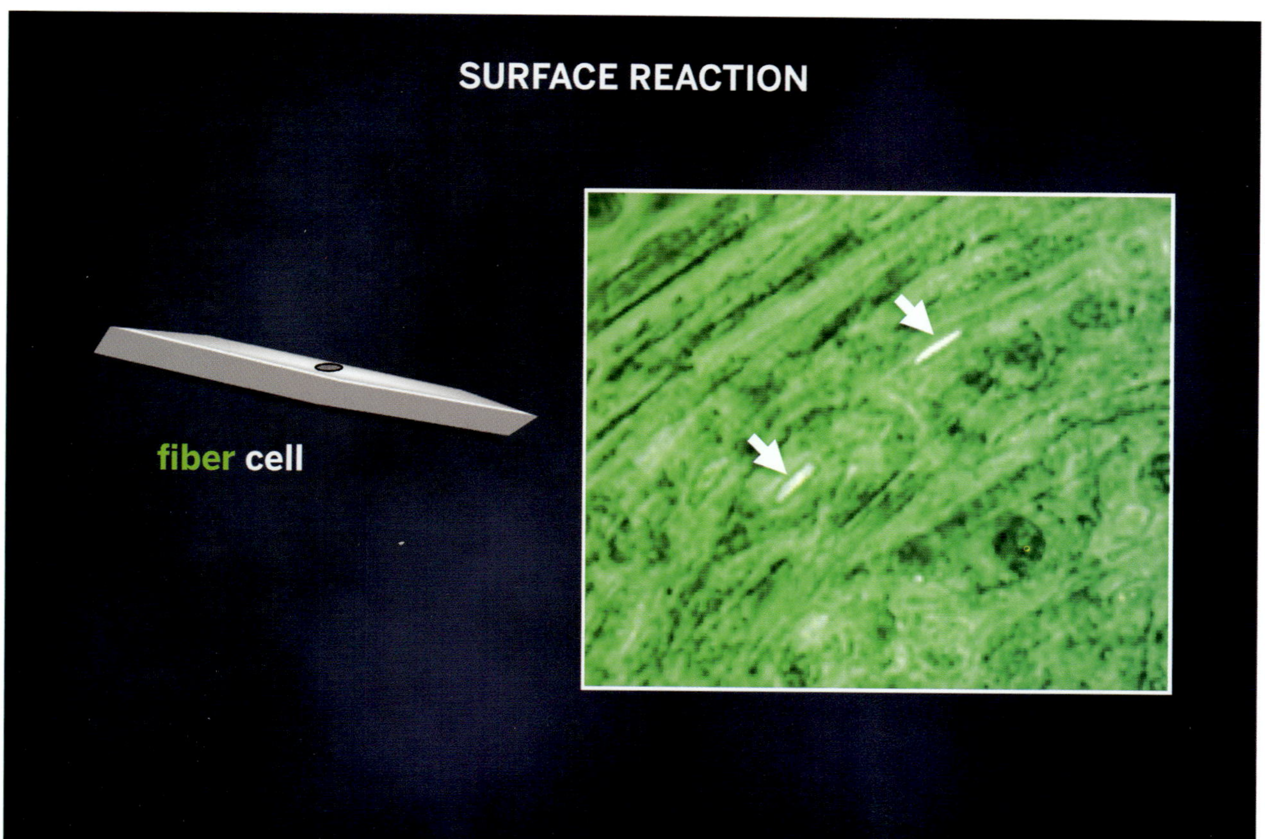

Figure 27 - Fiber cell.

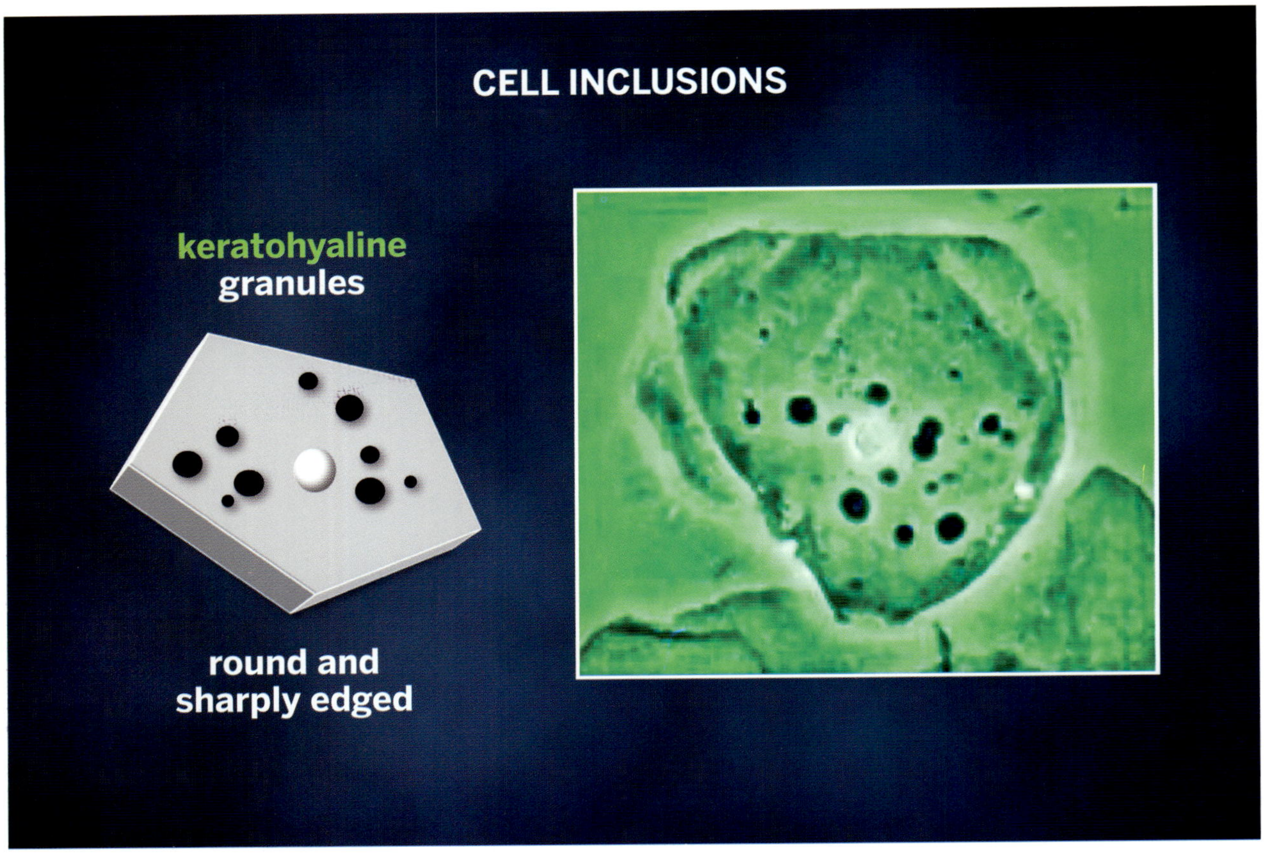

Figure 28 - Keratohyaline granules.

Some other cells can be encountered in a cervico-vaginal wet mount:

- *horny* cell
- *parakeratotic* cell
- *endocervical* cell
- *endometrial* cell.

Horny cells characterize hyperkeratosis whereas parakeratotic cells define parakeratosis. These flattened cells exhibit an excessive keratinization that usually involves their border and lack of cytoplasmic organelles (Figure 29).

Horny cells form the outermost layer of the epidermis, consisting of dead cells (corneocytes), but may also be present in the vagina. The horny cell (Figure 30) is anucleate or contains only a nuclear shadow (ghost nucleus). Keratinization could result from frequent infection, local irritation -as in uterine prolapse or in leukoplakia- or may be the consequence of an excessive estrogen stimulation. Horny cells frequently show bacterial adhesion.

The *parakeratotic* cell is highly keratinized and still contains a viable nucleus (Figure 31). Parakeratosis is usually associated with inflammatory conditions or with Human Papilloma Virus infection.

The uterine cervix consists of an outer ectocervix covered by a nonkeratinized stratified squamous epithelium and an endocervical canal lined with a single layer of columnar cells (Figure 32).

The *endocervical cells* may be secretory or ciliated. This epithelium begins at the squamocolumnar junction and lines the endocervix and the endocervical crypts. It consists of a single layer of mucus-producing columnar cells (*secretory cells*) (Figure 33). Secretory cells produce a mucus plug to prevent bacterial and fungal infection of the uterus. These cells are tall and cylindrical and are arranged in a "picket fence" alignment. Secretory cells contain abundant vacuolated cytoplasm, while nuclei show a finely granular and thin texture. Nucleoli are inconspicuous but become quite prominent in reactive conditions such as cervicitis. Endocervical cells vary greatly in their morphology. Nuclei may also vary in size, shape and position within the cell body. Nuclei are mostly situated basally, adjacent to the basement

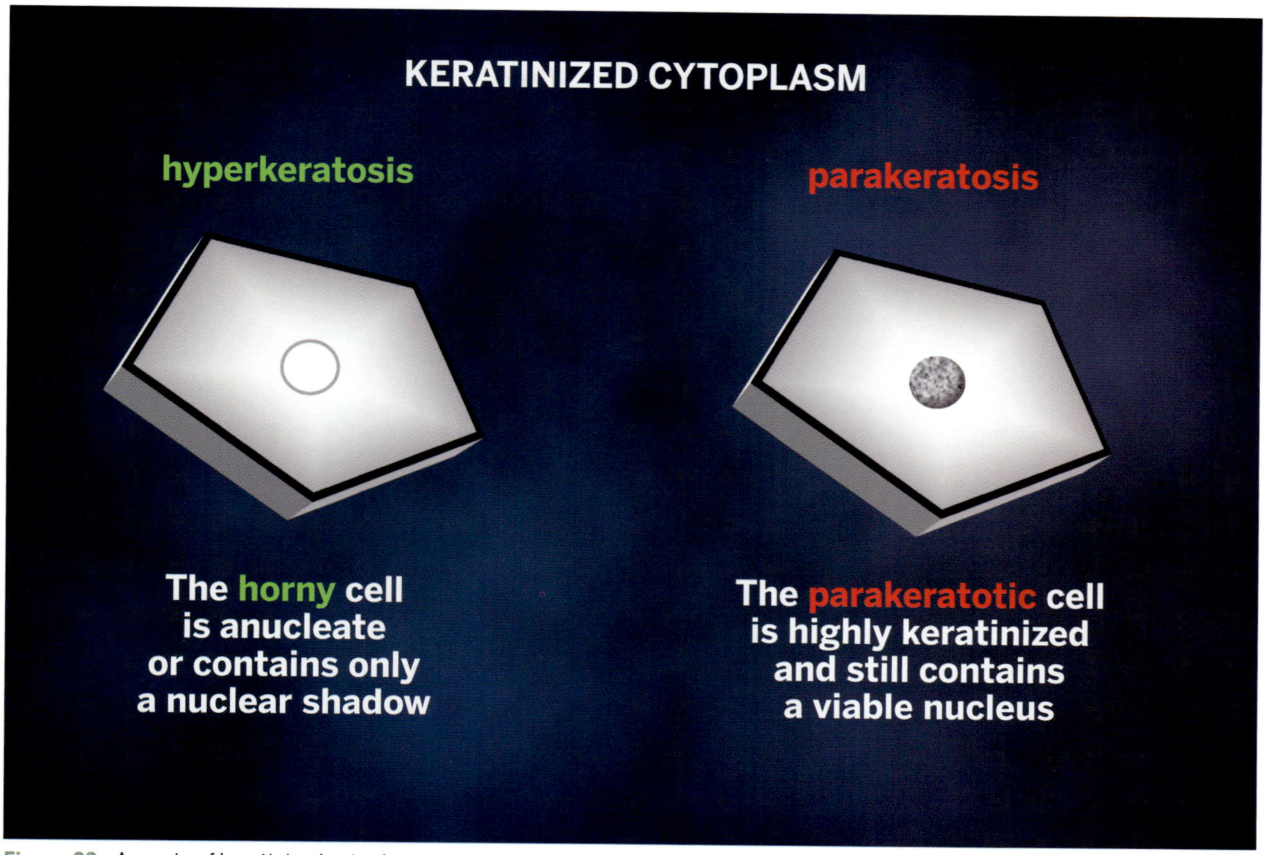

Figure 29 - Aspects of keratinized cytoplasm.

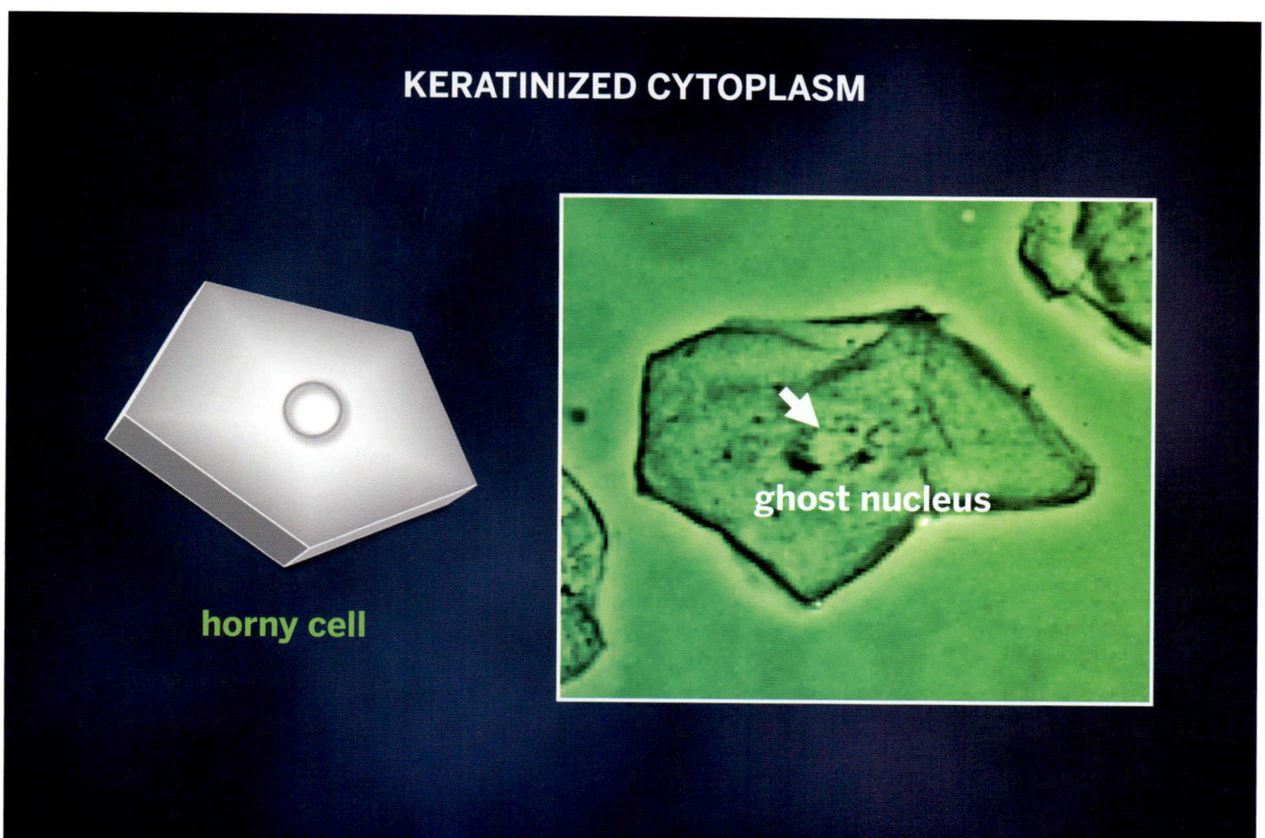

Figure 30 - Horny cell.

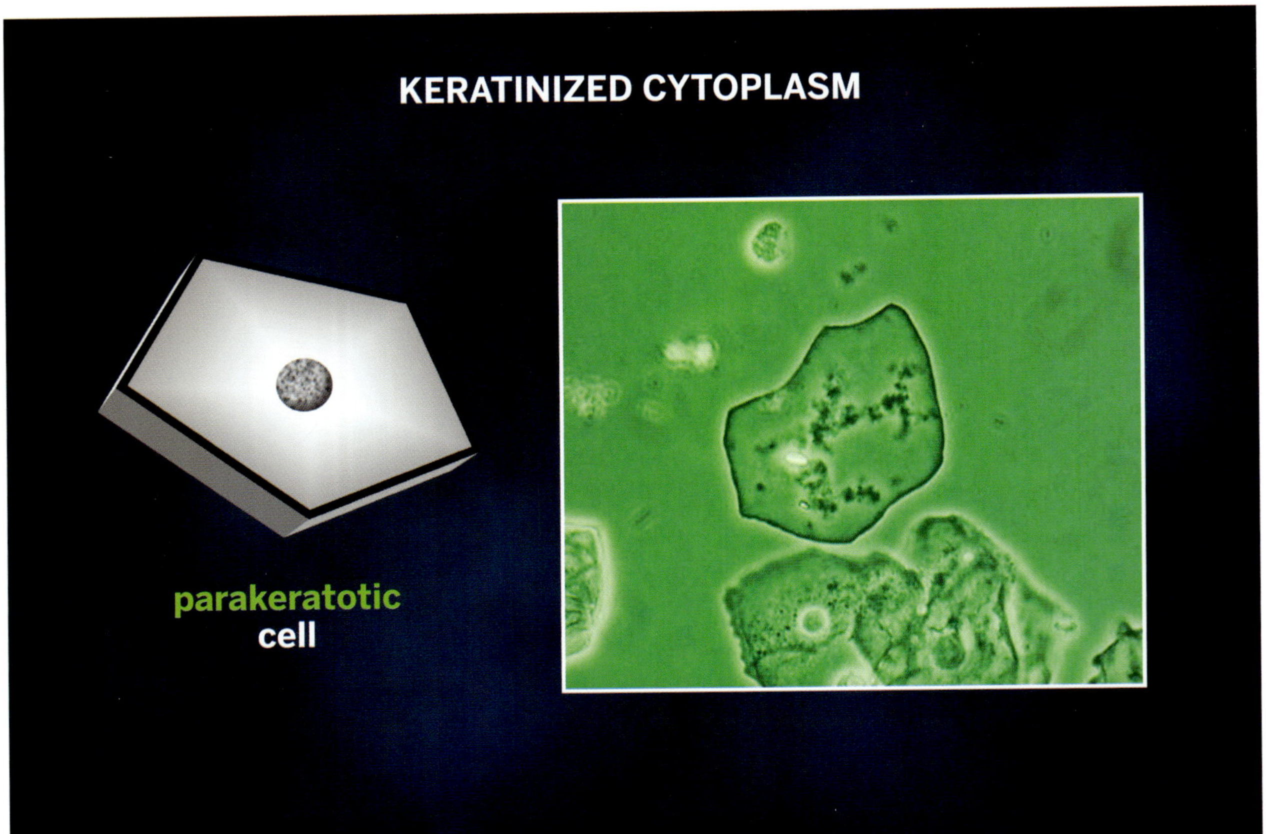

Figure 31 - Parakeratotic cell.

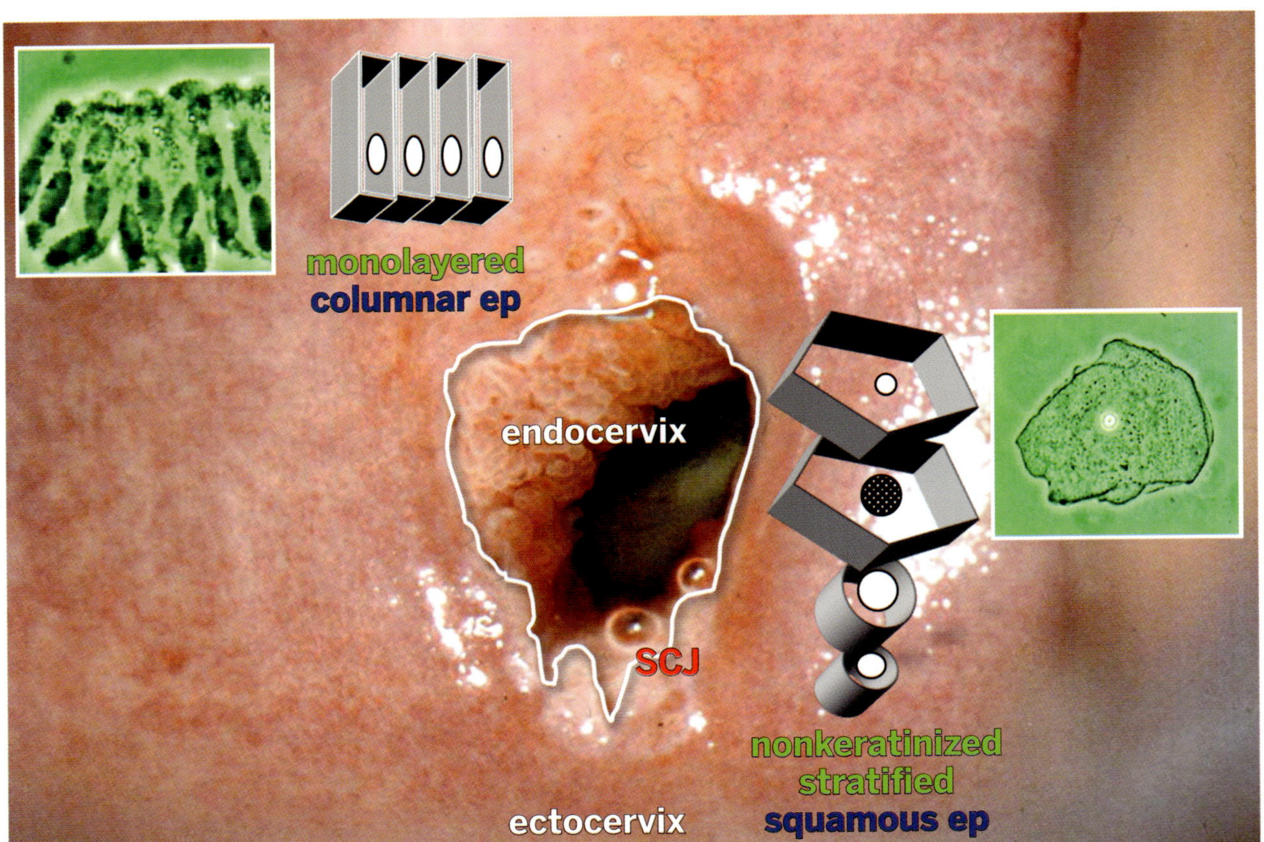

Figure 32 - Regions of the cervix and lining epithelia.

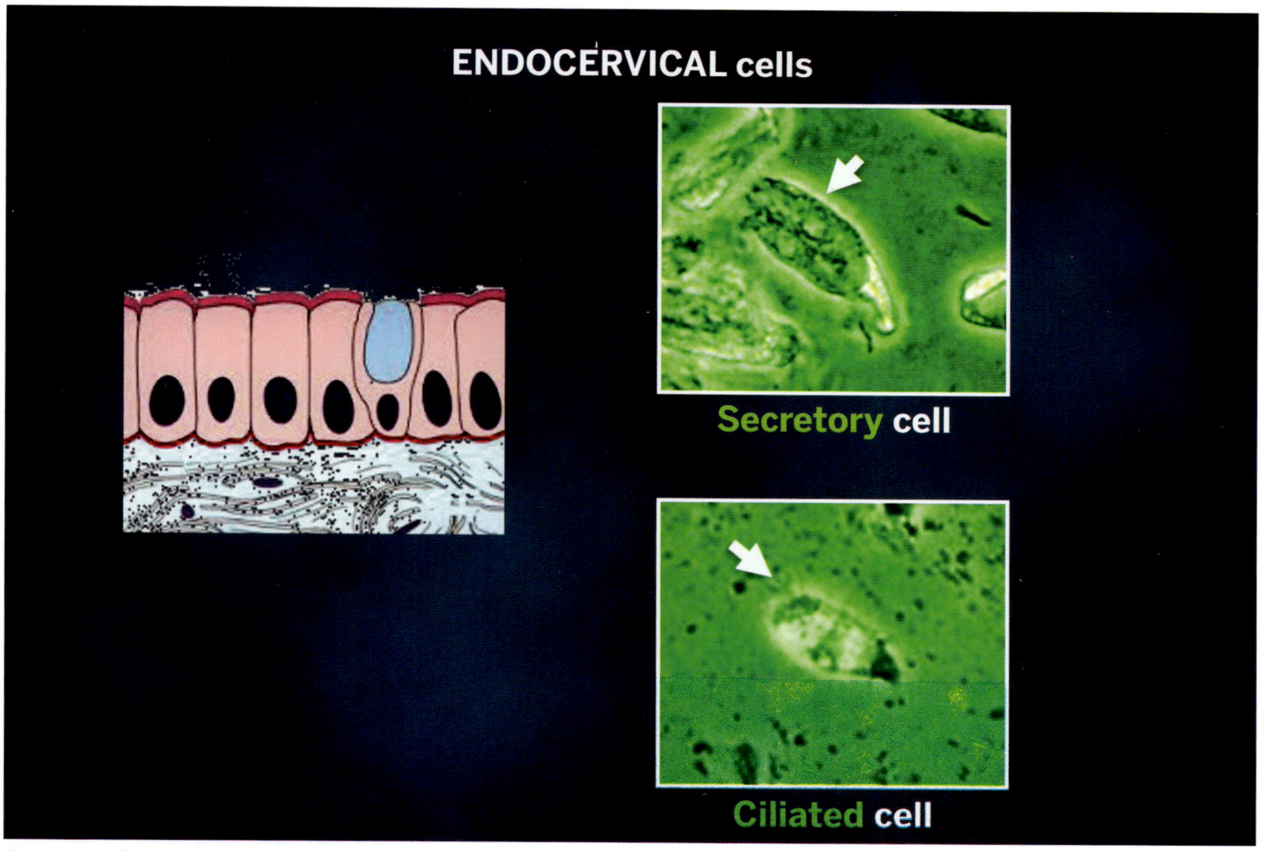

Figure 33 - Endocervical cells.

membrane, even though during active mucous secretion they can be displaced by the mucus and pushed towards the centre of the cell (Figure 34). In inflammatory conditions there may be mucus depletion (Figure 34), the endocervical cells are less tall and mitoses may occasionally be seen in the absence of neoplasia or pre-neoplasia.

The *ciliated cells* (Figure 33) are most numerous at the endometrial/endocervical junction. They may be present elsewhere in the endocervix as "tubal metaplasia", usually after surgery such as loop electrosurgical excision procedure (LEEP) or cone biopsy. Their main function is to actively carry the mucus along the mucous membrane. Ciliated cells may also contain mucus vacuoles.

When ciliated cells are shed isolated, they can move in water under microscopic examination and may be confused with mobile Trichomonas vaginalis. In case of doubt, the screener can observe the common emergence of the anterior flagella in Trichomonas, whereas apical cilia erase discretely from the top of the ciliated cell (Figure 35).

Endocervical cells are often observed in strips or sheets rather than as isolated cells. When arranged as strips, the cells have the appearance of a picket fence. When in sheets, they resemble a honeycomb because of the uniform cell arrangement and the well-defined cell borders (Figure 36).

Endometrial cells may have a columnar or cuboid (Figure 37) appearance. Ciliated glandular cells can be identified in a few cases, often in estrogen-stimulated conditions. Endometrial cells show scant cytoplasm and round, ovoid or elongated nuclei, appearing as pale or dark in case of dense chromatin. Isolated cells are common. Endometrial cells can be observed in sheets or cohesive groups, although rarely with a honeycomb pattern. When cell clusters with a honeycomb pattern are encountered, it is not easy to indicate with certainty whether the cluster originates from endometrium or endocervix, even if endometrial cells are generally smaller than endocervical cells and show ill-defined cell borders. Occasionally, endometrial cell clusters consist of a dual cell population with small, dark stromal cells

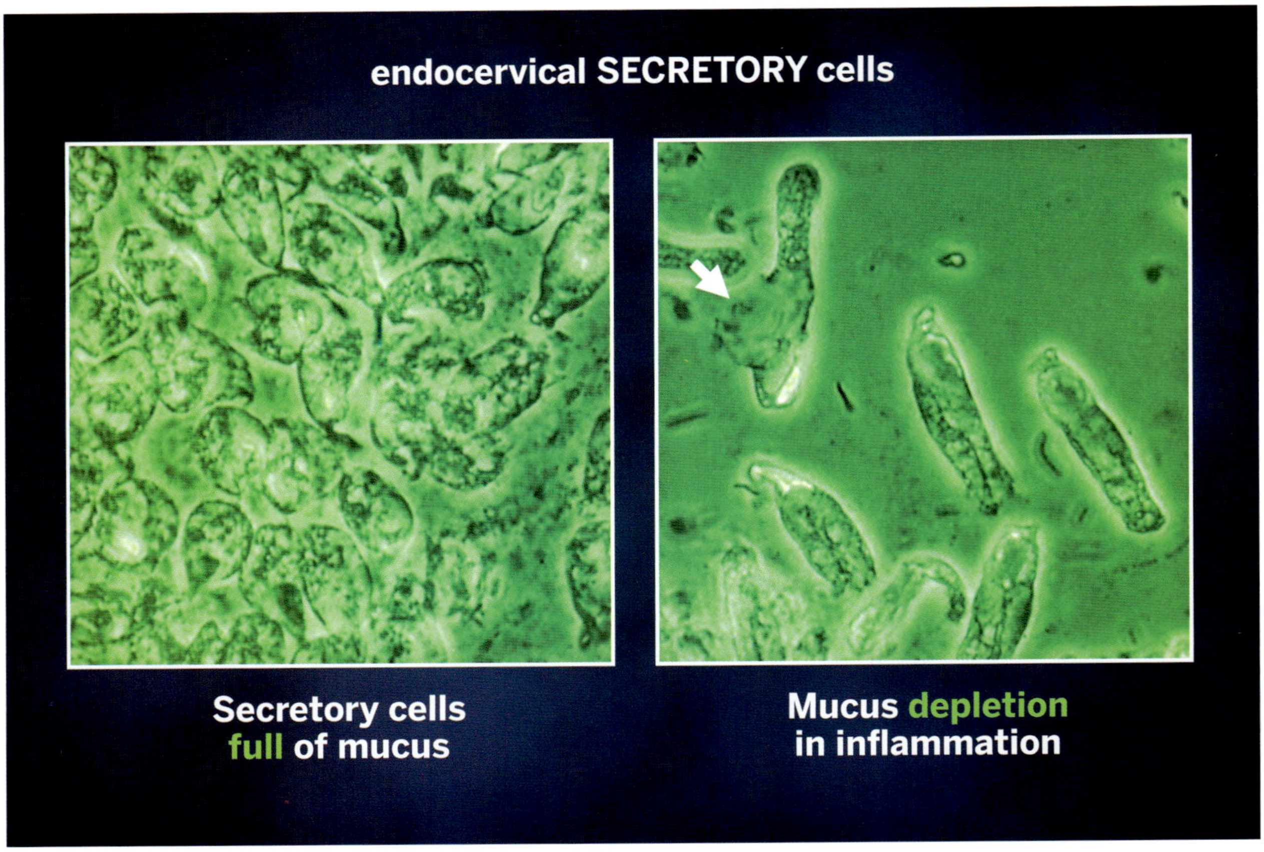

Figure 34 - Endocervical secretory cells.

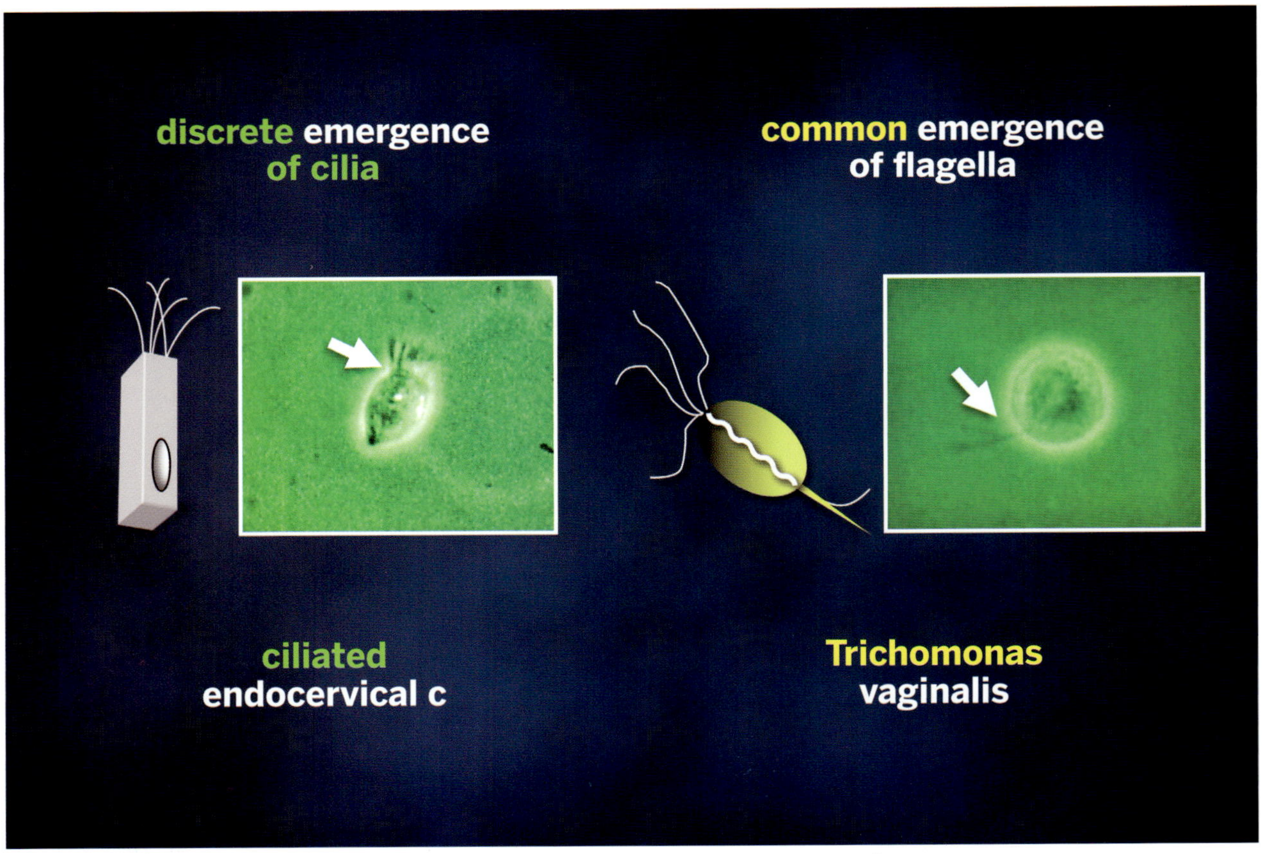

Figure 35 - Differential diagnosis between ciliated endocervical cell and Trichomonas vaginalis.

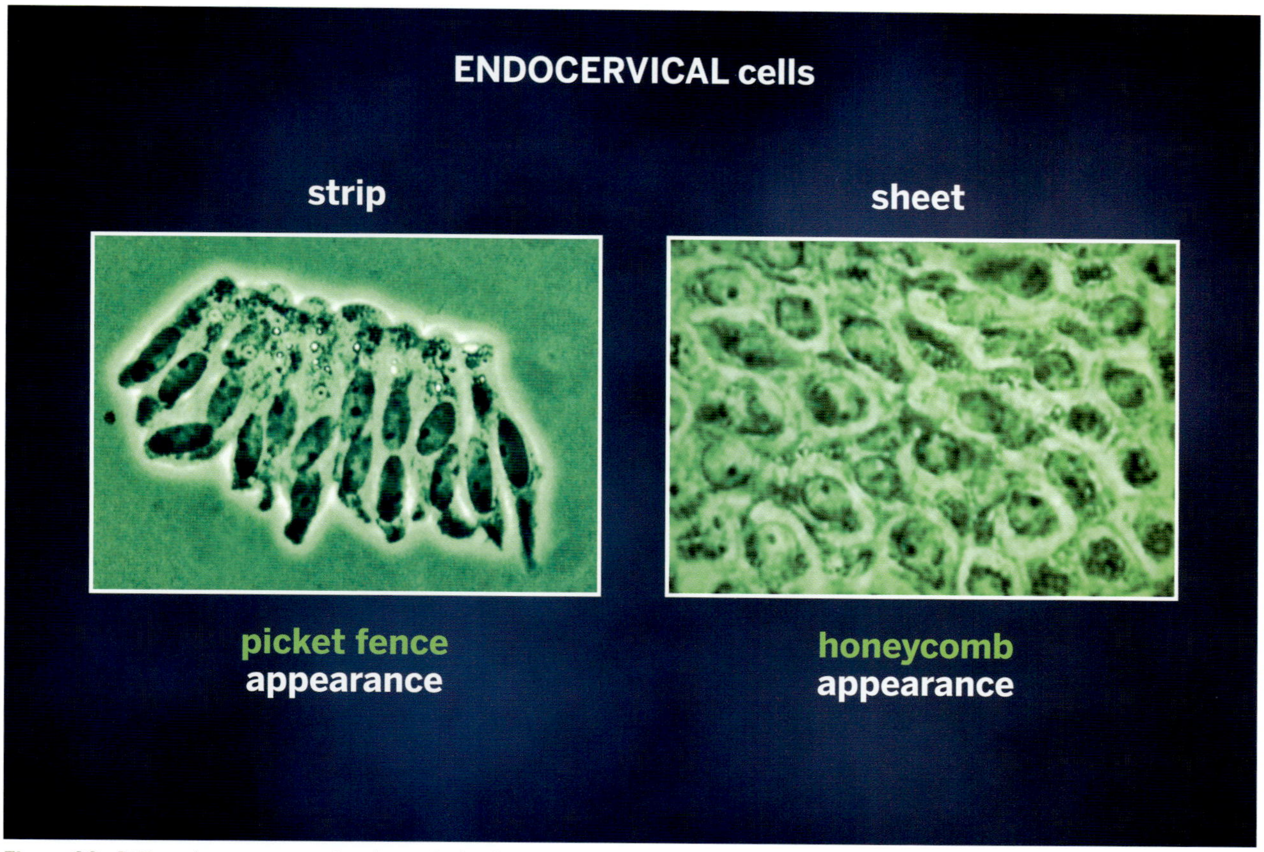

Figure 36 - Different appearance of endocervical cells.

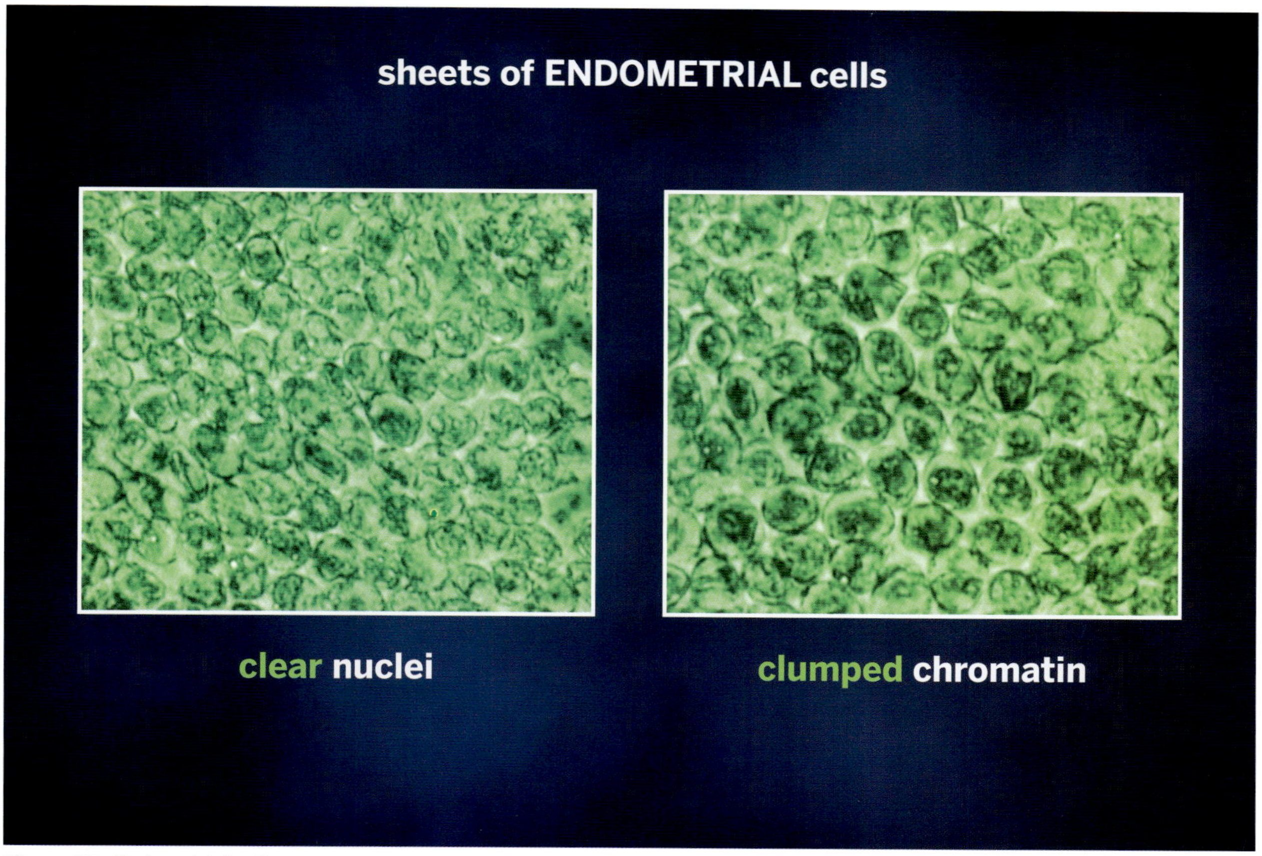

Figure 37 - Endometrial cells.

in the center and large glandular cells around the edges. Most endometrial clusters, however, do not show dual population.

Endometrial cells are notorious for their ability to be diagnostically challenging, because a variety of neoplastic cells resemble endometrial cells, particularly in the first 12 days of the menstrual cycle when scant endometrial shedding is normal. However, atypical cells that can mimic endometrial cells are usually bigger, vary more in size and have denser cytoplasm. Unfortunately, some poorly differentiated squamous cell carcinomas are composed of small dark cells that mimic endometrial cells to perfection.

The vaginal epithelium varies physiologically in response to the hormonal climate at different times of life and it reflects the changes recurring with each menstrual cycle (Table 1).

TABLE 1 - **Cellular changes in different times of life**
NEWBORN INFANT: prevalent intermediate cells and superficial cells.
WITHIN A WEEK AFTER DELIVERY: appearance of some parabasal cells.
THREE WEEKS AFTER DELIVERY AND DURING CHILDHOOD: basal and parabasal cells along with leukocytes and amorphous debris (*atrophic smear*).
PUBERTY: appearance of large superficial cells and Lactobacilli.
MESTRUAL CYCLE • **Menstruation**: erythrocytes, histiocytes, granulocytes and intermediate cells. Clusters of endometrial cells can be observed. • **Early proliferative phase**: slight desquamation of clumped small intermediate cells with folded cell margins along with fewer flattened and solitary superficial cells. Some leukocytes. • **Advanced proliferative phase**: predominant superficial cells are largely isolated and flattened. Rare leukocytes. • **Late proliferative phase**: initial tendency to clustering and folding up of superficial cells with the highest karyopiknotic index. • **Early secretory phase**: copious shedding of large intermediate cells with marked clustering. Leukocytes increase in number. • **Advanced secretory phase**: intermediate cells show a pronounced folding and rolling-up of their margins. Bare nuclei, cytoplasmic debris, numerous granulocytes and copious Döderlein flora (*cytolytic smear*). • **Late secretory phase**: dirty and faded smear for striking cellular breakdown.
PREGNANCY: predominant intermediate cells with frequent cytolysis and pronounced folding and rolling-up of cell margins (navicular cells).
PUERPERIUM • **Early** phase: basal and parabasal cells (atrophic smear) associated with bacteria, numerous granulocytes and macrophages. • **Advanced** phase: wide range of cell maturation with all cell types being present.
CLIMACTERIUM: estrogenic smear with predominance of superficial cells.
MENOPAUSE: semi-atrophic smear showing a maturation range from basal to intermediate cells. Some polymorphs.
POSTMENOPAUSE • **Atrophic** smear: basal and parabasal cells. Numerous polymorphs. • **Intermediate** (androgenic) smear: predominantly intermediate cells, but also some parabasal cells lying separately. • **Superficial** (estrogenic) smear: largely solitary and flattened superficial cells.

In the ***newborn infant*** (Figure 38) the high concentration of maternal blood estrogen transmitted across the placental membrane is responsible for the presence of intermediate cells (progestinic smear) and, to a lesser extent, of superficial cells (estrogenic smear).

Within a week the estrogen stimulation regresses and some basal cells appear. Three weeks after delivery the vaginal smear contains basal and parabasal cells associated with leukocytes and amorphous debris (atrophic smear).

This cell pattern, typical of an atrophic condition, will typify the vaginal smear during ***childhood*** (Figure 39) when the slow cell regeneration, the lack of protective action by the large squamous cells and the absence of Lactobacilli make vaginal mucosa fragile and liable to infection.

During this age of life, the screener may immediately detect, by a direct observation of a vaginal wet mount, any condition of estrogen stimulation revealed by the predominance of superficial cells (Figure 40). Most of the times, the early symptom is represented by a "sterile" watery discharge. This condition should be a warning signal requiring additional diagnostic evaluation of ovarian and suprarenal activity. In fact, an estrogenic smear can reveal an unsuspected precocious puberty. It must be pointed out that cytologic evidence of estrogen stimulation may appear long before Rx and magnetic resonance imaging.

A physiological estrogen stimulation on the vaginal mucosa accompanies the onset of ***puberty*** (Figure 41) and is responsible for the appearance of large superficial cells mixed with Lactobacilli in the vaginal smear.

When ***reproductive age*** is reached, peripheral effects exerted by different hormones on the vaginal mucosa are responsible for all four cellular smears (Figure 42).

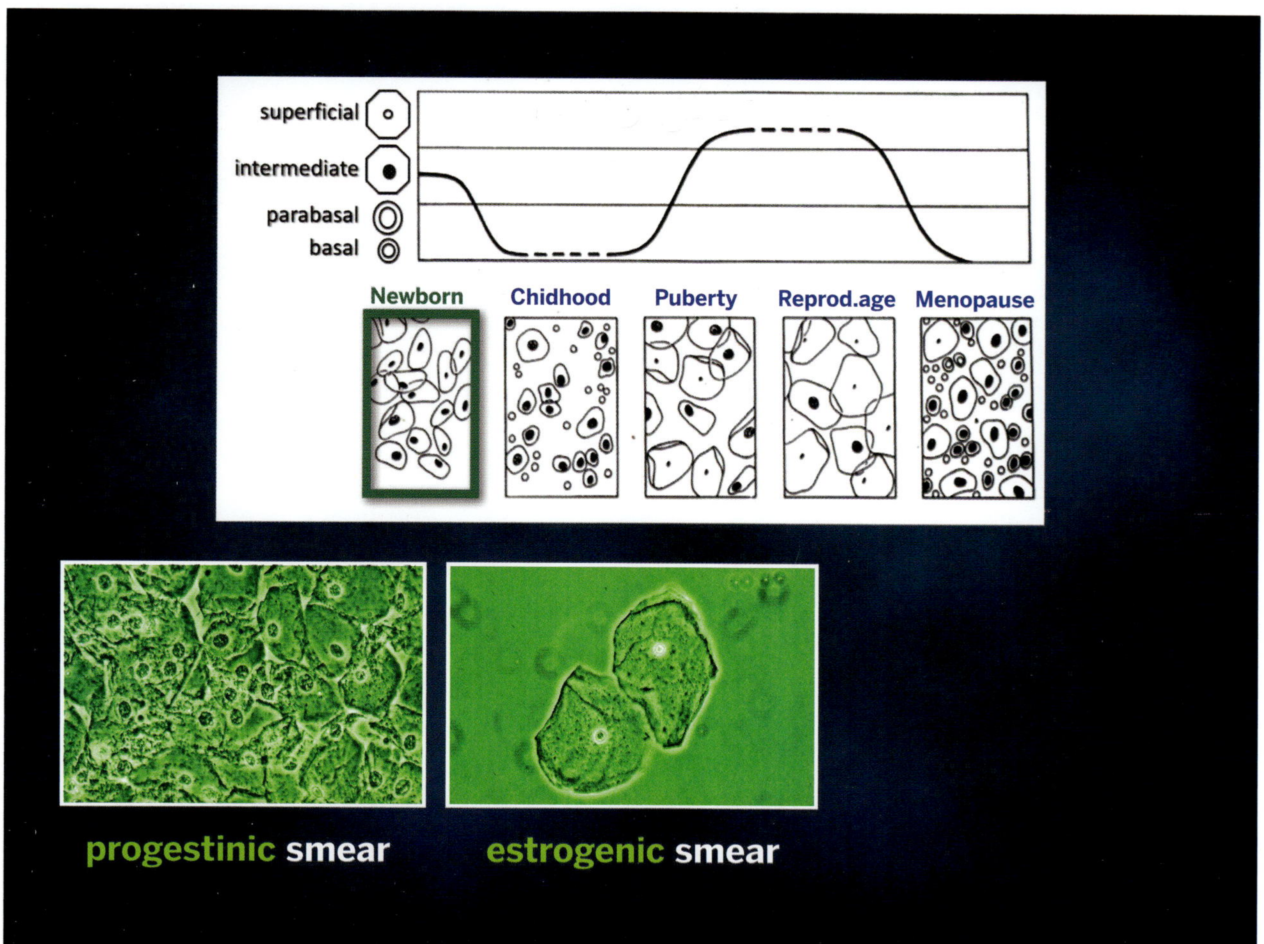

Figure 38 - Progestinic or estrogenic smear in newborn.

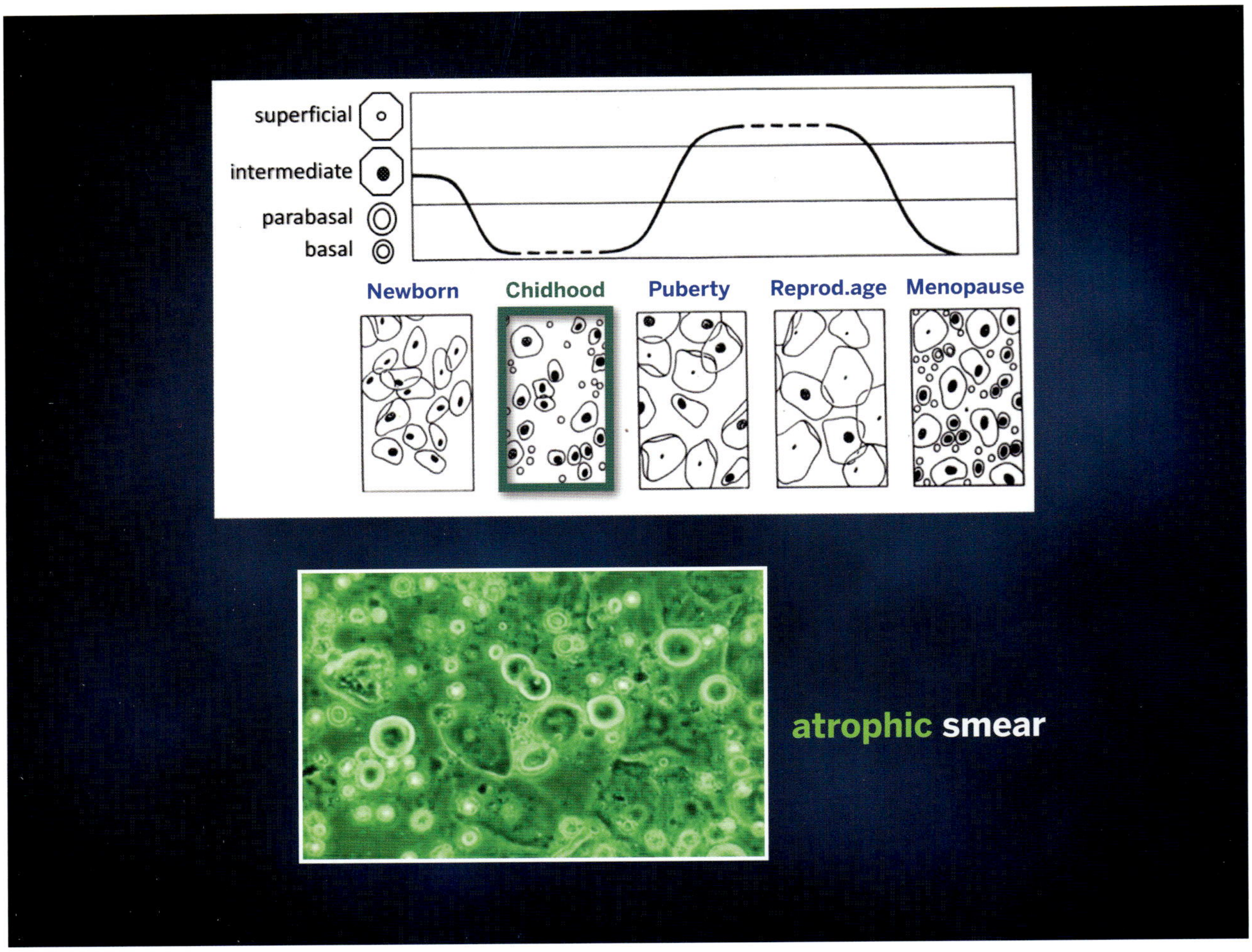

Figure 39 - Atrophic smear in childhood.

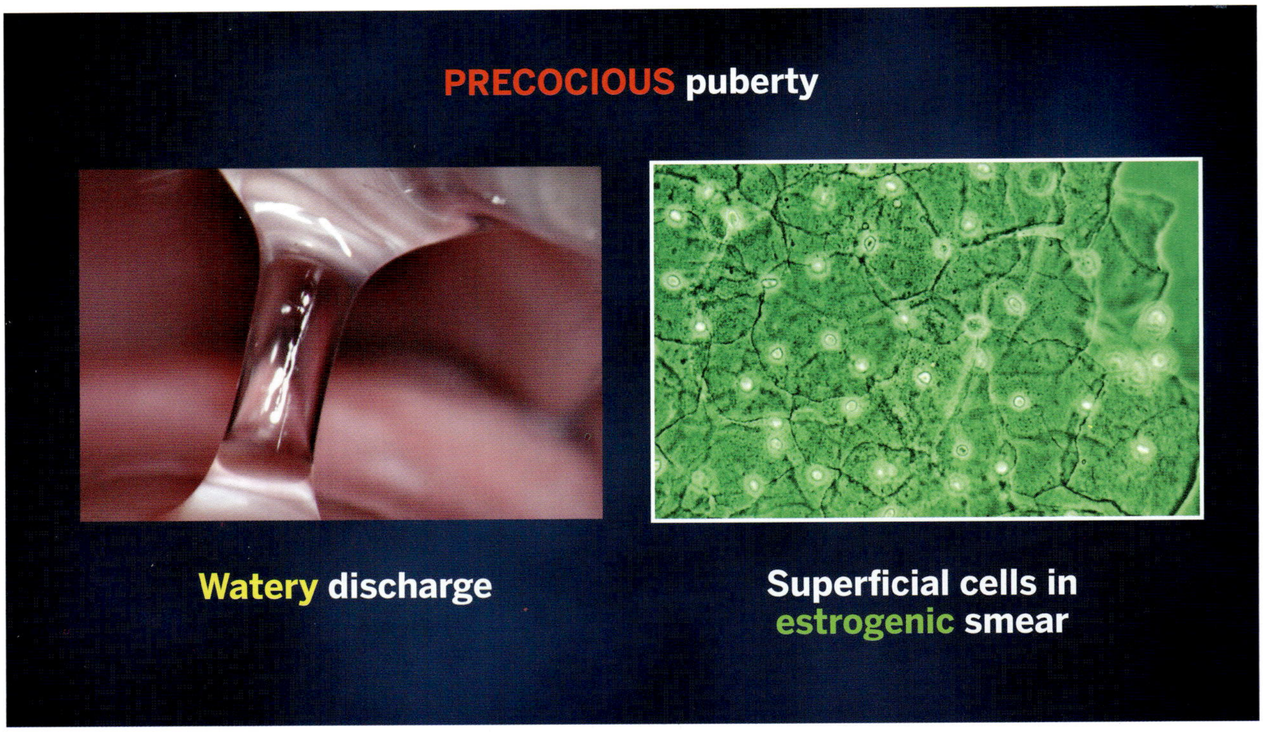

Figure 40 - Clinical and cytologic aspects in precocious puberty.

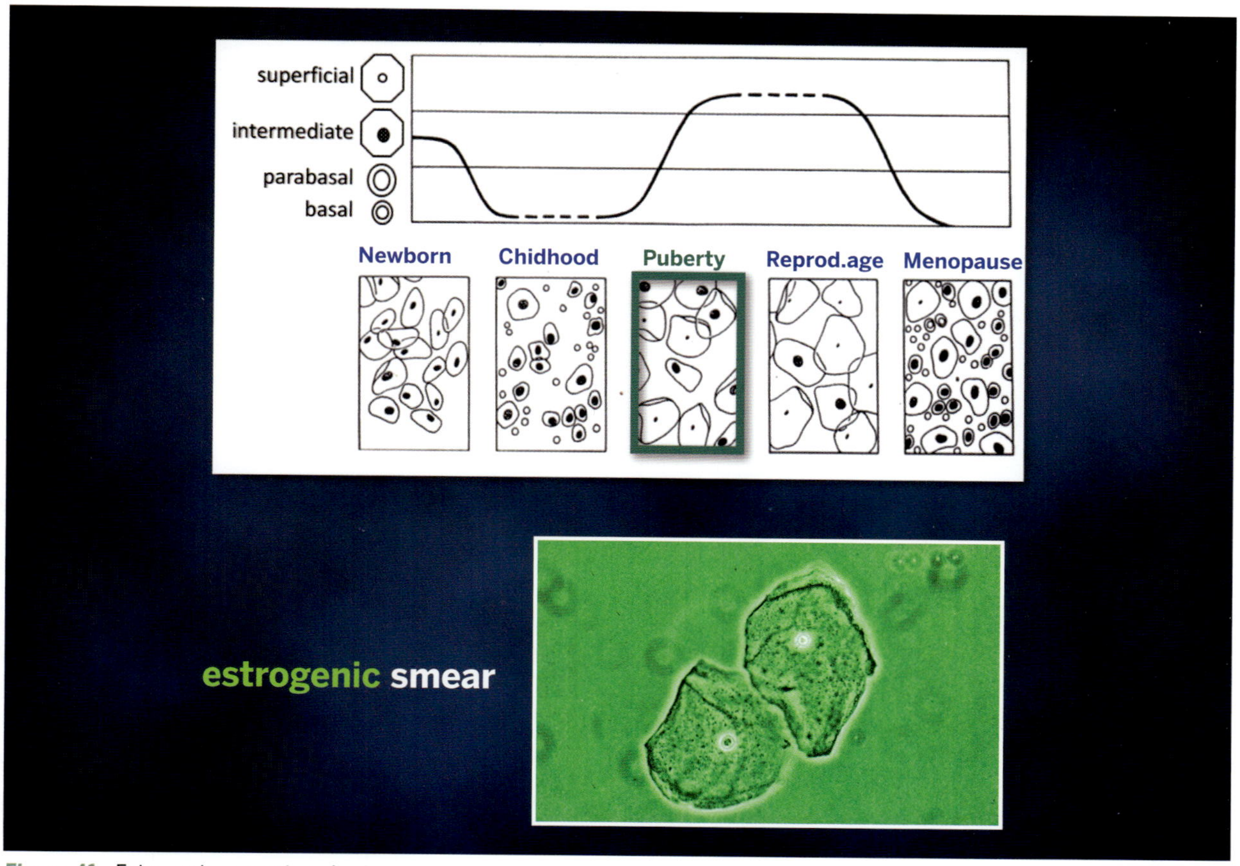

Figure 41 - Estrogenic smear in puberty.

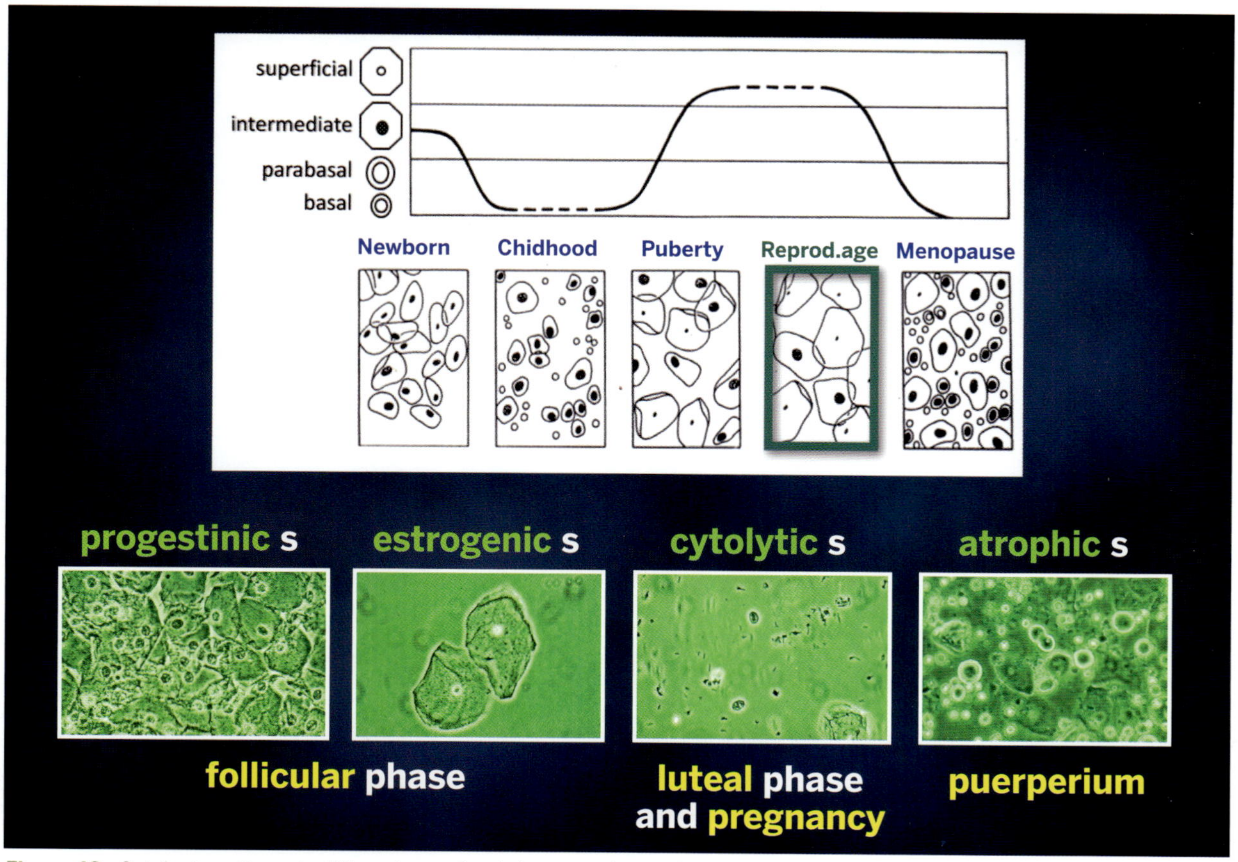

Figure 42 - Cytologic patterns in different menstrual phases and periods of reproductive age.

During *menstruation* (Figure 43) the vaginal smear shows a great amount of viable and dysmorphic erythrocytes, macrophages, many polymorphonuclear leukocytes and bacteria. Vaginal epithelium is predominantly represented by intermediate cells which appear as flat and discrete.

Endometrial cells tightly clumped in clusters are normally detected during menstruation, but they may also be observed in the first 12 days of the menstrual cycle and in women wearing an IUD (Figure 44). With the exception of these conditions, the presence of endometrial cells in vaginal smear makes further investigation advisable, even when the cells look normal. In fact, shedding endometrial cells after day 12 ("out of phase") may be associated with endometritis and endometrial polyps. Women older than 40 must be further investigated to exclude glandular hyperplasia and endometrial adenocarcinoma. Abnormal shedding of endometrial cells in young women hardly ever results from endometrial adenocarcinoma.

During *early follicular phase* (Figure 45) in post-menstrual period, desquamation of intermediate and fewer superficial cells is slight; superficial cells are flattened and lie separately, while intermediate cells appear clumped with folded-up cytoplasmic margins. Some leukocytes persist from the menstrual period.

Under the increasing estrogenic stimulation the nucleus progressively becomes smaller and densely piknotic; around the 11th-12th day of cycle (*advanced follicular phase*) (Figure 46) predominant superficial cells are largely isolated and flattened, and almost no granulocyte can be observed.

The *late follicular phase* (14th day of cycle) (Figure 47) is characterized by superficial cells with the highest karyopyknotic index and good cytoplasmic turgor, but showing an initial tendency to clustering and folding-up of the edges. Scattered leukocytes can be found in the vaginal smear.

Daily vaginal smears allow to recognize the time of *ovulation* by the sudden change of the cell pattern.

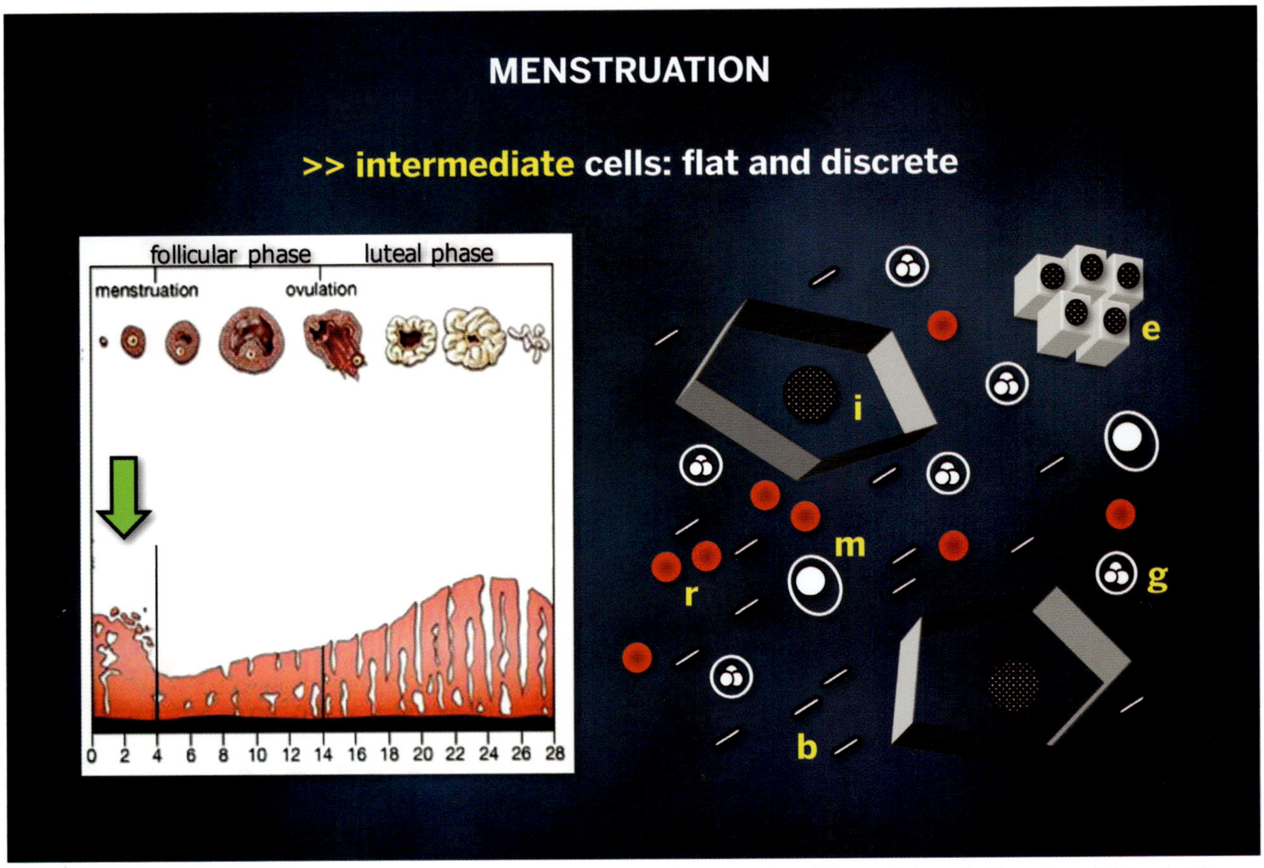

Figure 43 - Diagrammatic representation of cell predominance during menstruation: intermediate cells (i), endometrial cells (e), red blood cells (r), granulocytes (g), macrophages (m) and bacteria (b).

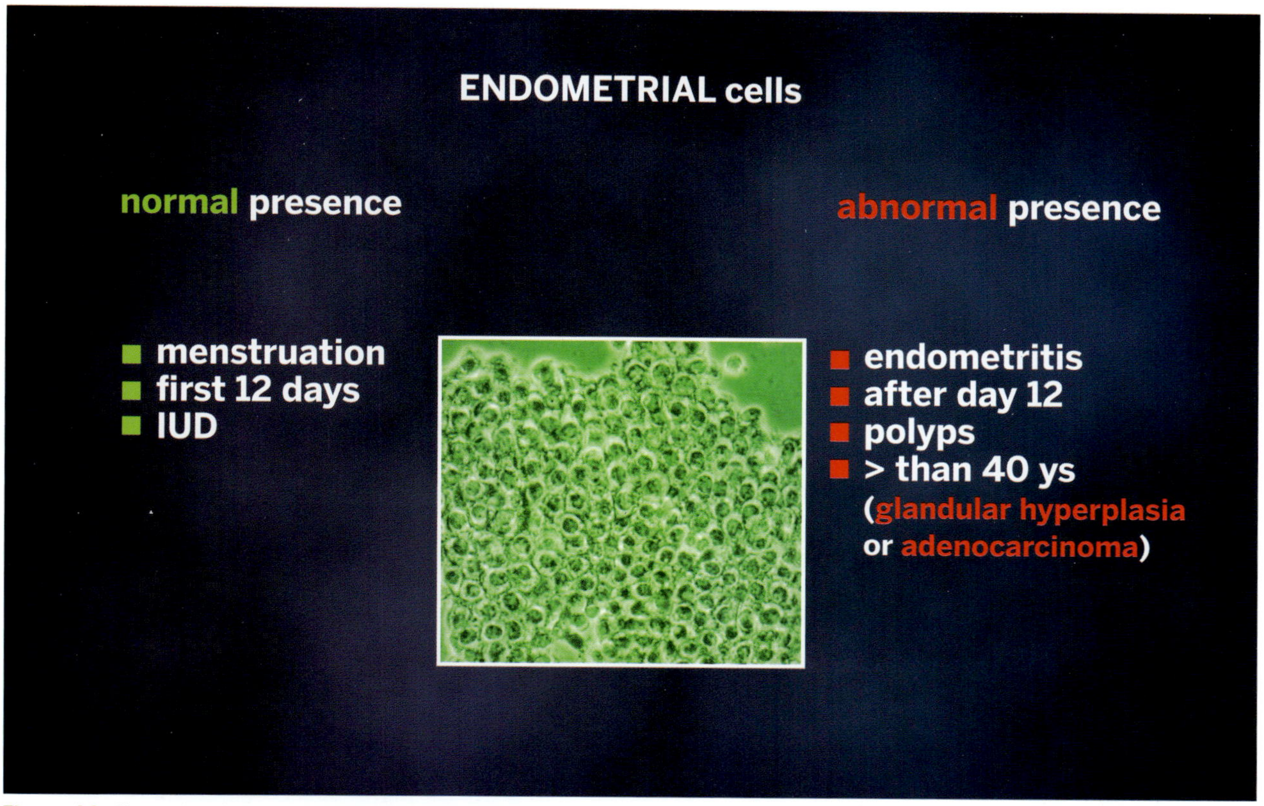

Figure 44 - Normal and abnormal detection of endometrial cells.

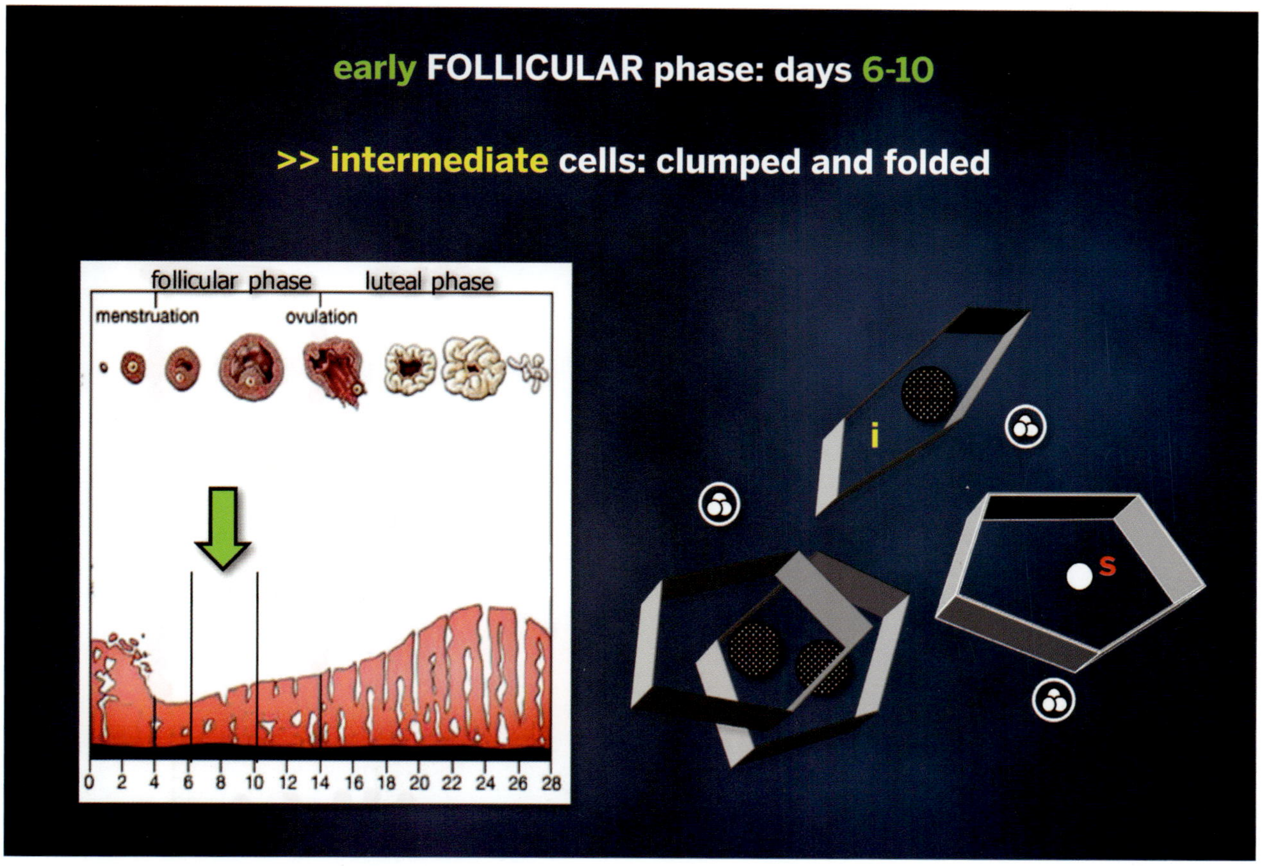

Figure 45 - Diagrammatic representation of cell distribution during early follicular phase: intermediate cells (i) predominate on superficial cells (s).

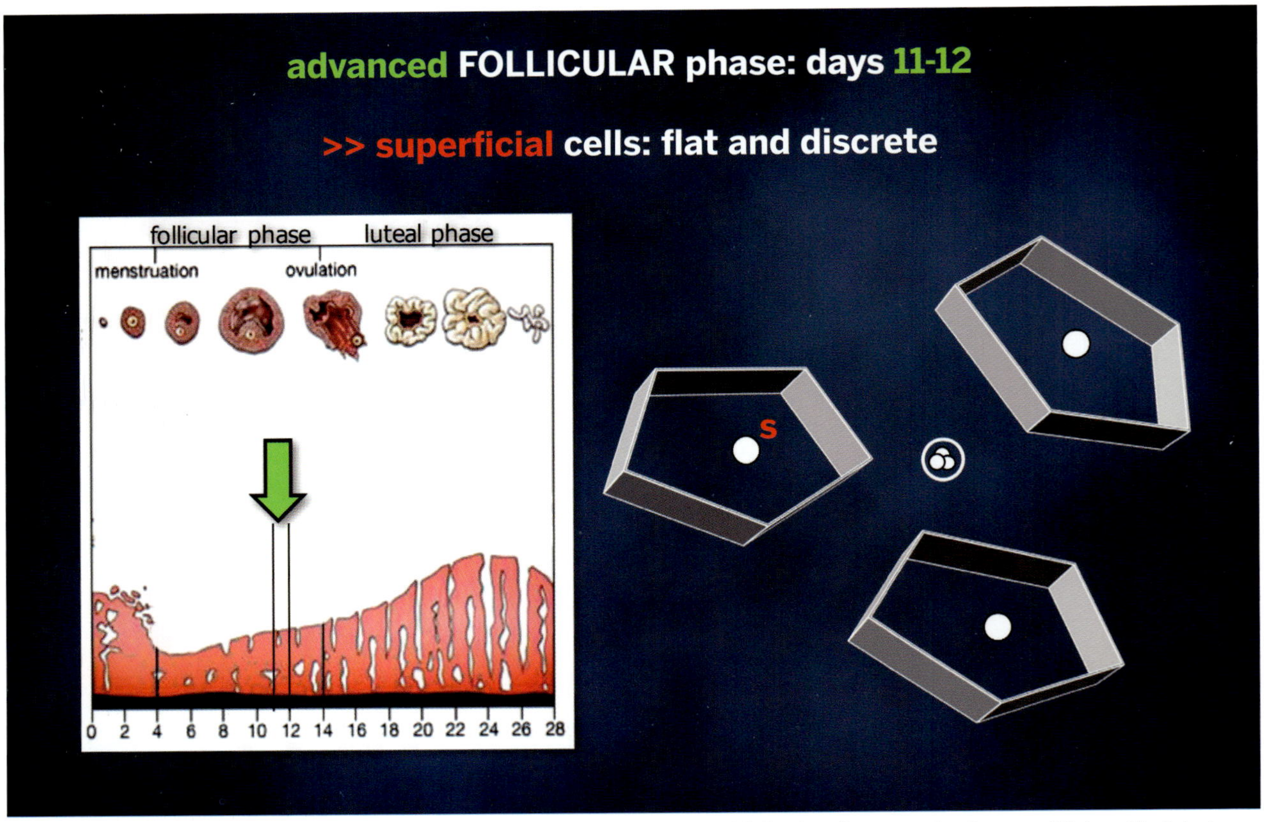

Figure 46 - Diagrammatic representation of cell distribution during advanced follicular phase: predominance of flat and isolated superficial cells (s).

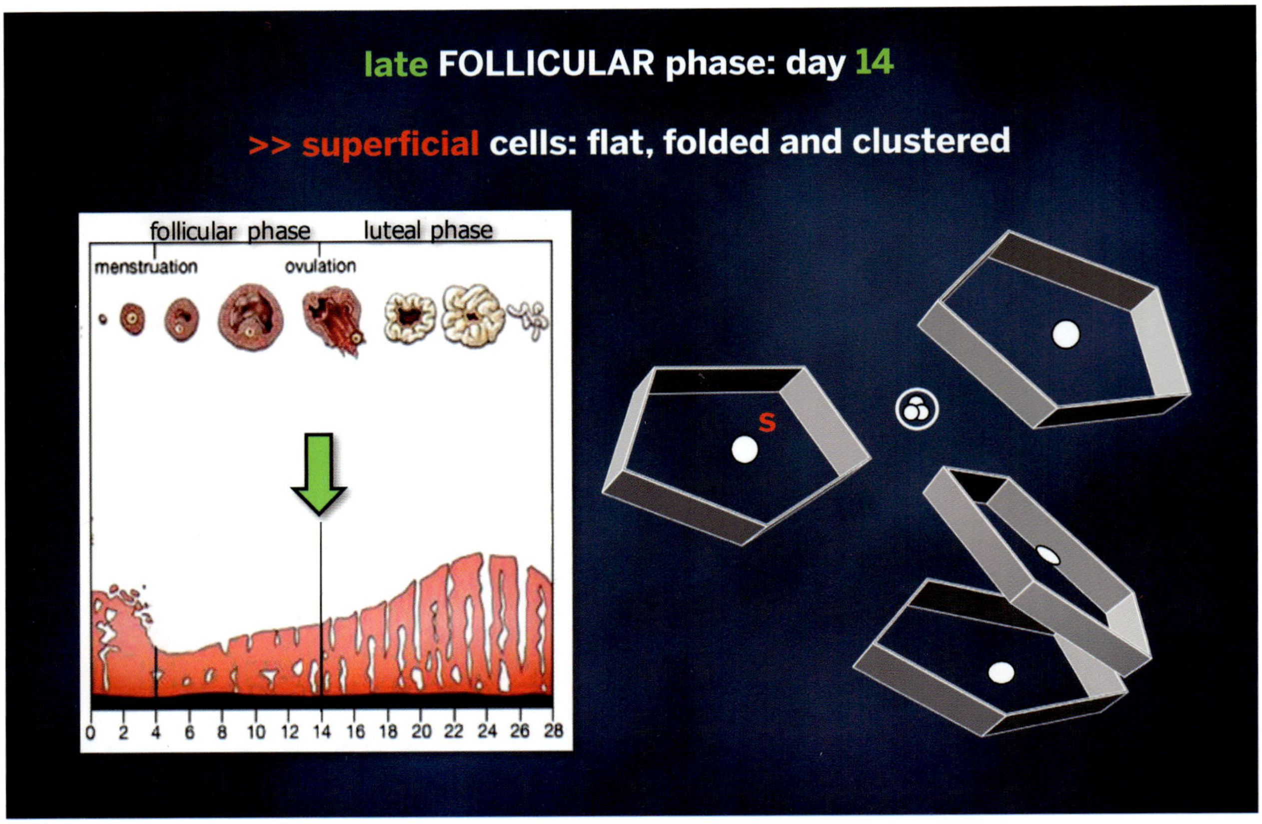

Figure 47 - Diagrammatic representation of cell distribution during late follicular phase: predominance of superficial cells (s) in different behavior.

In fact, production of progesterone from the rapidly forming corpus luteum is responsible for an epithelial regression towards intermediate cells (Figure 48).

The *early* stage of *luteal phase* (days 15-17) (Figure 49) is characterized by an increasing number of intermediate cells. In contrast to early proliferative phase, intermediate cells appear larger, clustering of cells is more marked, cell shedding is copious and leukocytes increase in number.

During the *advanced luteal phase* (days 20-22) (Figure 50) clumping of intermediate cells, associated with folding and rolling-up of their margins, is very pronounced; moreover, a great amount of Lactobacilli and numerous granulocytes can be seen. Progesterone causes cytoplasmic frying with release of bare nuclei and cytoplasmic debris (cytolytic smear).

Two or three days before the onset of menstruation (*late luteal phase*) (Figure 51) the degree of cell desquamation and cellular breakdown reaches its peak, therefore the overall appearance is that of a "dirty" and poorly defined smear.

The presence of viable or dysmorphic erythrocytes indicates the imminent menstruation.

A more or less pronounced cytolysis, induced by the increasing progesterone stimulation during advanced and late luteal phases, confirms that ovulation took place. On the other hand, the evidence of an estrogenic smear in advanced and late luteal phases is a precious tool for the screener to diagnose the lack of ovulation or at least progesterone insufficiency (Figure 52).

Cytolytic smear can be observed in different conditions (Figure 53):

- advanced and late luteal phase
- pregnancy
- androgen stimulation
- oral contraceptive intake.

During the early months of ***pregnancy*** the vaginal smear simulates the cell pattern of the secretory phase, with predominant intermediate cells with marked folding and rolling-up of cytoplasmic edges (navicular cells) and frequent cytolysis, as a result of

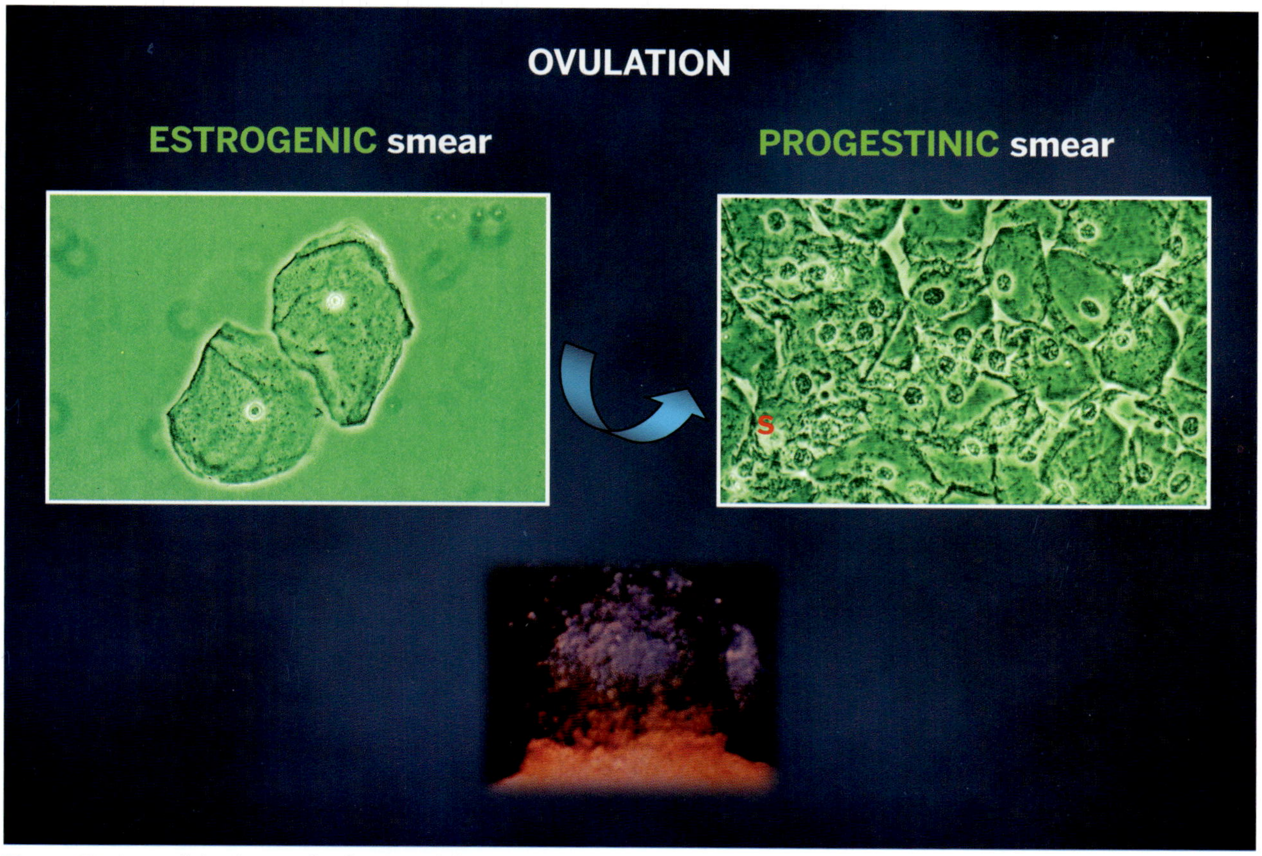

Figure 48 - Immediate change of cell pattern following ovulation.

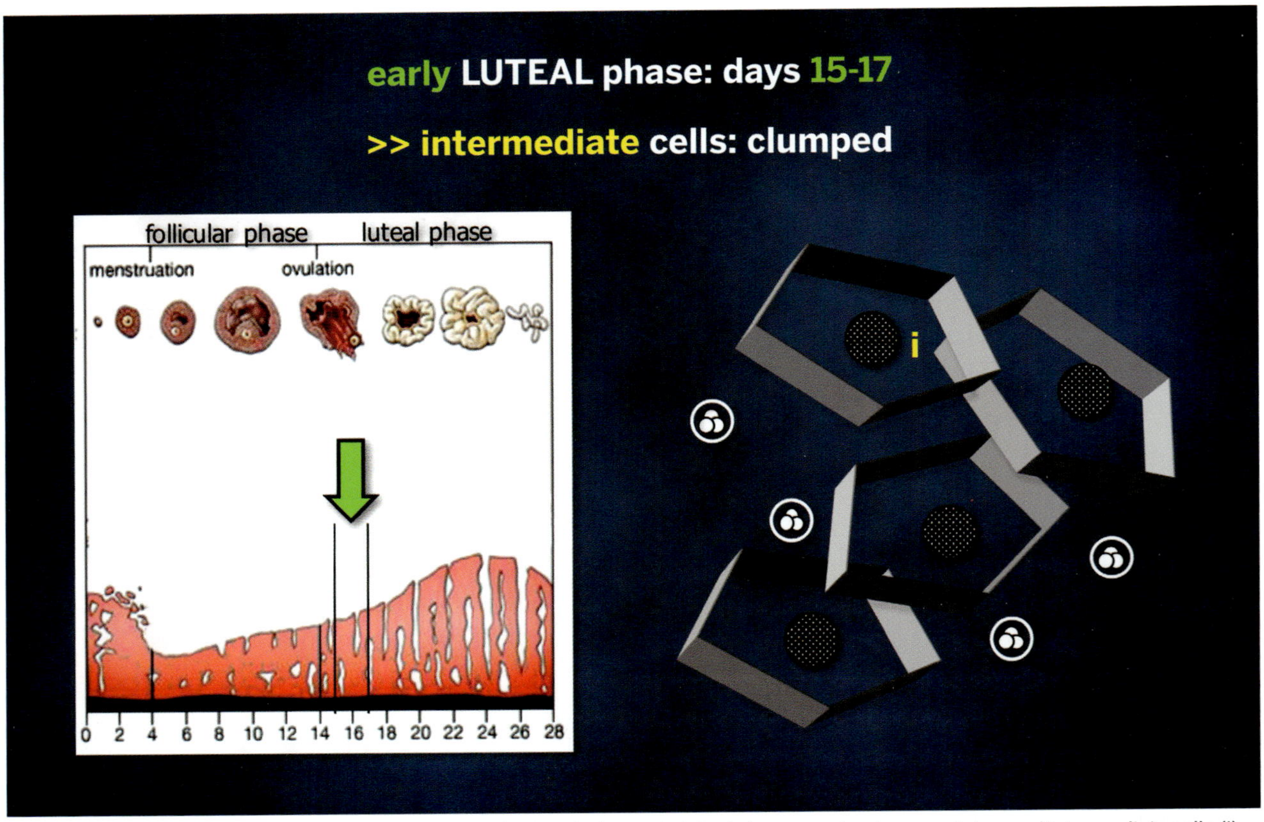

Figure 49 - Diagrammatic representation of cell distribution during early luteal phase: predominance of clumped intermediate cells (i).

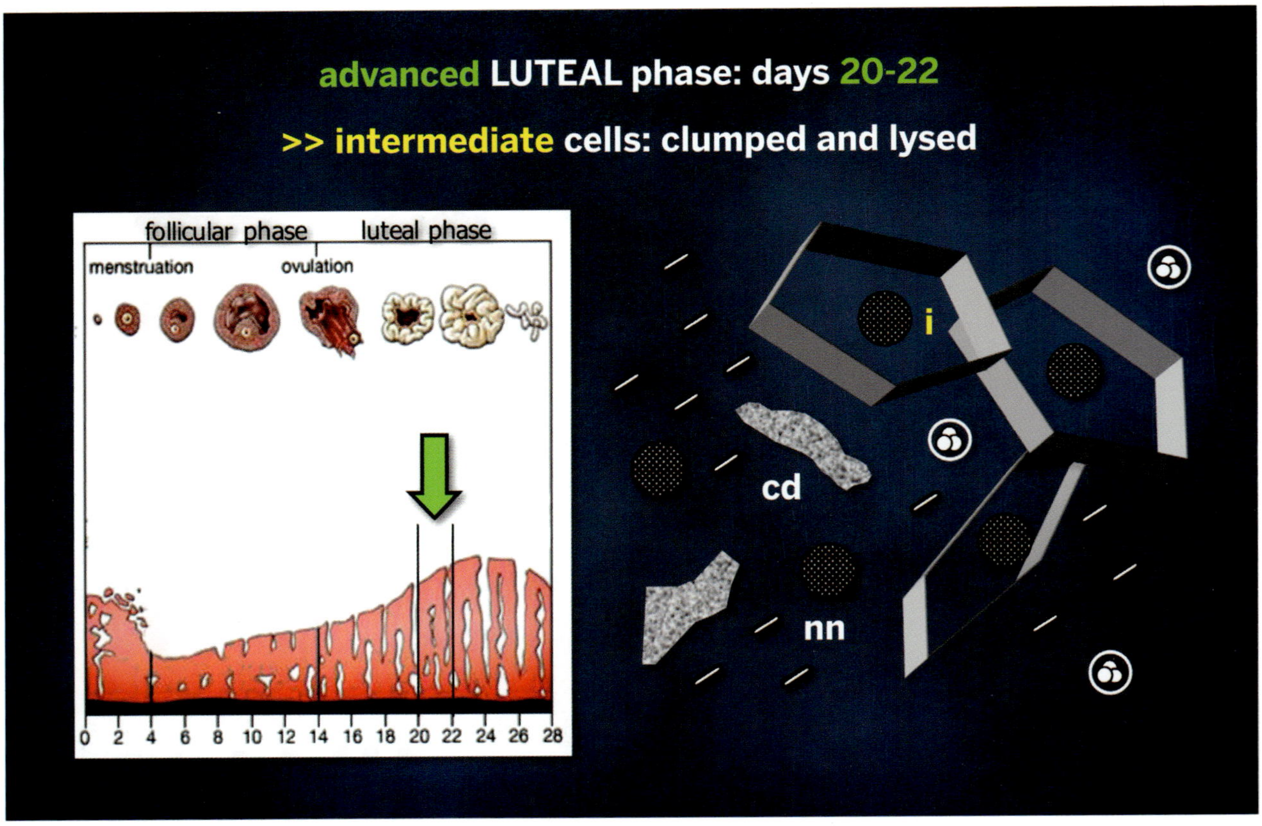

Figure 50 - Diagrammatic representation of cell distribution during advanced luteal phase: predominance of clumped and lysed intermediate cells (i), associated with naked nuclei (nn) and cytoplasmic debris (cd).

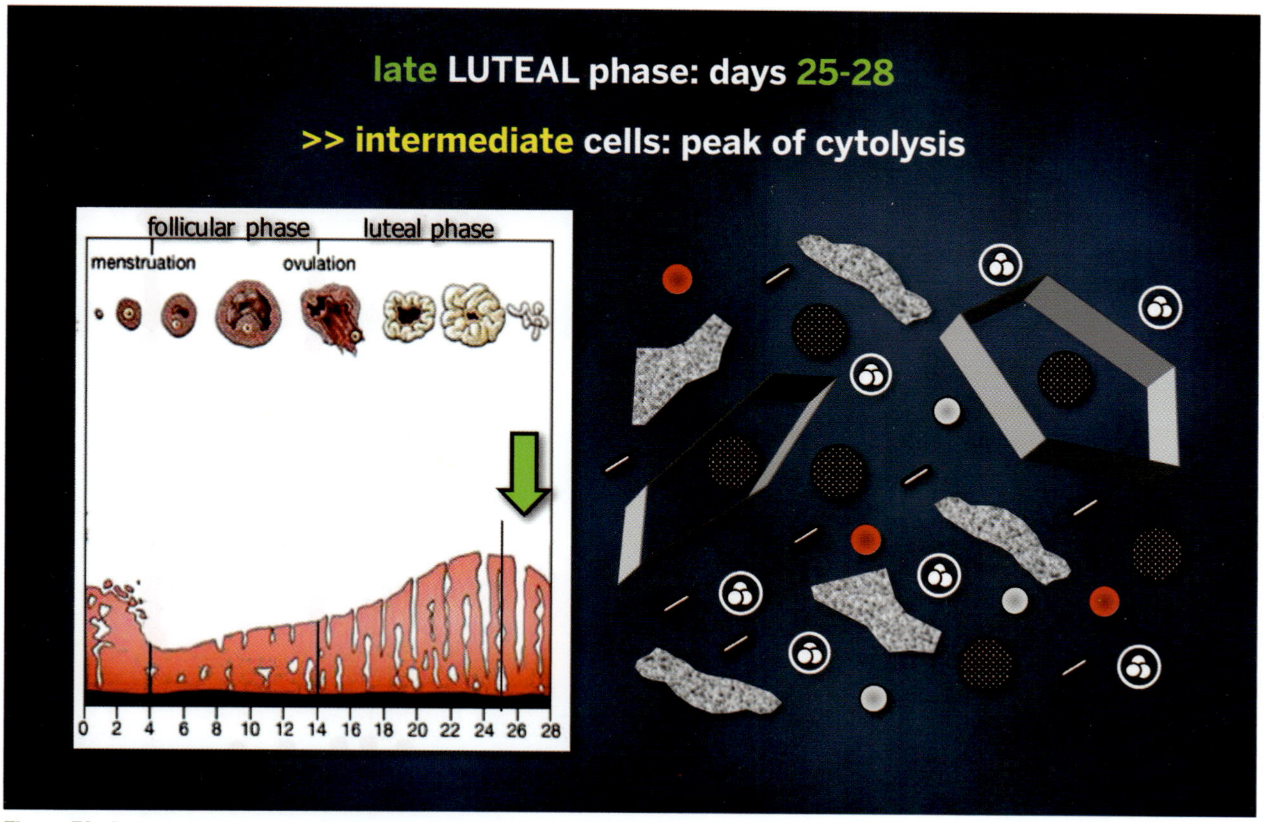

Figure 51 - Diagrammatic representation of cell distribution during advanced luteal phase: intermediate cells undergo peak of cytolysis.

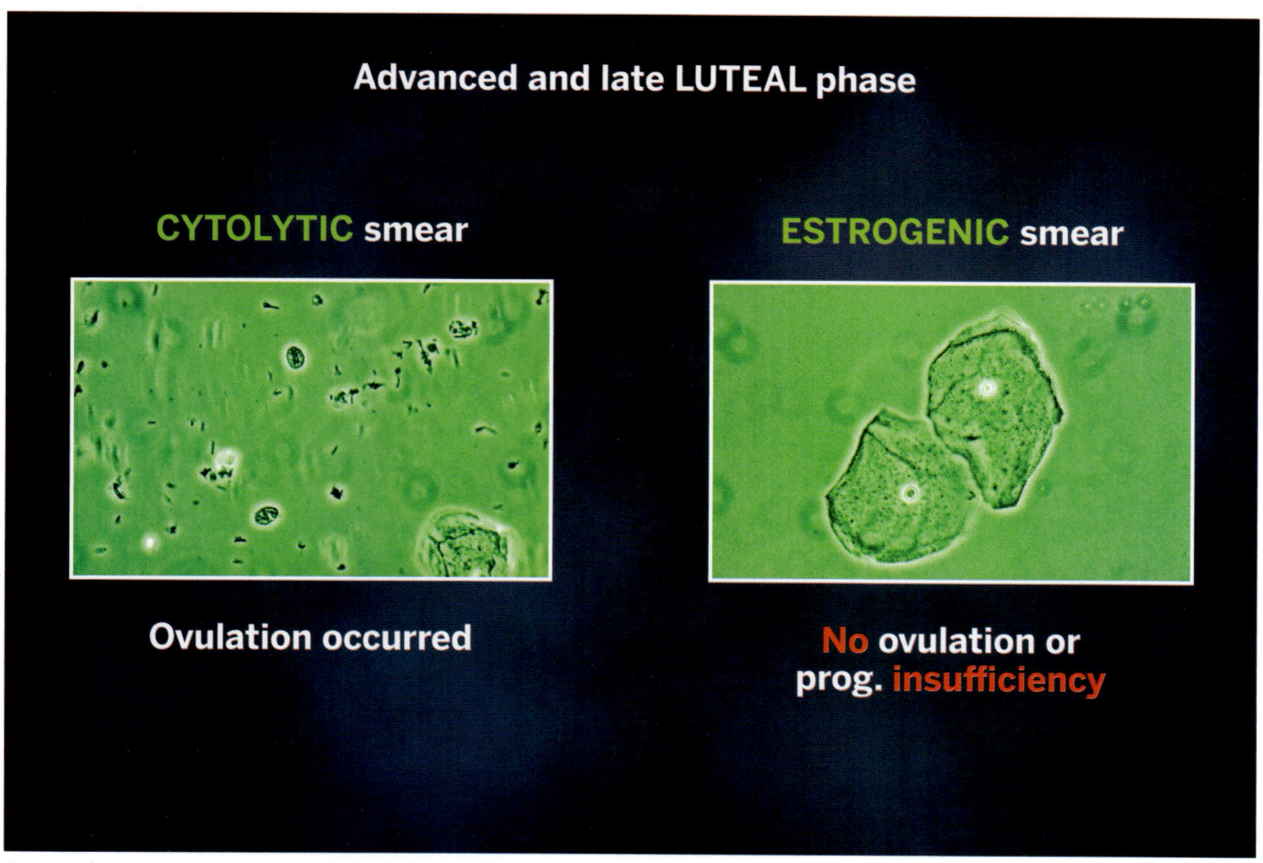

Figure 52 - Clinical significance of different cytologic patterns during advanced and late luteal phase.

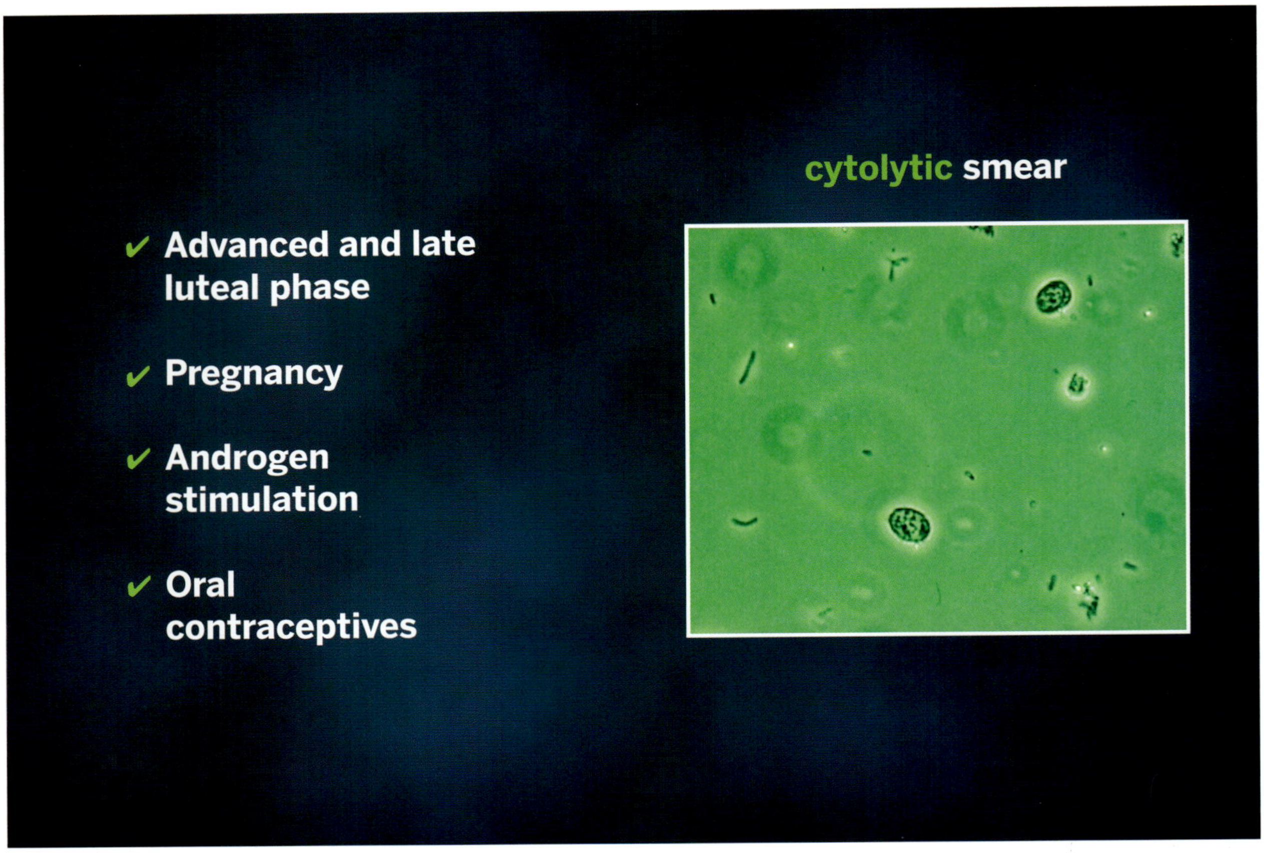

Figure 53 - Cytolytic smear in different conditions.

high levels of both estrogen and progesterone. If cell desquamation is very low and the majority of cells is represented by flat and discrete superficial cells, the cell pattern may indicate a placental failure (Figure 54), suggesting the administration of progesterone in order to avoid a threatened abortion.

Peripheral effects of ***androgen*** stimulation is revealed by the detection of a cytolytic smear during follicular phase (Figure 55), when usually estrogen is responsible for progestinic and estrogenic smears. The vaginal cytogram of women taking ***oral contraceptives*** is characterized by a cytolytic smear (Figure 56); on the contrary, when wet mount microscopy shows an estrogenic smear, it is advisable to reduce the estrogen content of the contraceptive pill, if possible.

Different physiological, clinical and therapeutic settings associated with a low estrogen state may be responsible for an atrophic smear (Figure 57):

- premenarche
- puerperium
- amenorrhea
- LH-RH analogues
- tamoxifen
- Turner syndrome
- postmenopause
- status post bilateral oophorectomy.

The atrophic smear characterizes the early phase of ***puerperium*** when parabasal and fewer small intermediate cells are seen together with bacteria, a high number of granulocytes and macrophages (Figure 58). The advanced phase of puerperium is characterized by a wide range of cell maturation with all cell types being present. Lastly, vaginal wet mount enables to detect imminent recurrence of normal cyclic changes by observing progestinic or estrogenic smears.

In patients affected by ***amenorrhea*** (Figure 59), the direct evaluation of exfoliated vaginal cells can differentiate hypothalamic and pituitary defects or ovarian failure (atrophic smear) from ovarian dysfunction (estrogenic smear).

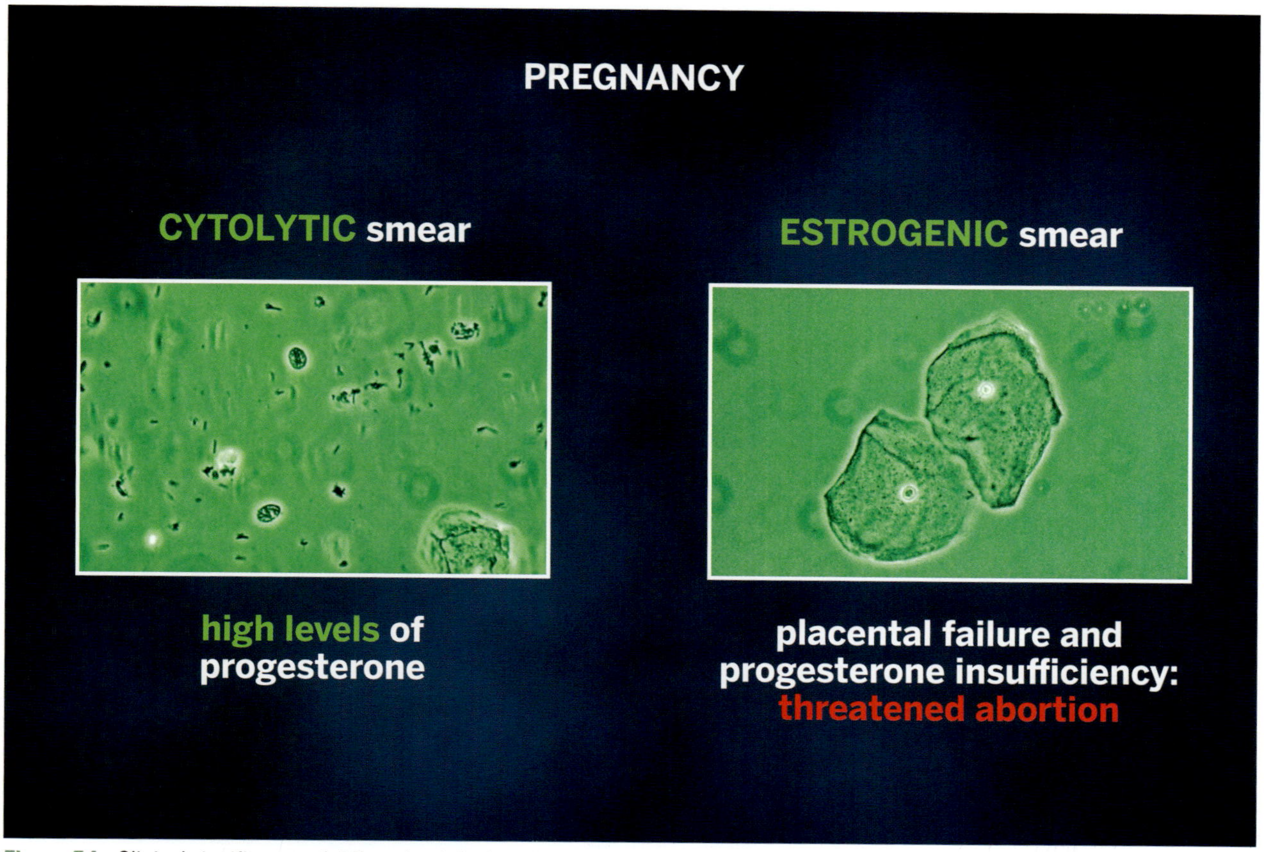

Figure 54 - Clinical significance of different cytologic patterns during pregnancy.

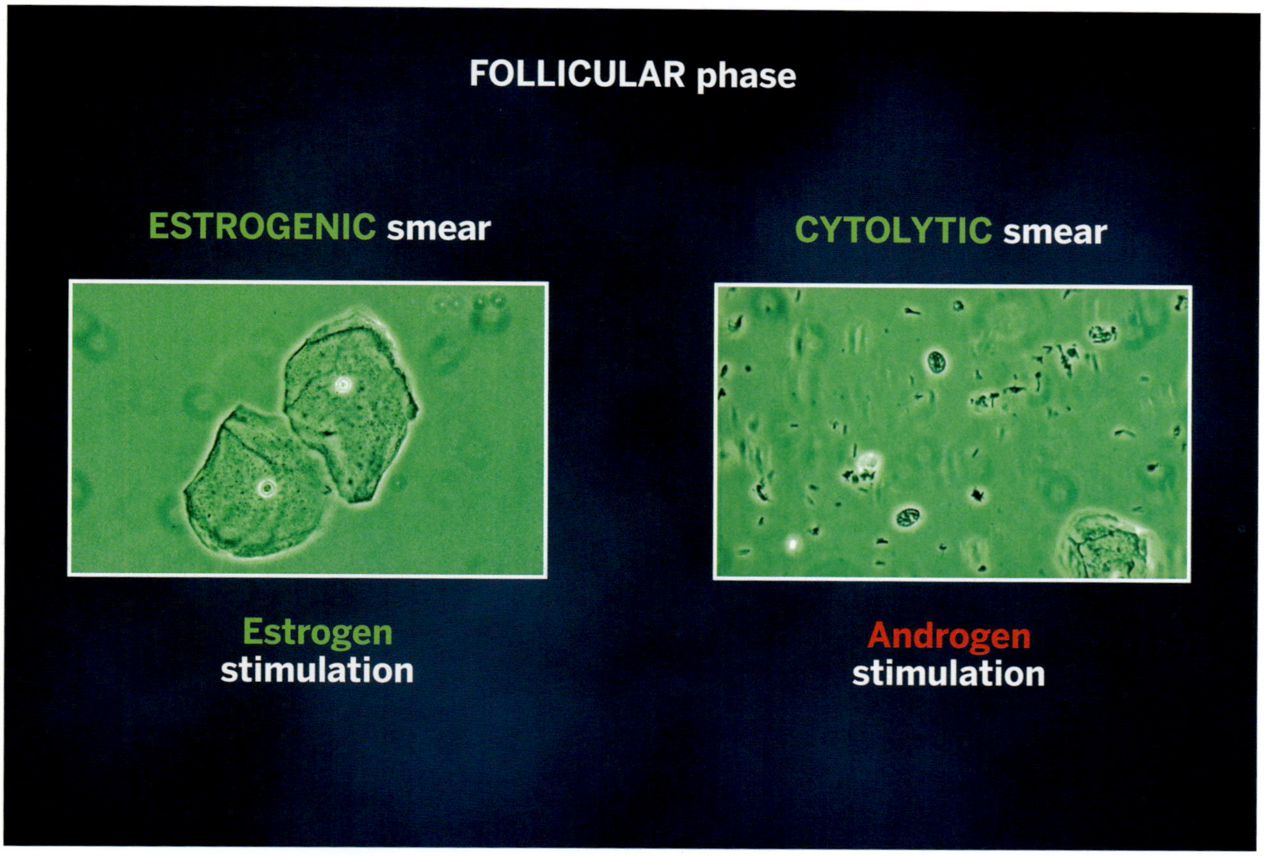

Figure 55 - Clinical significance of different cytologic patterns during follicular phase.

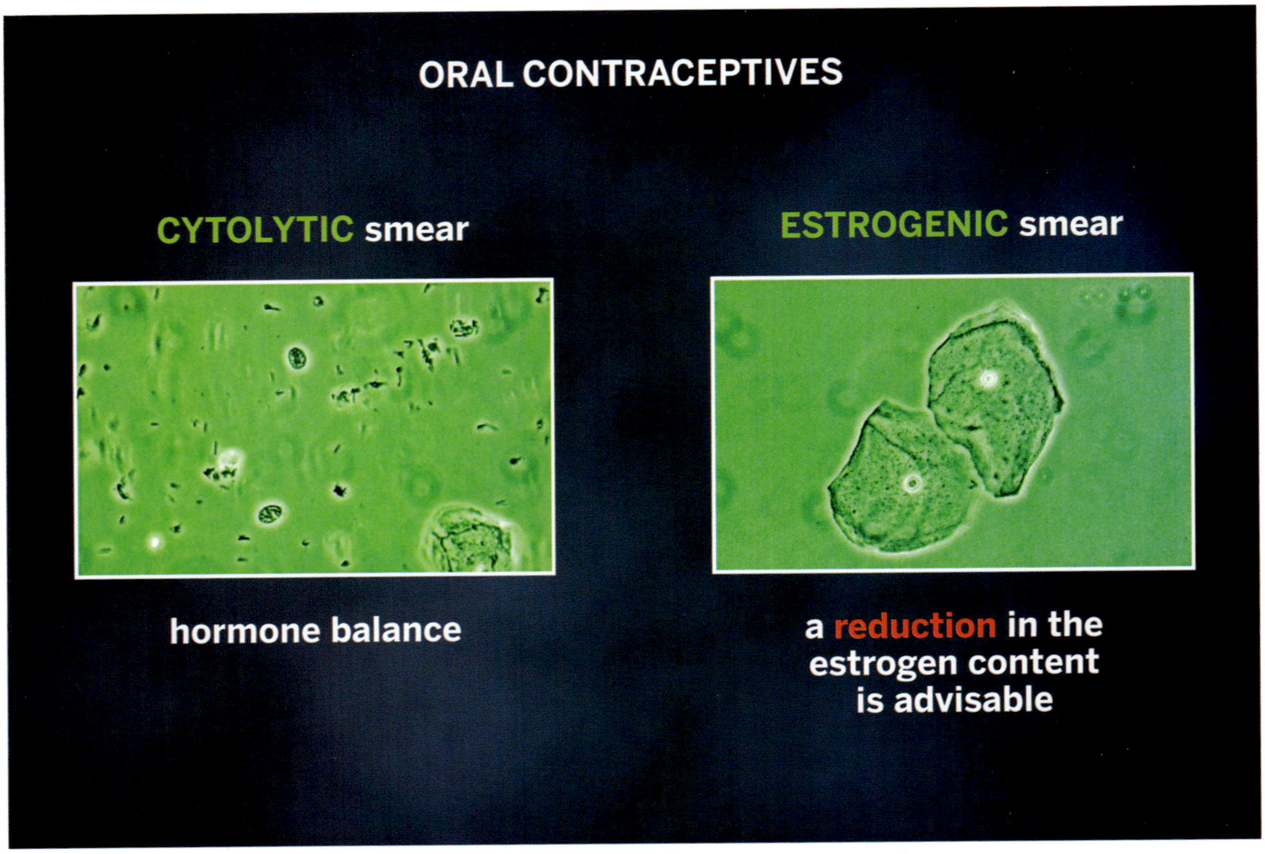

Figure 56 - Clinical significance of different cytologic patterns in women taking oral contraceptives.

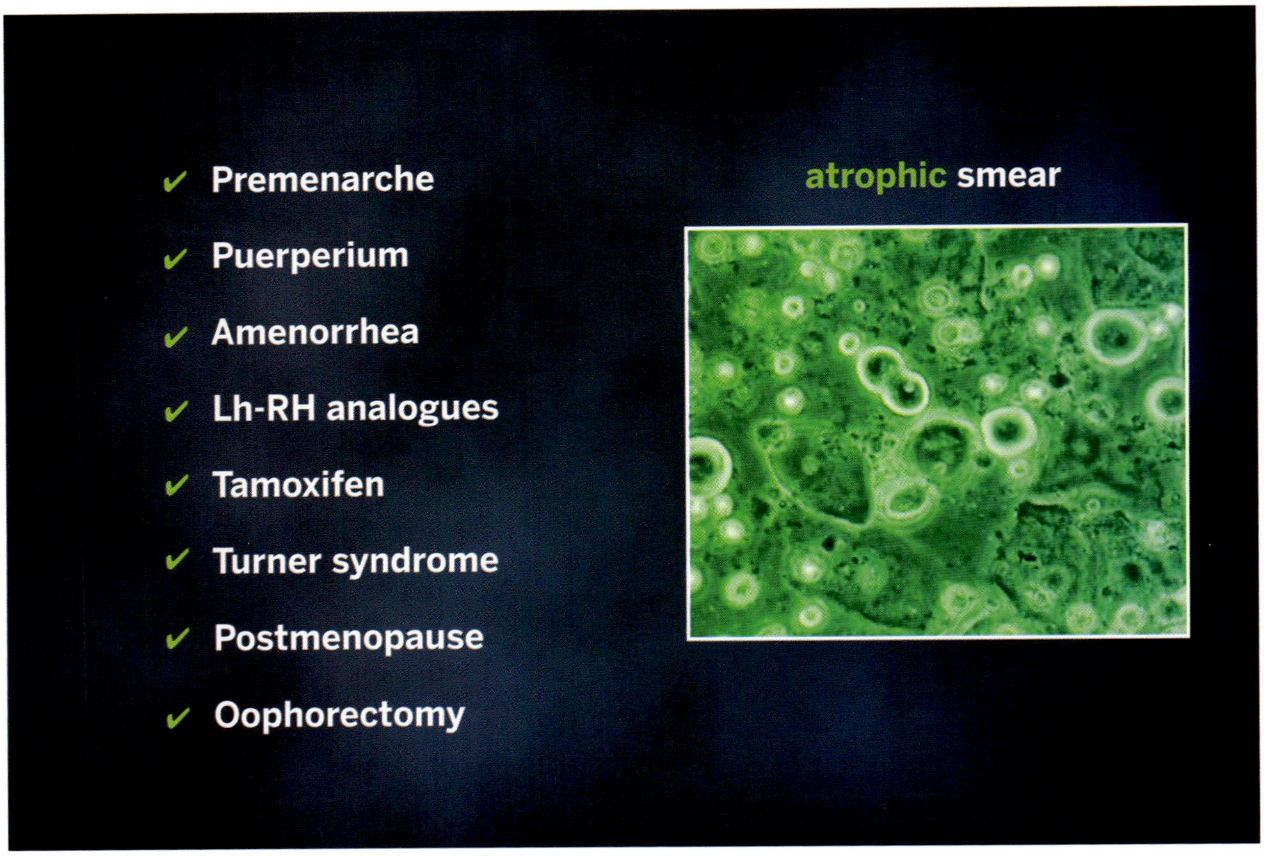

Figure 57 - Atrophic smear in different conditions.

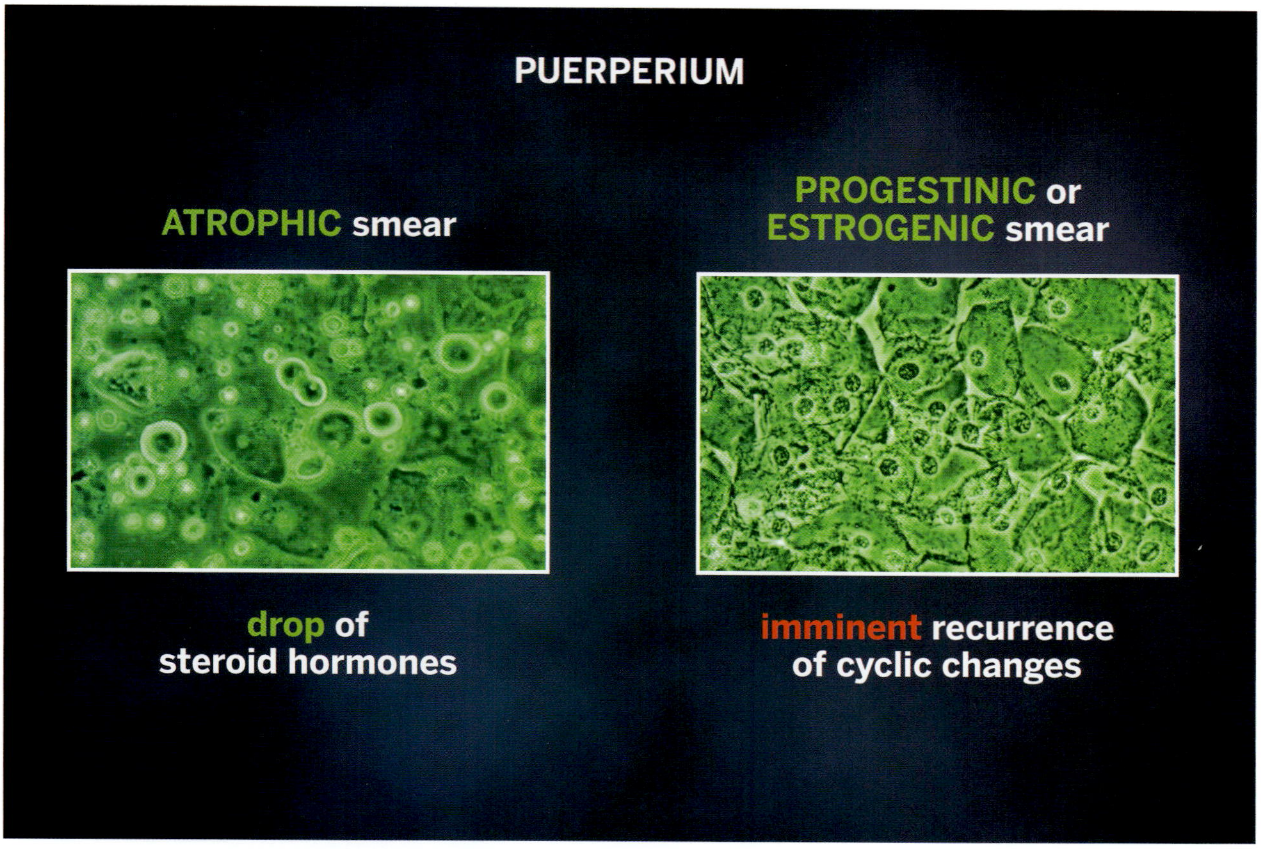

Figure 58 - Clinical significance of different cytologic patterns during puerperium.

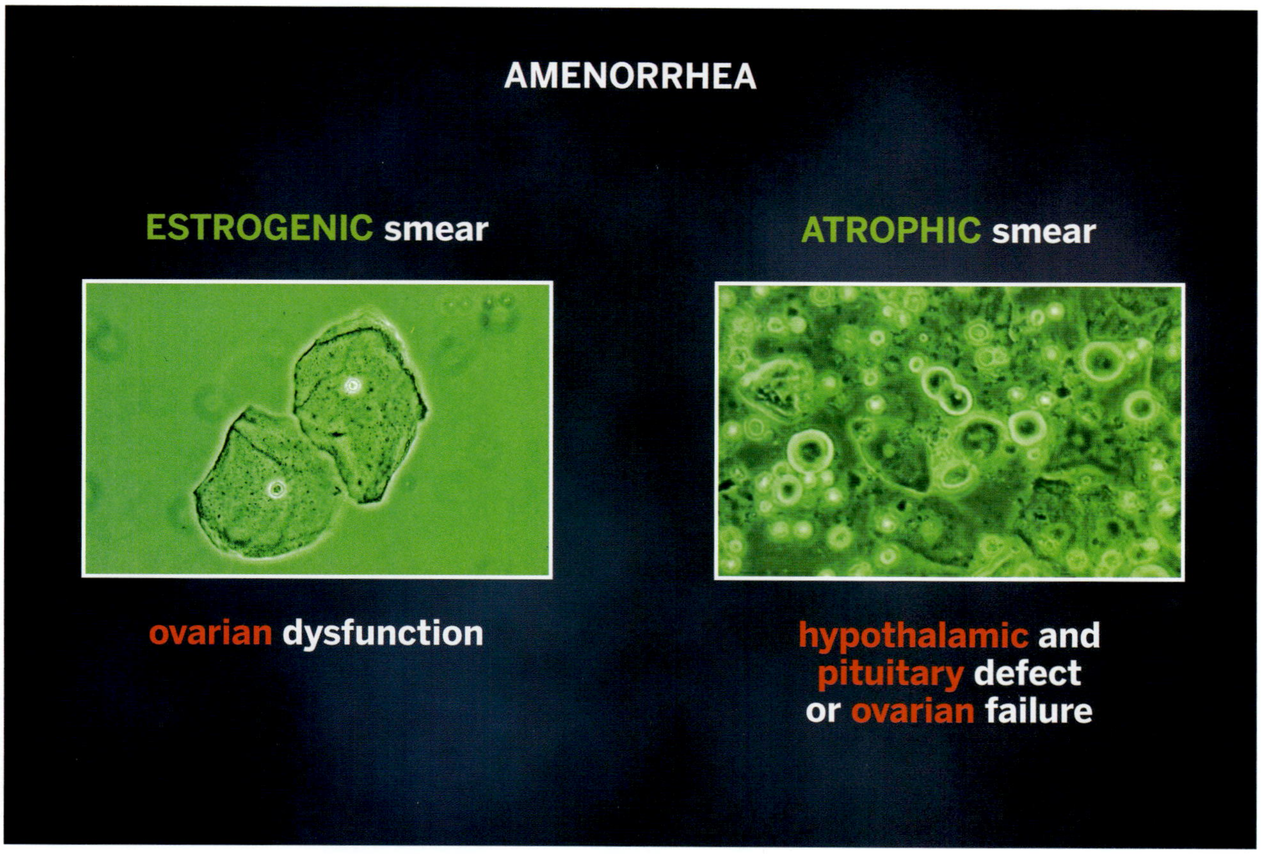

Figure 59 - Clinical significance of different cytologic patterns during amenorrhea.

In women undergoing ***LH-RH analogues*** therapy, phase contrast microscopy of the vaginal smear provides a reliable monitoring of iatrogenic cellular changes, so that several cycles of therapy may be used, according to the needs of the patients; the appearance of a severe atrophic smear may suggest suspension of the treatment or the concomitant administration of trophic therapy.

Tamoxifen is a nonsteroidal antiestrogen drug widely used for the management of patients with breast cancer and to prevent breast cancer recurrence. Tamoxifen is also FDA approved as a chemopreventive agent in healthy women at risk for breast cancer. Consequently, a large number of women will be subjected to both the benefits and the potential risks of long-term tamoxifen therapy.

This drug works by competing with estrogen to bind to estrogen receptors in breast cancer cells. By blocking the actions of estrogen in the breast tissue, tamoxifen helps slowing the growth and reproduction of breast cancer cells. The antiestrogen effects of tamoxifen are responsible for an atrophic vaginal smear (Figure 60) and for the genito-urinary syndrome of menopause (GSM), previously known as atrophic vaginitis.

Although primarily an antiestrogen, tamoxifen may also exhibit some mild estrogenic effects. Recently, several reports have implicated tamoxifen treatment in the development of endometrial polyps and hyperplasia. One of the most significant potential complications is the development of endometrial cancer. The estimated annual risk of endometrial cancer in tamoxifen-treated patients is approximately 2 per 1,000. In these cases, an estrogenic smear (Figure 60) and/or a vaginal discharge can be an indication of a more serious conditions, and may require further investigation.

The ***climacterium*** is the time period between normal cycles and menopause, it usually lasts 1 or 2 years and is characterized by irregular cycles. At the end of the female reproductive activity, a complex of endocrine, somatic and psychic changes occurs. The residual estrogen stimulation on the epithelium, not contrasted by progesterone, is responsible for an estrogenic smear (Figure 61).

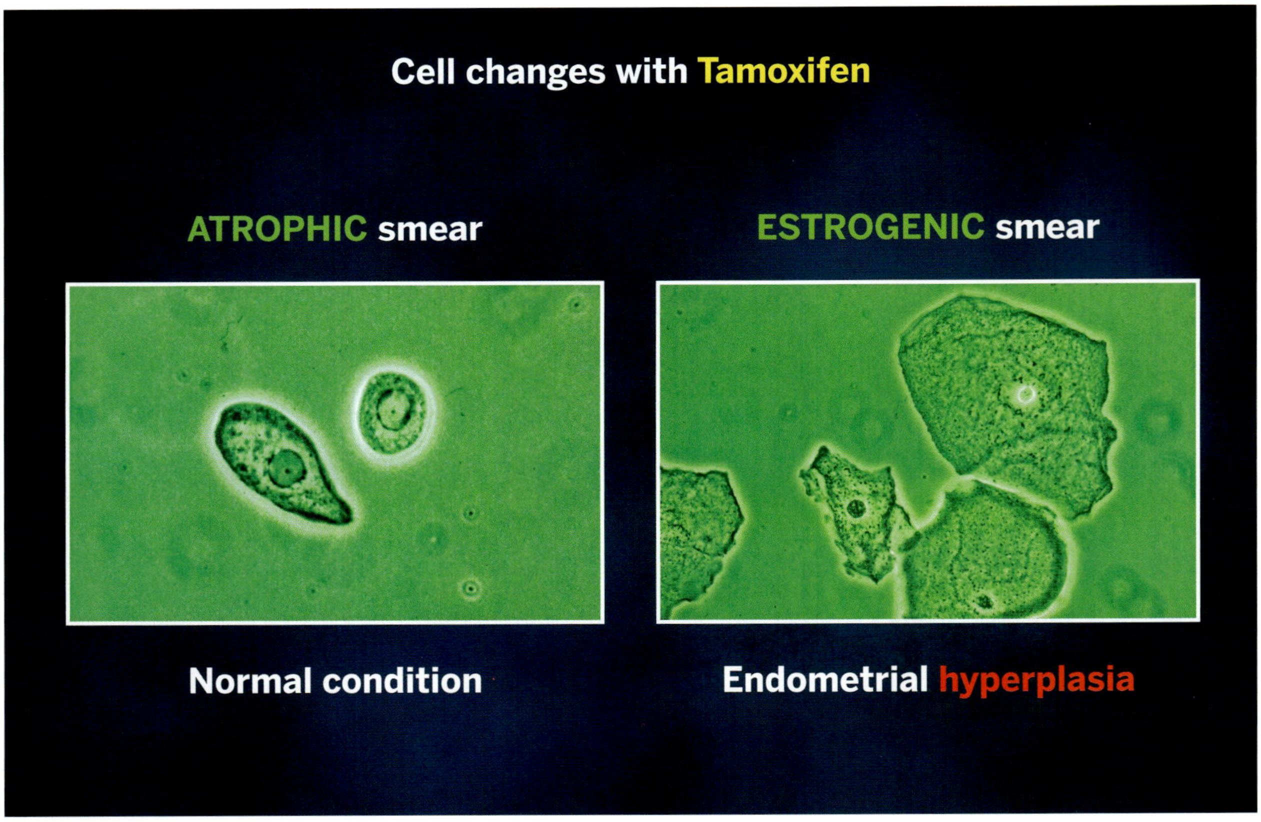

Figure 60 - Clinical significance of different cytologic patterns in women taking Tamoxifen.

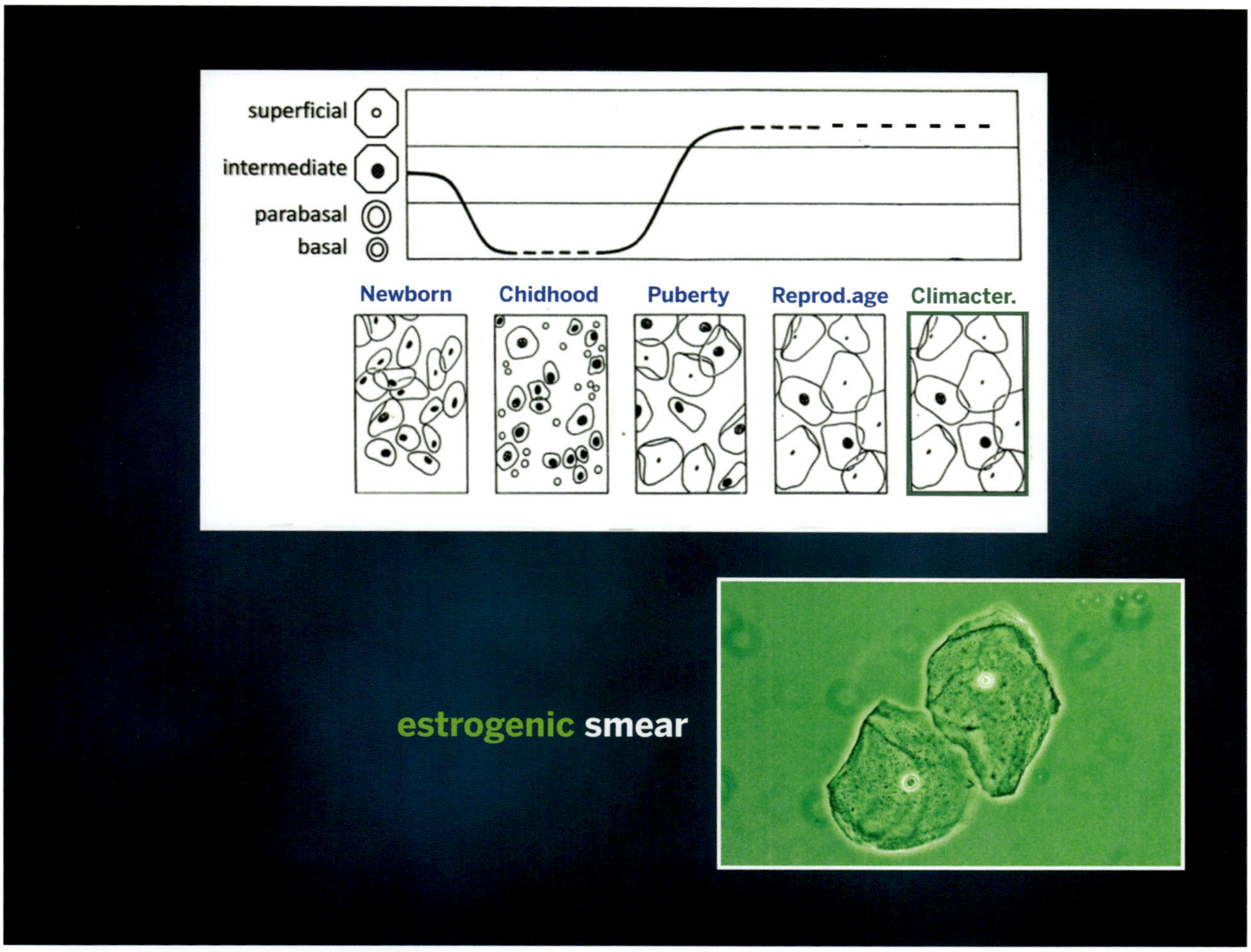

Figure 61 - Estrogenic smear in climacterium.

During ***menopause***, the aging of ovaries causes a definitive interruption of menstruation. Cells with a maturation degree ranging from basal to intermediate can be observed (Figure 62). Some polymorphs are usually present.

The ***postmenopausal period*** is characterized by tranquillity in gonadal activity; nevertheless, the variable function of the adrenal cortex ("third gonad") and/or the persistence of ovarian activity may be responsible for different degrees of epithelial maturation, with corresponding postmenopausal cell patterns:

- *atrophic* smear
- *progestinic* (androgenic) smear
- *estrogenic* smear.

The *atrophic* pattern accounts for about 25% of the smears in early postmenopause. This percentage, however, increases when hormonal stimulation is lacking during senility (Figure 63). Basal and parabasal cells do not produce glycogen so that Lactobacilli cannot survive but are substituted by mixed bacterial flora, with predominance of cocci. Microscopic background may appear dirty due to cellular fragments and presence of polymorphs, even in absence of active inflammation (atrophic vaginitis).

Atrophic epithelium, particularly in postmenopausal women often shows a spectrum of changes that must be recognized as normal and not confused with a significant lesion. In fact, the sheets of immature cells are crowded and syncytium-like, mimicking the crowded cells of an H-SIL. Nevertheless, in atrophic conditions, the chromatin is finely stippled, evenly distributed, and nuclear contours are mostly thin and smooth.

During senility, a freshly mounted preparation can immediately indicate uro-genital atrophy, responsible for vaginal dryness, dyspareunia and/

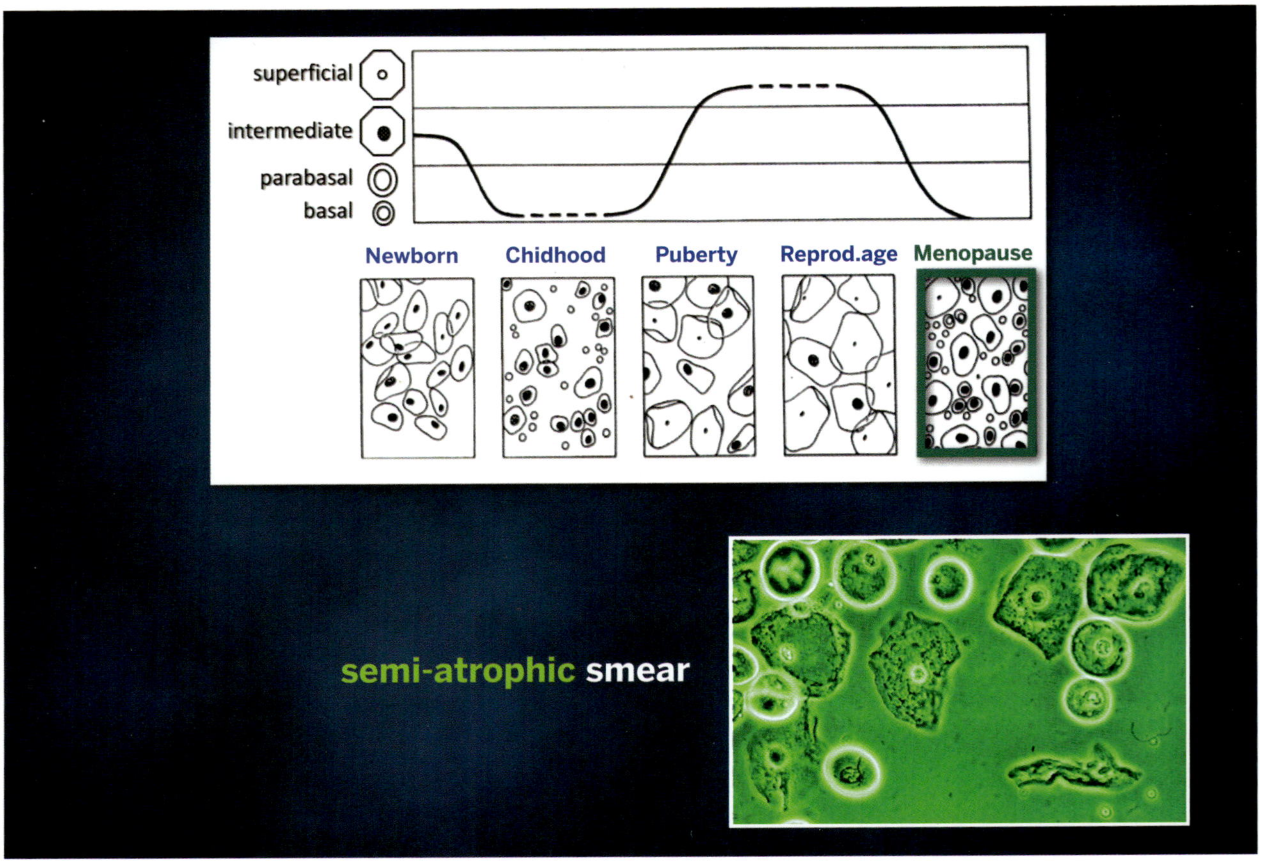

Figure 62 - Semi-atrophic smear during menopause.

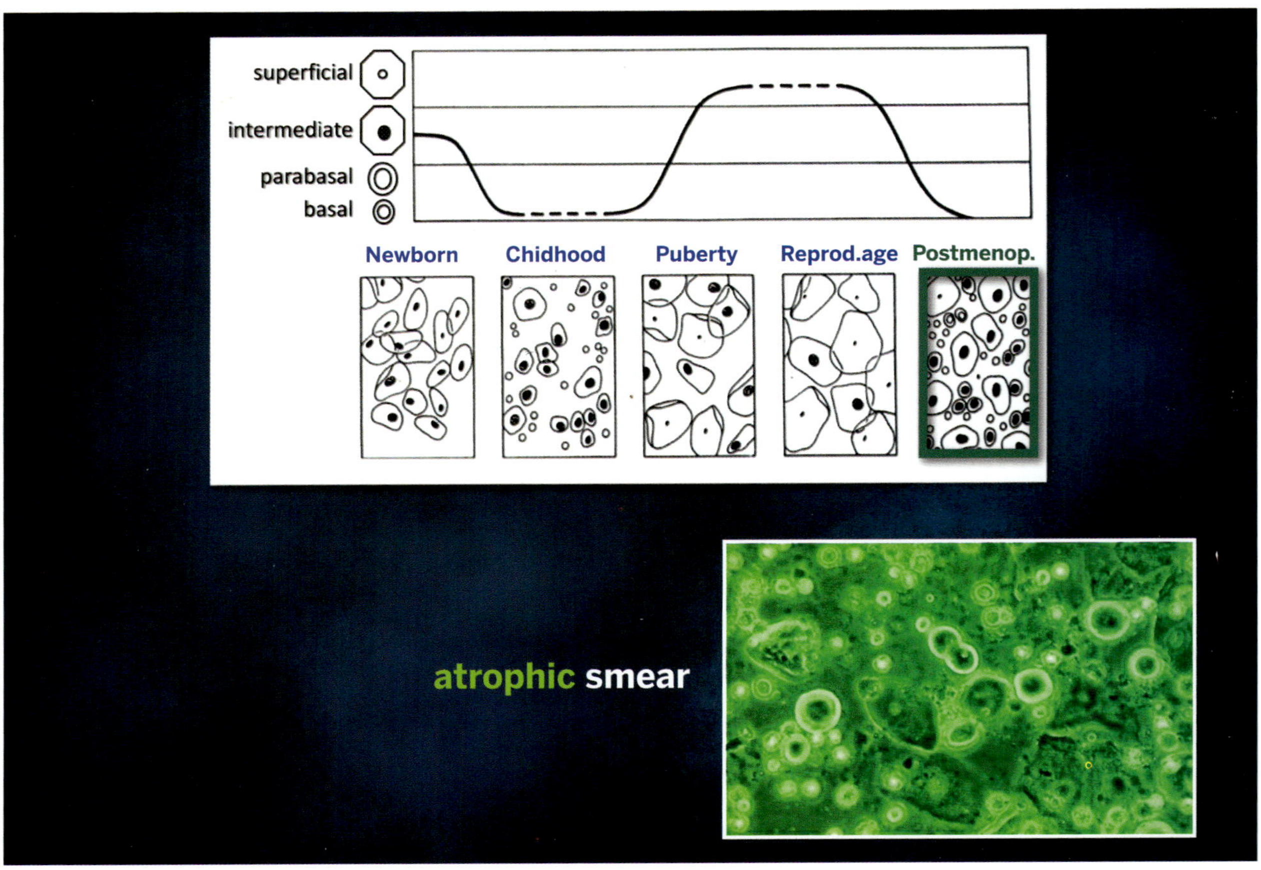

Figure 63 - Atrophic smear in postmenopause.

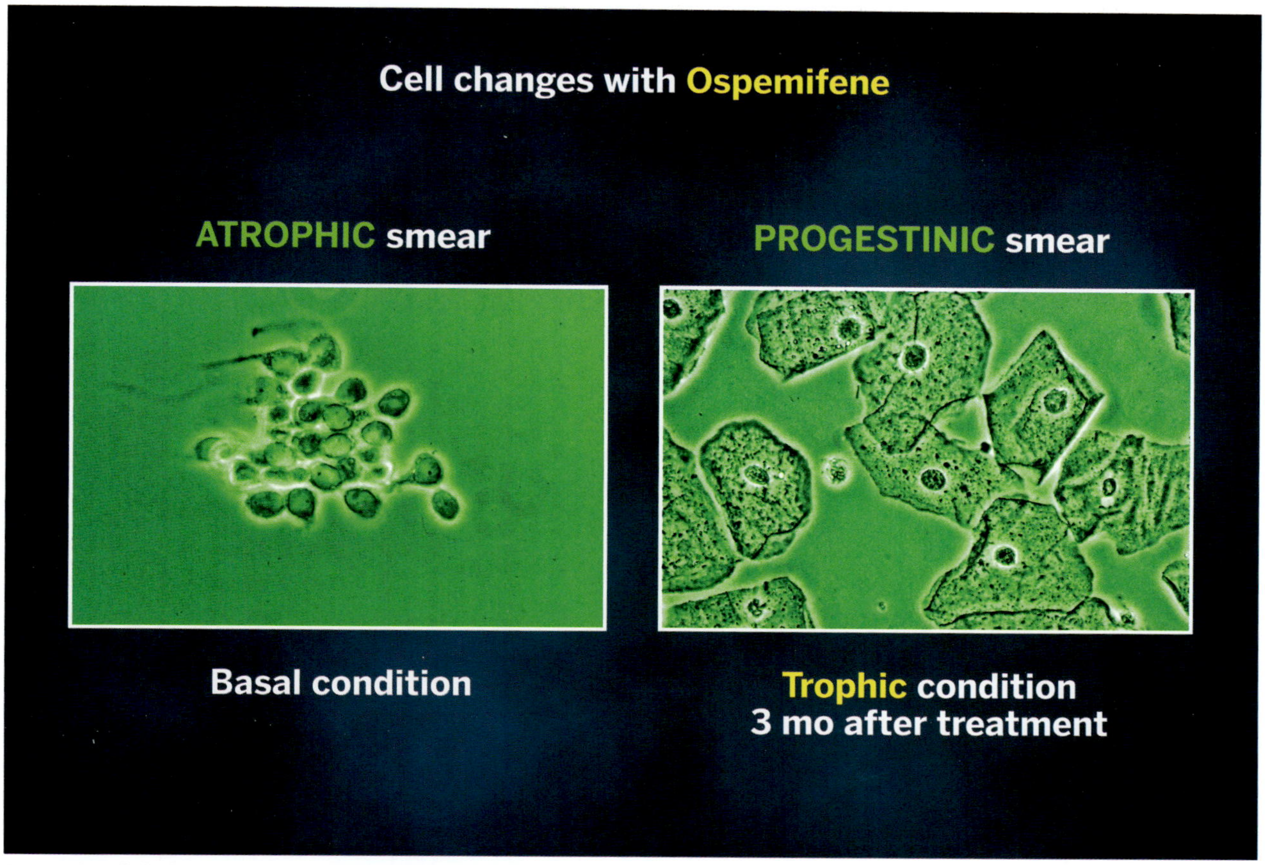

Figure 64 - Cell changes in women taking Ospemifene.

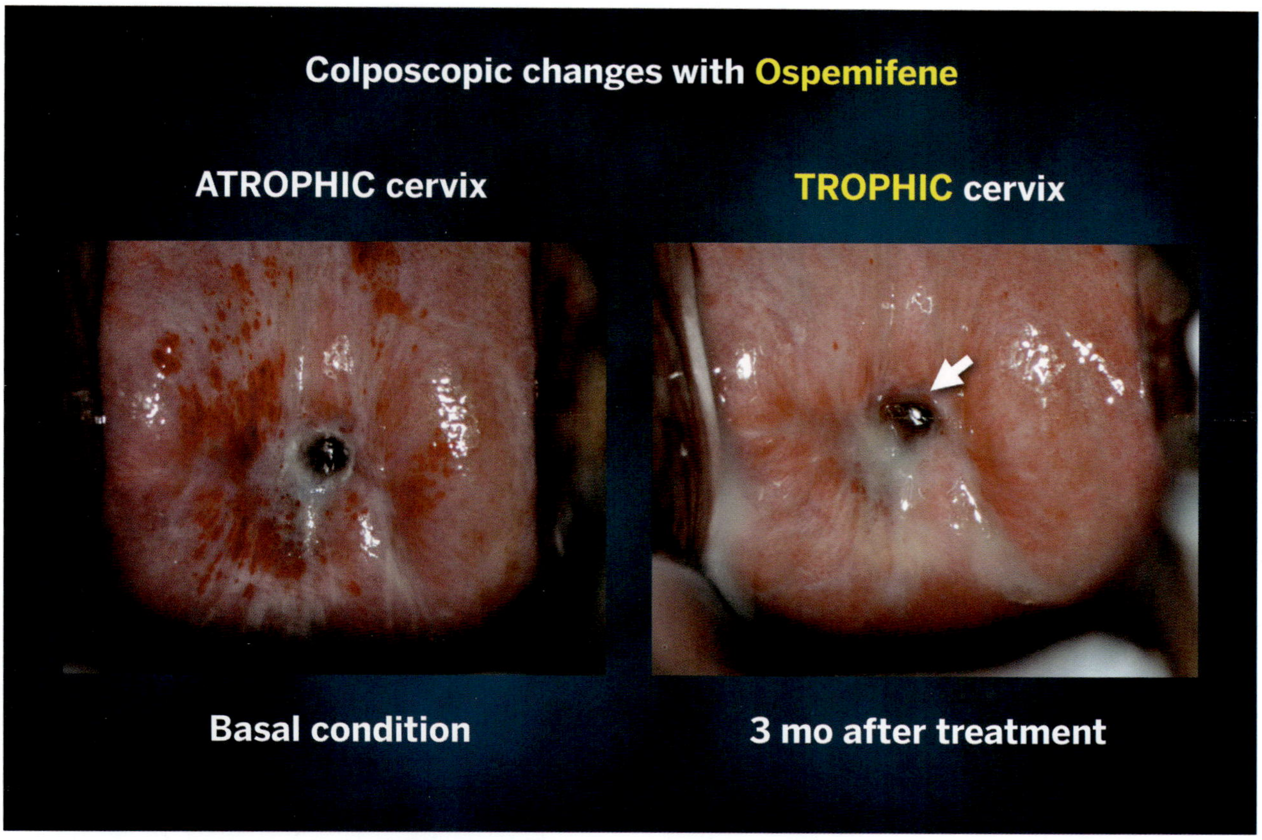

Figure 65 - Severe atrophic cervix with subepithelial petechiae and on the right trophic cervix without eversion of the SCJ (→) and normal vaginal fluor after treatment with Ospemifene

or dysuric symptoms (GSM), thus suggesting the prescription of a non hormonal therapy with phytoestrogens or estrogen agonist/antagonists increasing the maturation indices of vaginal cells like the karyopycnotic index (KI) and maturation value (MV). It must be stressed that the clinical data supporting many of the currently claimed health benefits of phytoestrogens remain to be established definitively. When a hormonal replacement therapy (HRT) is chosen, follow-up by phase contrast microscopy is extremely useful to assess the effects of HRT and, more importantly, to suggest its eventual suspension.

In the *progestinic* or androgenic smear, the adrenal cortex and an eventual residual ovarian function are responsible for a proliferative effect on vaginal epithelium, which characteristically matures only at the intermediate cell level. The cells in the androgenic pattern range from basal to intermediate cells, which usually lie separately and are accompanied by polymorphs.

The *estrogenic* smear indicates any condition of estrogen stimulation. Vaginal wet mount shows largely solitary and flattened superficial cells with rare leukocytes.

Every estrogenic smear in postmenopause requires an additional diagnostic evaluation; it must be pointed out, in fact, that an estrogen overstimulation may depend on long-term treatment with tranquillizers, disturbed hormonal breakdown in hepatic diseases, accumulation for increased estrogen conversion in fatty tissue in presence of adiposity, and even on ovarian, endometrial and breast tumors. In the case of estrogenic smears, Ph microscopy proved to be a precious diagnostic tool to avoid prescribing an unnecessary or even dangerous hormonal replacement therapy (HRT). It is useful to stress that a dystrophic cervix can be associated with an estrogenic smear (cytologic-colposcopic dissociation).

Lastly, the direct evaluation of the epithelial trophyc status enables the clinician to establish the appropriate dosage of estrogen during HRT, in order to reach the desired cytologic pattern. When non-hormonal therapy is more advisable in presence of postmenopausal moderate-to-severe dyspareunia due to vulvar and vaginal atrophy, wet mount is a precious diagnostic tool to appreciate the maturation of the epithelium obtained by the administration of non-estrogen drugs like estrogen agonist/antagonists (Ospemifene) (Figures 64, 65).

Cervico-vaginal infections

Vaginal discharge is highly variable in quality and quantity among different individuals, and even in the same individual during different periods of life. Non-infectious causes of vaginal discharge are quite rare (10% non-infectious as compared to 90% infectious causes).

Cervico-vaginal infections represent the most frequent cause of gynaecological consultation. In the diagnostic work-up of this pathology, direct microscopy may decisively contribute to define the causative microorganism; on the other hand, when a particular infective agent is only suspected, wet mounts can indicate other cytologic, histologic, or immunohistochemical investigations to perform.

Phase contrast microscopy enables the direct observation of viable microorganisms, both physiologic and pathogenic, which can be easily distinguished in bacteria, yeasts and protozoas, even when cultures give false negative results or clinical symptoms are lacking. Some etiological agents such as viruses and Chlamydia trachomatis are too tiny for phase contrast microscope resolution, but they may cause some specific cell tracks, that are easily recognizable under direct microscopic observation.

Most bacteria and fungi present characteristic shapes and sizes and their microscopic detection enables a prompt therapy. It must be pointed out that a definitive diagnosis of bacterial and fungal species rests upon isolating pathogens on appropriate culture media.

Under normal conditions, the predominant bacterial flora of the vagina consists of hydrogen peroxide-producing Lactobacilli (Figure 66). Hydrogen peroxide is toxic to a wide variety of organisms, since its interaction with oxygen produces a toxic hydroxyl radical. Lactobacilli may adhere to the squamous cells by their whole length or may be anchored by only one tip (Figure 67), causing the cell break (cytolysis) and the following release of glycogen, which is converted in lactic acid. The large amount of lactic acid is responsible for the normal vaginal pH, whose values range between 3.8 and 4.4.

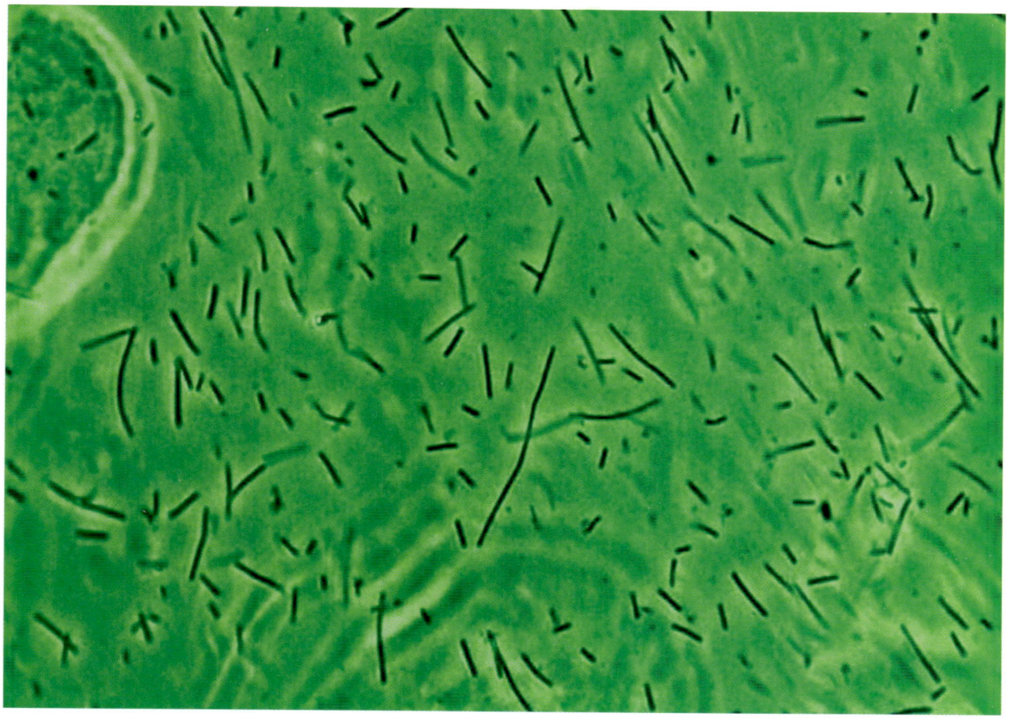

Figure 66 - Lactobacilli.

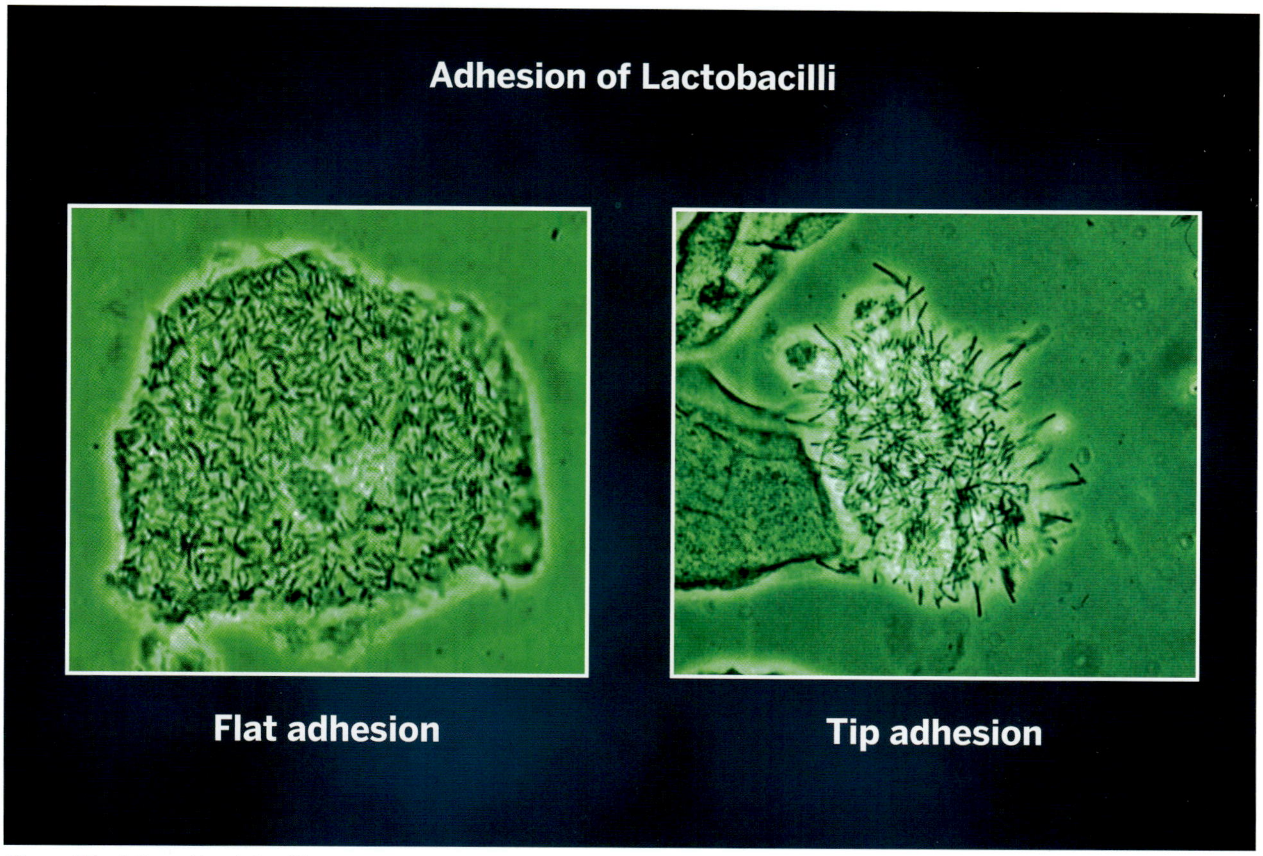

Figure 67 - Adhered Lactobacilli.

Vaginal lactobacillosis

In some of the patients who have symptoms and signs of vaginal candidiasis, which is unresponsive to antifungal drugs, a diagnosis of vaginal lactobacillosis may be suspected. Vaginal lactobacillosis is also known as Lactobacillus overgrowth syndrome o cytolytic vaginosis. It is manifested as a very annoying, profuse white and creamy vaginal discharge (Figure 68), with the sensation of incessantly having wet the underwear, often associated with vulvar and vaginal itching. The etiology is unknown and the prevalence is approximately 15%.

Vaginal lactobacillosis is characterized by the presence of abundant and extremely longer (filamentous) than normal Lactobacilli in vaginal wet mount preparations (Figure 69), resulting in lysis of vaginal epithelial cells. If vaginal lactobacillosis is misinterpreted as a fungal infection, allergic reactions to antimycotic therapy may result in continuation of symptoms that are incorrectly thought to be caused by yeast. Wet mount microscopy offers an immediate distinction between the two opposite conditions and enables to avoid unnecessary and even harmful pharmacological treatments.

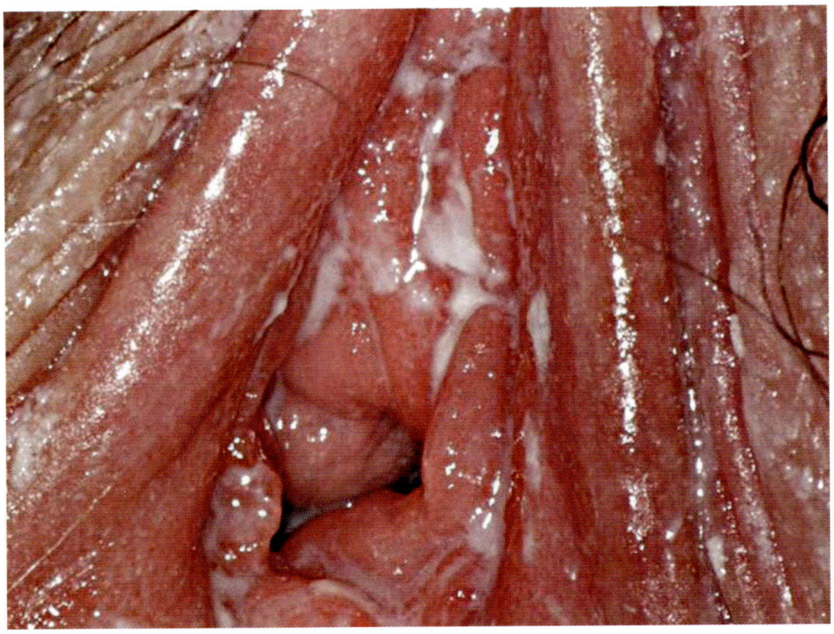

Figure 68 - Creamy discharge in vaginal lactobacillosis.

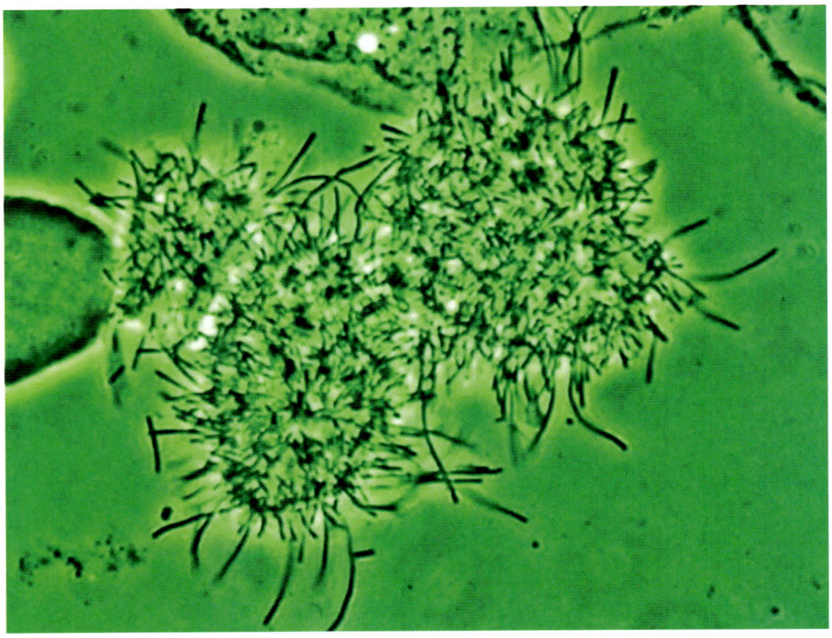

Figure 69 - Adhered filamentous Lactobacilli.

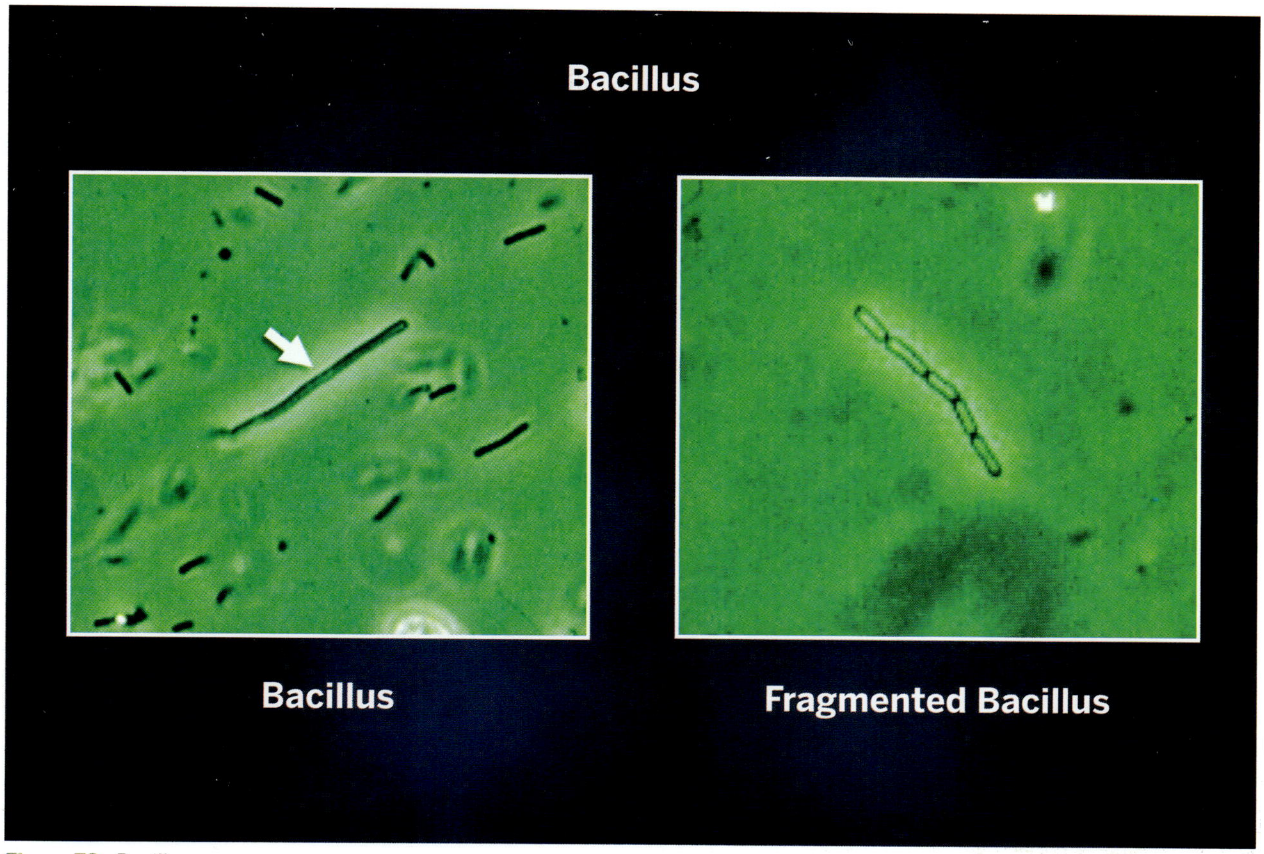

Figure 70 - Bacillus.

Some rod-shaped bacteria members of the genus *Bacillus* may resemble Lactobacilli. They are easily distinguishable from Lactobacilli because they appear longer, wider and often subdividing in fragments (Figure 70). Bacillus belongs to normal intestinal microbiota and its presence in the vaginal wet mount usually indicates a fecal contamination.

Bacterial vaginosis

Bacterial vaginosis (BV) is the most common cause of vaginal discharge in women of childbearing age, accounting for 40 to 50 percent of cases.

Bacterial vaginosis increases a woman's risk of acquiring HIV, is associated with increased adverse pregnancy outcomes, may be involved in the pathogenesis of pelvic inflammatory disease (PID) and may be responsible for the impairment of sperm mobility and quantity in males. Since BV produces carcinogenic nitrosamines, it could be in some way associated with the development of cervical intraepithelial neoplasia (CIN), as a cofactor to HPV.

This common infection is the result of a complex change in the vaginal flora: with the reduction in concentration of the normally dominant hydrogen-peroxide producing Lactobacilli, pH rises and massive overgrowth of vaginal anaerobes occurs. The major anaerobes detected in BV are: *Gardnerella vaginalis, Prevotella species, Bacteroides species, Peptostreptococcus species, Porphyromonas species, Mycoplasma hominis, Ureaplasma urealyticum, Mobiluncus species, Fusobacterium species, Atopobium vaginae.* These anaerobes appear as elongated cocci resembling rugby balls or as rods with irregular morphology. For this reason they are defined pleomorphic bacteria. The evaluator of the wet mount examination can observe different distributions of pleomorphic bacteria:

- free floating (Figure 71)
- arranged in clusters (Figure 72)
- adhered to exfoliated vaginal cells (clue cells) (Figure 73).

Anaerobes produce large amounts of proteolytic carboxylase enzymes, which break down vaginal

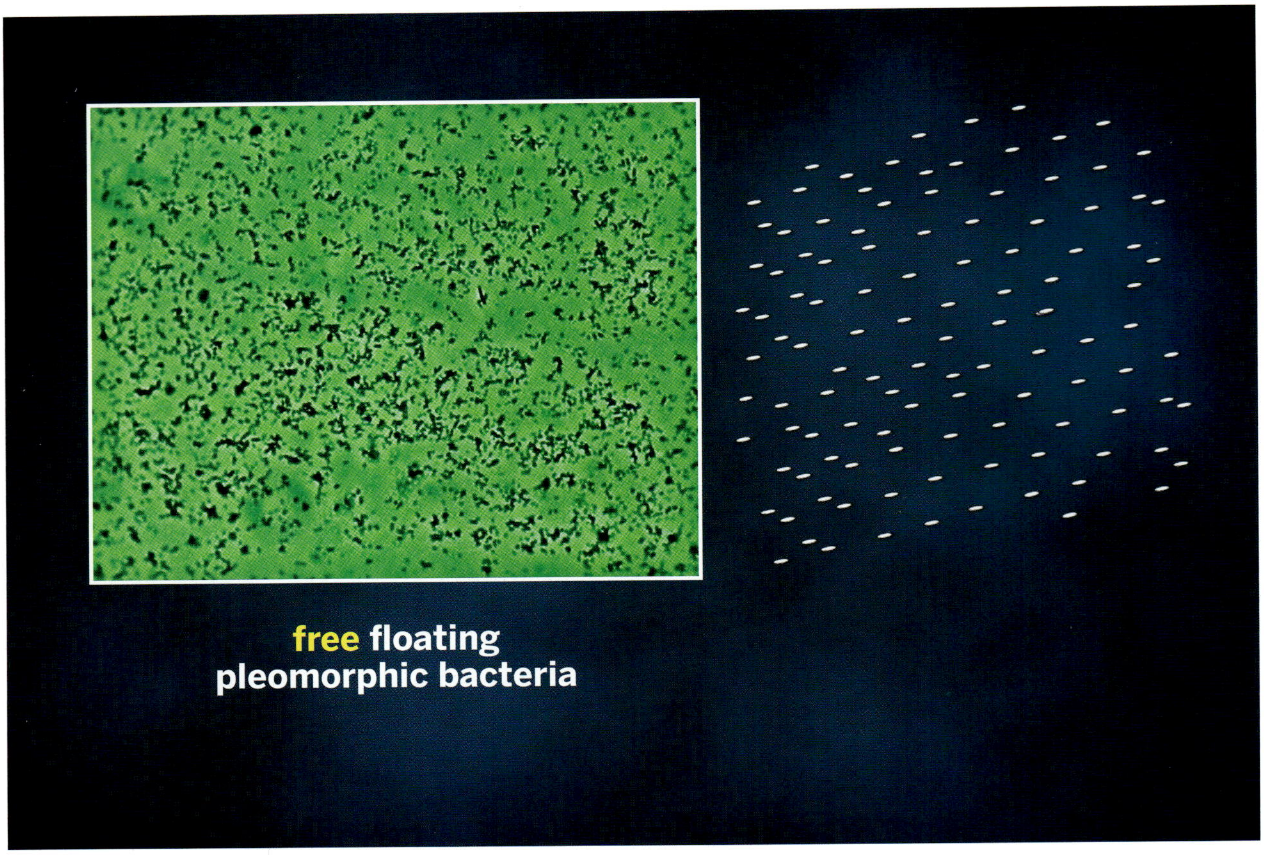

Figure 71 - Free-floating pleomorphic bacilli.

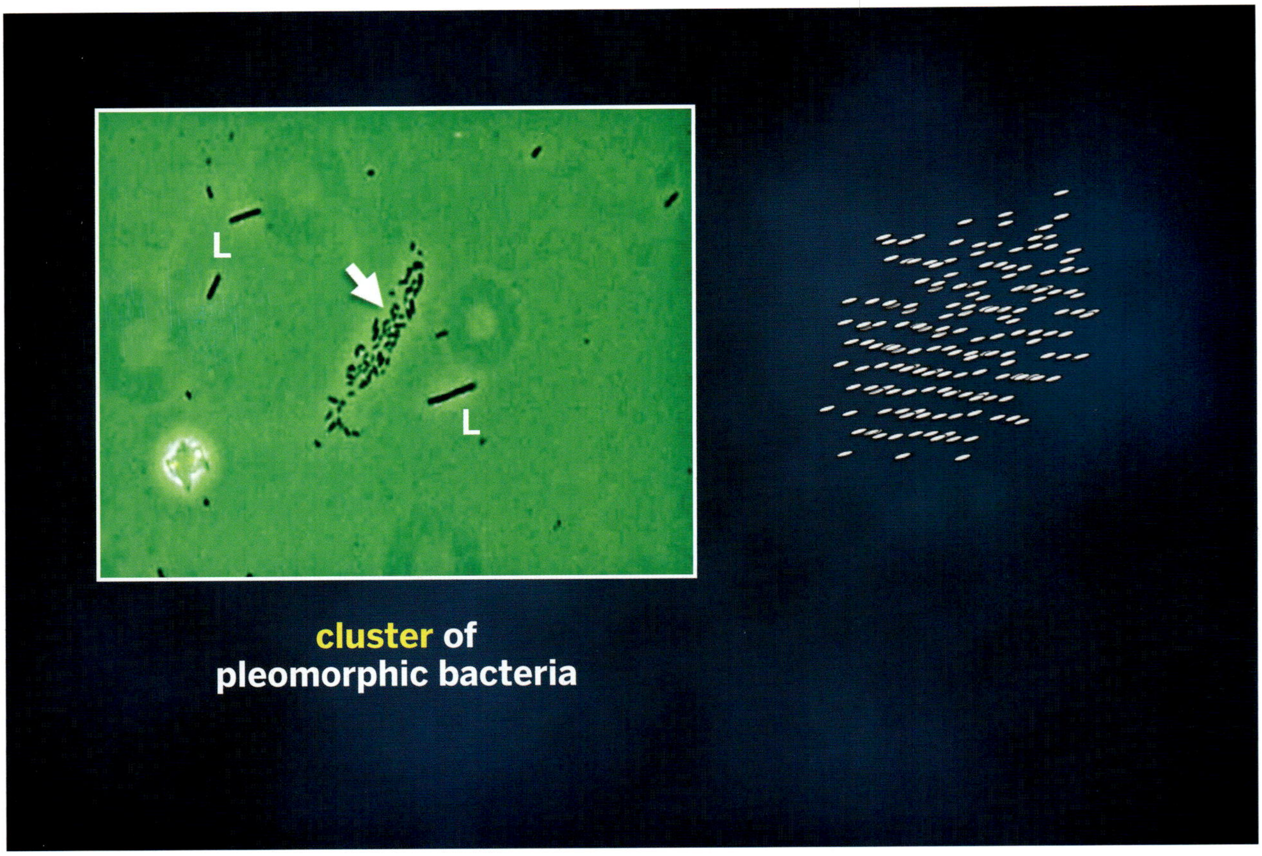

Figure 72 - Cluster of pleomorphic bacilli (→) surrounded by Lactobacilli (L).

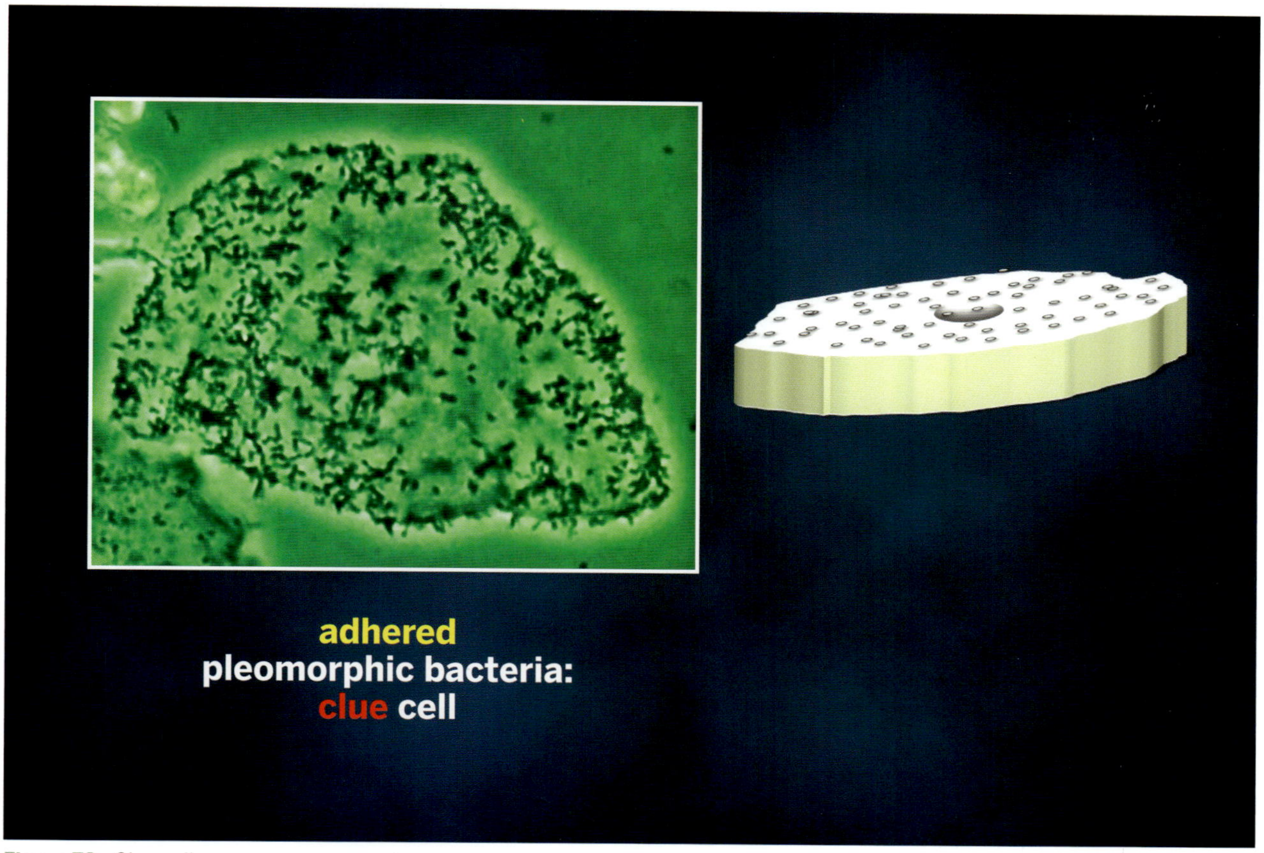

Figure 73 - Clue cell.

peptides into a variety of amines that are volatile, malodorous, and associated with increased vaginal transudation and squamous epithelial cell exfoliation, resulting in the typical clinical features observed in patients with BV.

The rise in pH also facilitates adherence of *G. vaginalis*, formerly known as Haemophilus vaginalis and Corynebacterium vaginale, to the exfoliating epithelial cells that appear coated with coccobacillary organisms and are called clue cells (Figure 73). The etymology behind the term "clue" cell derives from the original research article by Gardner and Dukes describing the characteristic cells. The name was chosen for its brevity in describing the sine qua non of bacterial vaginosis.

Diagnostic criteria of Bacterial vaginosis include:

- clue cell
- white, homogeneous, frothy and malodorous discharge
- "whiff test"
- vaginal pH > 4.5.

The white, abundant, homogeneous and frothy discharge (Figure 74), with a foul or fishy odour, resembles a cup of milk poured into the vagina (Figure 75). Many women show no symptoms and discharge is often scant.

To perform "whiff test", several drops of a potassium hydroxide solution are added to a sample of the vaginal discharge. A strong fishy odour from the mix usually indicates the presence of Bacterial vaginosis.

Bacterial vaginosis, aerobic vaginitis, trichomoniasis, and atrophic vaginitis often cause a vaginal pH higher than 4.5.

All the above criteria are common to trichomoniasis, except for the clue cell which is pathognomonic for Bacterial vaginosis. BV-associated anaerobes produce a substance called succinate. This substance suppresses the normal inflammatory reaction otherwise caused by this huge influx of bacteria. Only few white blood cells (WBCs) can be observed in the wet mount.

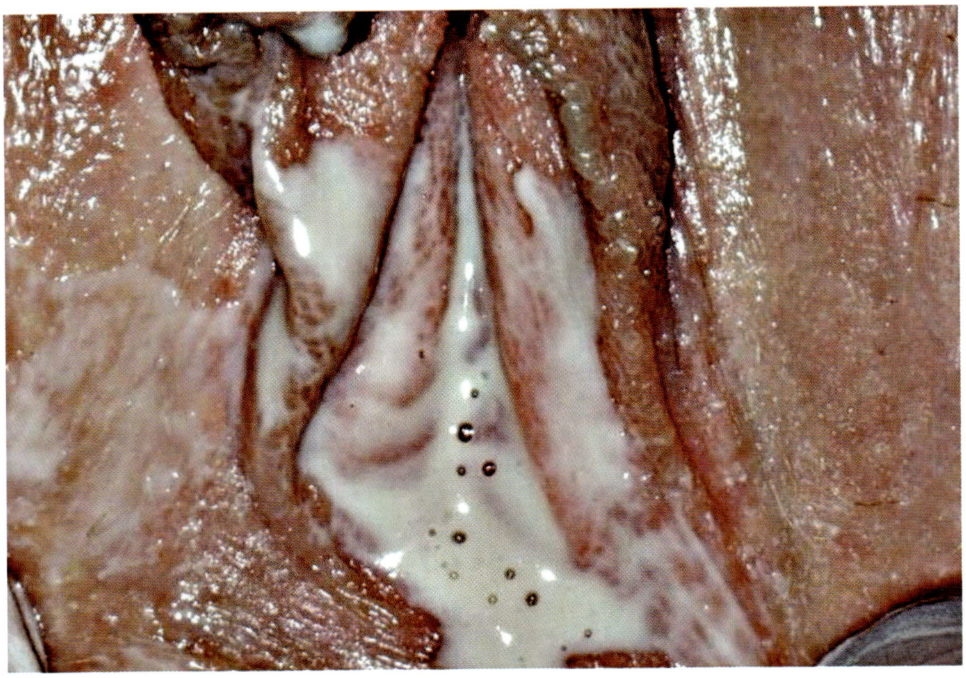

Figure 74 - White copious, homogeneous and frothy discharge in Bacterial vaginosis.

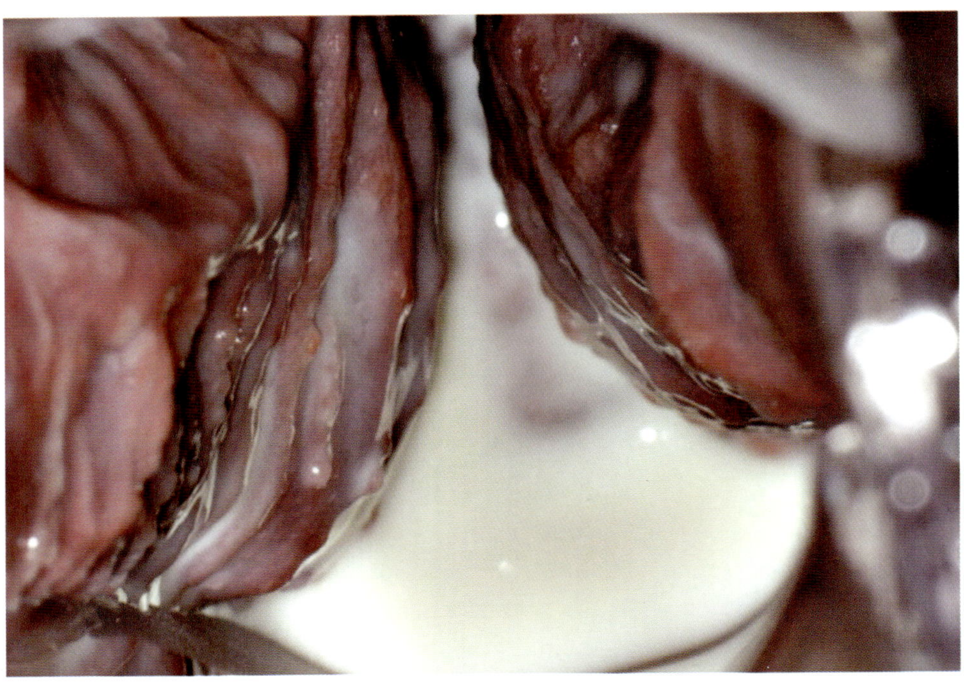

Figure 75 - The white copious and homogeneous discharge resembles a cup of milk poured into the vagina.

Unfortunately male patients are asymptomatic and nearly half of the affected women complain no discomfort. In their turn, urinary and vaginal cultures for laboratory confirmation of Bacterial vaginosis show excellent sensitivity but a less than 50% predictive value , therefore cultures are not recommended. On the other hand, when confidence in microscopic examination is good, a direct observation of pleiomorphic bacilli sticking to the cell surface ("clue cells") has a 90% sensitivity, a 98% specificity and a PPV ranging from 76% to 100%. For this reason, microscope is the most valuable diagnostic support.

In their famous report on Haemophilus vaginalis vaginitis (BV) of 1955, Gardner and Dukes stated: "a correct diagnosis could be made in practically every instance on the basis of wet mount findings alone".

Aerobic vaginitis

Aerobic vaginitis (AV) is a new unclassifiable pathology that is neither specific vaginitis nor Bacterial vaginosis. Although many studies state that the frequency of AV is still unknown, the frequency in pregnant women amounts to 25%. Given the increased local production of interleukin (IL)-1, IL-6 and IL-8 associated with AV during pregnancy, AV is not surprisingly associated with an increased risk of preterm delivery, chorioamnionitis and funisitis of the fetus. Elevated pH value of the vaginal environment (pH higher than 4,5) has been found in 94,10% of the cases. Enhanced and changed vaginal secretion can be observed in all of the patients suffering from aerobic vaginitis. Vaginal discharge (Figure 76) is often yellowish (70%), sometimes frothy or malodorous and may be associated with itching.

Escherichia coli is cited as one of the most common causes of this type of vaginitis and sometimes is isolated alone, even though Enterococcus faecalis, Staphylococcus sp. and group B of streptococcus are also involved. It must be pointed out that the presence itself of an organism in the culture does not denote causation. Therefore, how can we distinguish infection from vaginal contamination that is not necessary to treat? Aerobic vaginitis is accompanied by an increased localized inflammatory reaction, as opposed to the suppressed immune response that is characteristic of Bacterial vaginosis (Figure 77). The diagnosis of "aerobic vaginitis" is essentially based on microscopic examinations using a phase contrast microscope.

Syphilis

Syphilis is a highly contagious venereal disease spread primarily by sexual activity, including oral and anal sex, and is responsible for long-term damage to different organs, if not properly treated. *Treponema pallidum*, a gram-negative spirochaete bacterium, is the aetiological agent.

Direct detection methods are not widely available and require specialized laboratories with trained technicians. Hence, false negative tests are relatively common, and amount to about 30% of the cases. Specimens for microscopic examination are best obtained from serous transudate of moist lesions such as a primary chancre. Treponema pallidum may be recognized in the microscopic field as a delicate, narrow and coiled bacillus (Figure 78).

Syphilis causes pustules which progress to ulcerated lesions, called chancres, characterized by an eroded center covered by a yellowish secretion (Figure 79). Other primary lesions may be condyloma latum

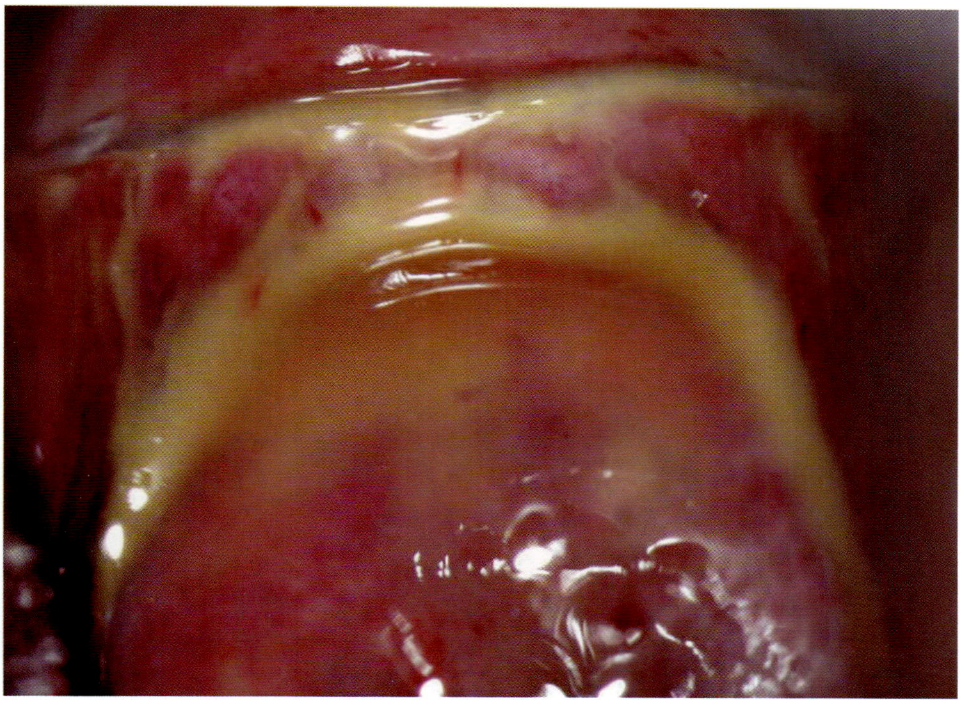

Figure 76 - Yellowish discharge in aerobic vaginitis.

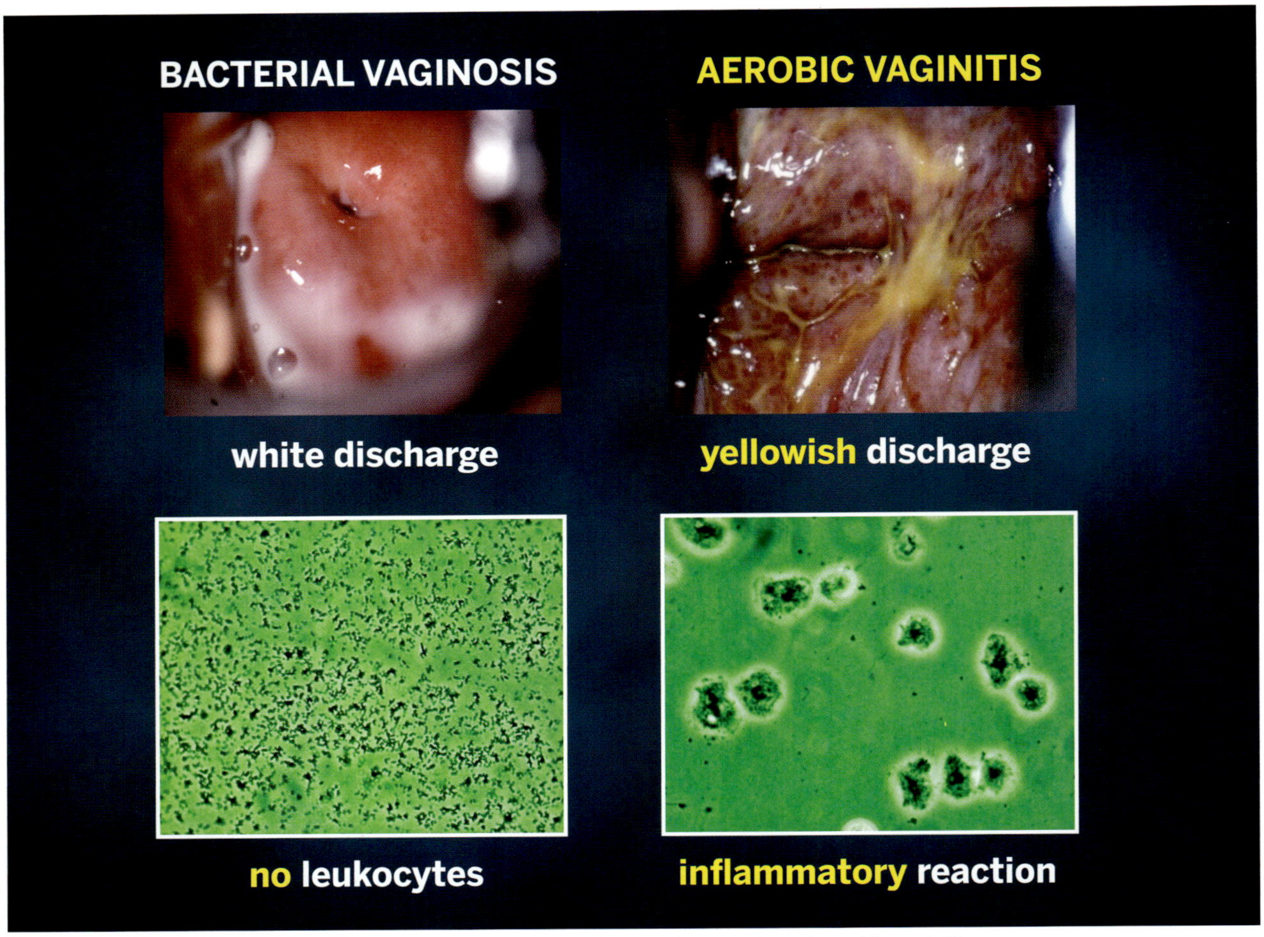

Figure 77 - Colposcopic and microscopic differences between Bacterial vaginosis and aerobic vaginitis.

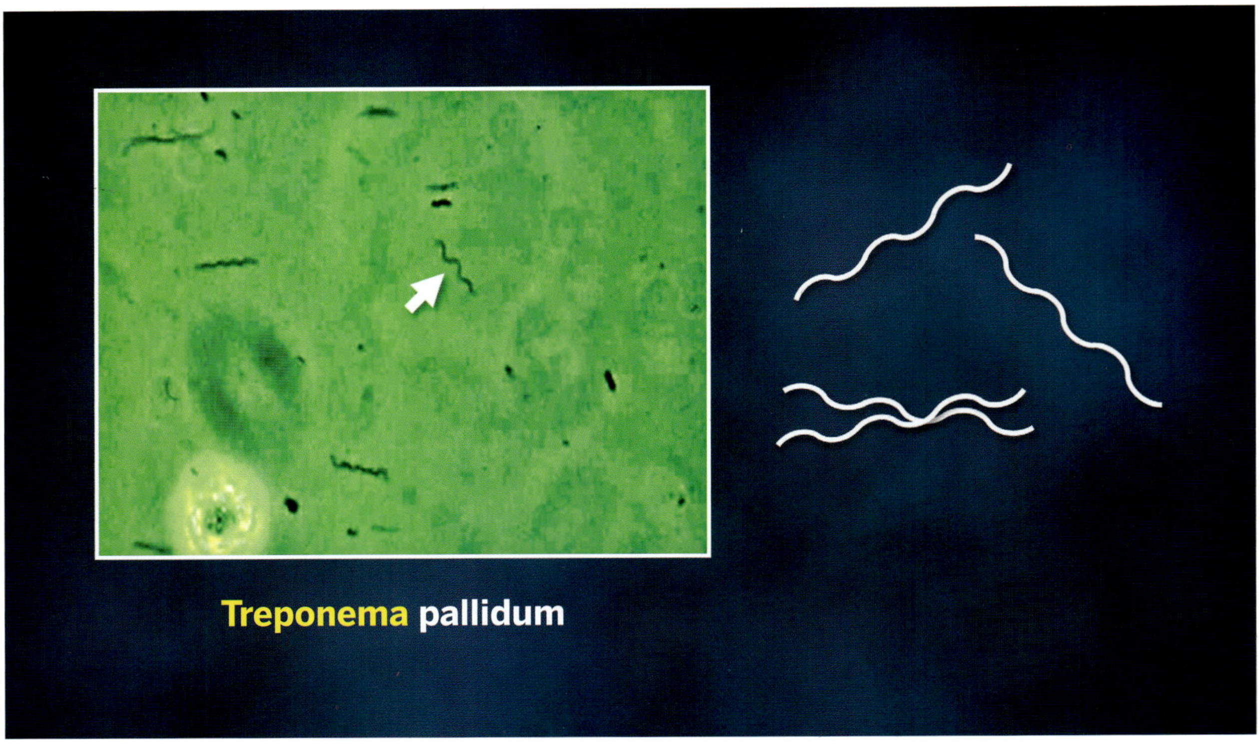

Figure 78 - Delicate, narrow and coiled bacilli (→) (Treponema pallidum).

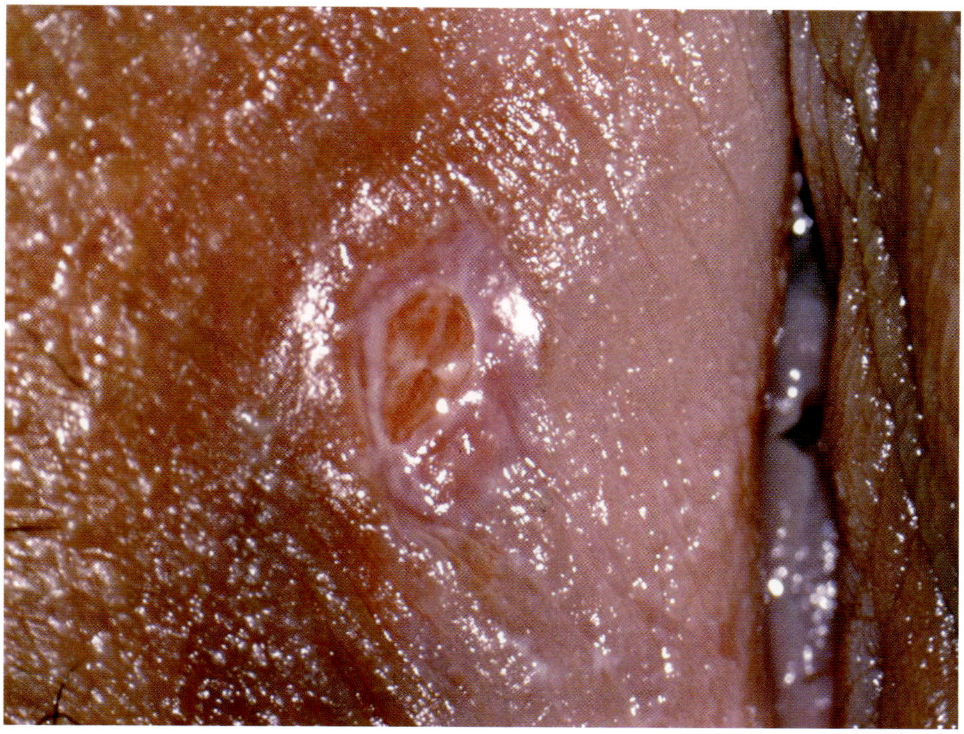

Figure 79 - Hard ulcer with an eroded center (chancre).

(wart-like lesions, sometimes extensive), or mucous patches (shallow ulcers on mucous membranes, non-painful unless secondarily infected). Primary chancre must be differentiated from chancroid, caused by Haemophilus ducrey. Both originate at the site of inoculation and are 1-2 cm in diameter. However, chancre is typically non exudative, whereas chancroid has a grey or yellow purulent exudate. Furthermore, chancre is typically painless and has a stiff edge, whereas chancroid is painful and shows a soft edge.

Chlamydia trachomatis

Chlamydia infection, often simply known as Chlamydia, is a sexually transmitted infection caused by the Chlamydia trachomatis (CT) bacterium. Chlamydia t. is found worldwide, infecting both females and males, adults as well as children.

People affected by Chlamydia often do not show outward symptoms in the early stages. This infection is easily spread because it often causes no symptoms and may be unknowingly transmitted to sexual partners. About 75% of infections in women and 50% in men show no symptoms. However, Chlamydia can cause health problems in the later stages, including pelvic inflammatory disease (PID) and damage to the fallopian tubes that can lead to future infertility and an increased risk of ectopic pregnancy. In addition, infection of the female genital tract during pregnancy may result in spontaneous abortion, premature labor, baby with low birth weight, postpartum endometritis, neonatal conjunctivitis or pneumonia.

In the later stages women can complain different symptoms such as abnormal vaginal discharge that may be bad smelling, bleeding between periods, painful periods, lower abdominal pain, possibly with fever, bleeding after sexual intercourse, painful intercourse, itching or burning in the genital area and burning or pain on urination.

As the infection progresses, both sexes complain an increased sebum production resulting in greasy sweat and more oily complexion. Such signs can be misdiagnosed as acne eruptions.

Chlamydia t. may be found in the form of an elementary body (EB) and a reticulate body (RB) (Figure 80). Chlamydia replication takes place inside of a host cell, exclusively within a vacuole known as the *inclusion*.

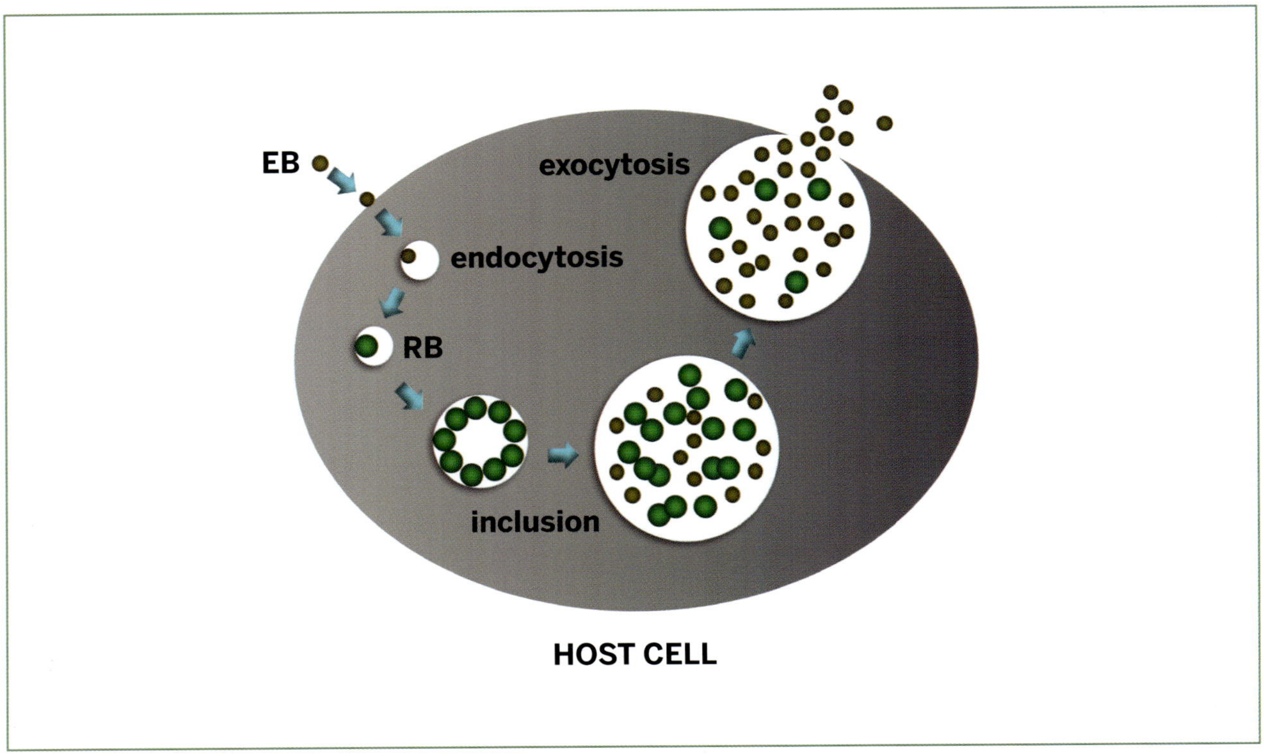

Figure 80 - Life cycle of Chlamydia trachomatis. (EB) Elementary Bodies, (RB) Reticulate Bodies.

The *elementary body* is the non-replicating infectious particle that enters the host cell via endocytosis. Upon entry, the EB converts into a non-infectious *reticulate body* (RB). The RB appears slightly larger than the elementary body and is metabolically active and highly involved in the process of replication and growth. The reticulate body replicates by binary scission. Once this biphasic developmental cycle is almost complete, the RBs form particles that develop into new infectious EB progeny after synthesis of the outer cell wall, stimulating exocytosis or host cell lysis. This process releases the infectious EBs into the extracellular space. These EBs then move on to infect other host cells.

During an infection, the inclusion expands to accommodate the increasing number of C. trachomatis, pushing progressively the nucleus towards the periphery of the infected cell. Microscopy observation enables to easily detect the inclusion which may contain a condensed body (Figures 81, 82) or a fragmented body (Figures 81, 83). It is also possible to observe the entire inclusion being ejected from the infected cell (Figures 84, 85, 86) or breaking to release the new infectious EBs (Figure 87).

Both PAP smear and wet mount microscopy (Figure 88) provide a high specificity with a poor sensitivity, due to the extreme fragility of the cells containing the inclusion. However, direct microscopy does not use laboratory processing, including dehydration, fixation and staining, so its sensitivity is higher than in Pap smear.

Chlamydia infection can be suspected in presence of characteristic colposcopic findings:

- fragile epithelium and congested cervix ($p<0.001$) (Figure 89)
- hypertrophic and congested exposed columnar epithelium (Figure 90)
- mucopurulent discharge at the os (62%) ($p<0.005$) (Figure 91).

Gonorrhea

Gonorrhea is a very common disease, especially among young people aged 15-24. This infection is caused by the Gram-negative cocci *Neisseria gonorrhoeae* and is transmitted by oral, anal, and vaginal sex. Gonococcal infection can also be transmitted

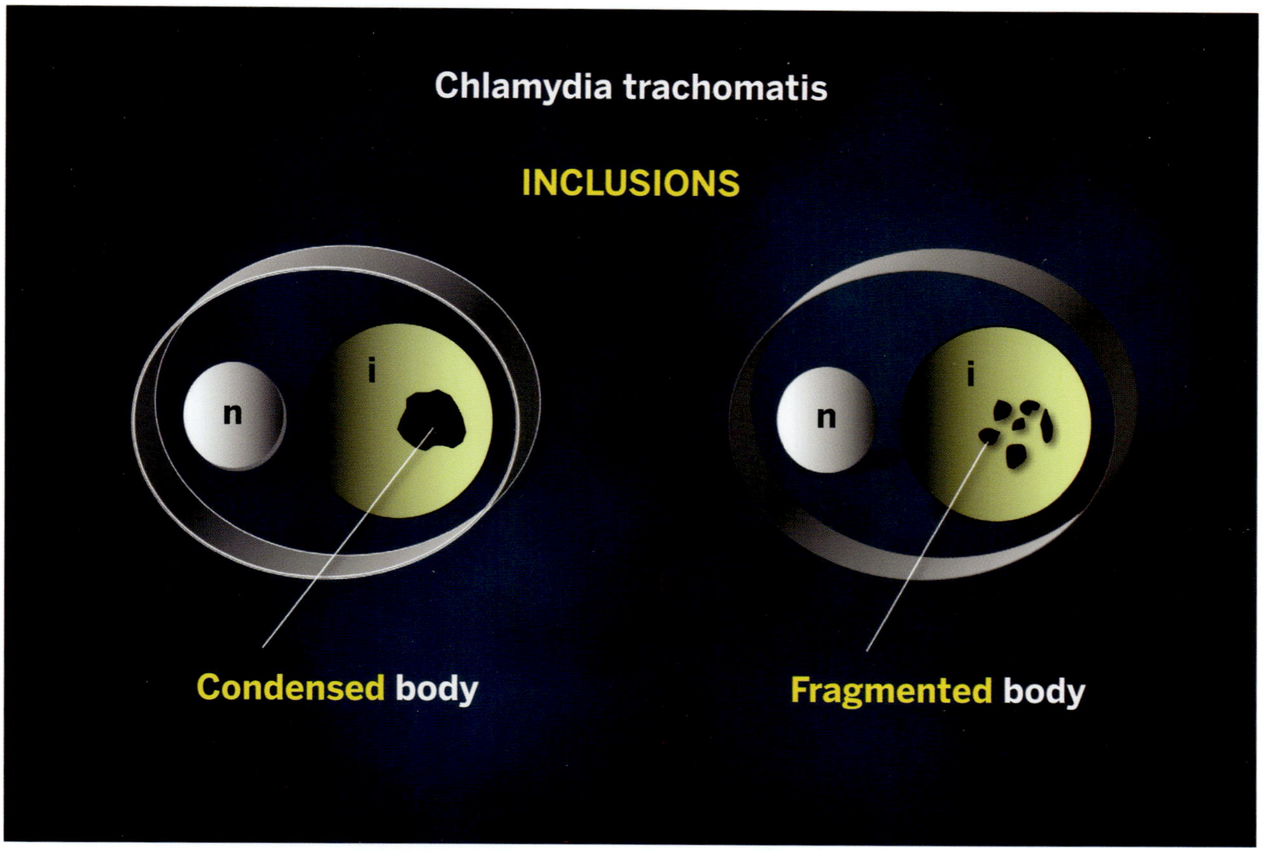

Figure 81 - Different types of bodies contained in inclusions (i) of Chlamydia trachomatis. (n) Nucleus.

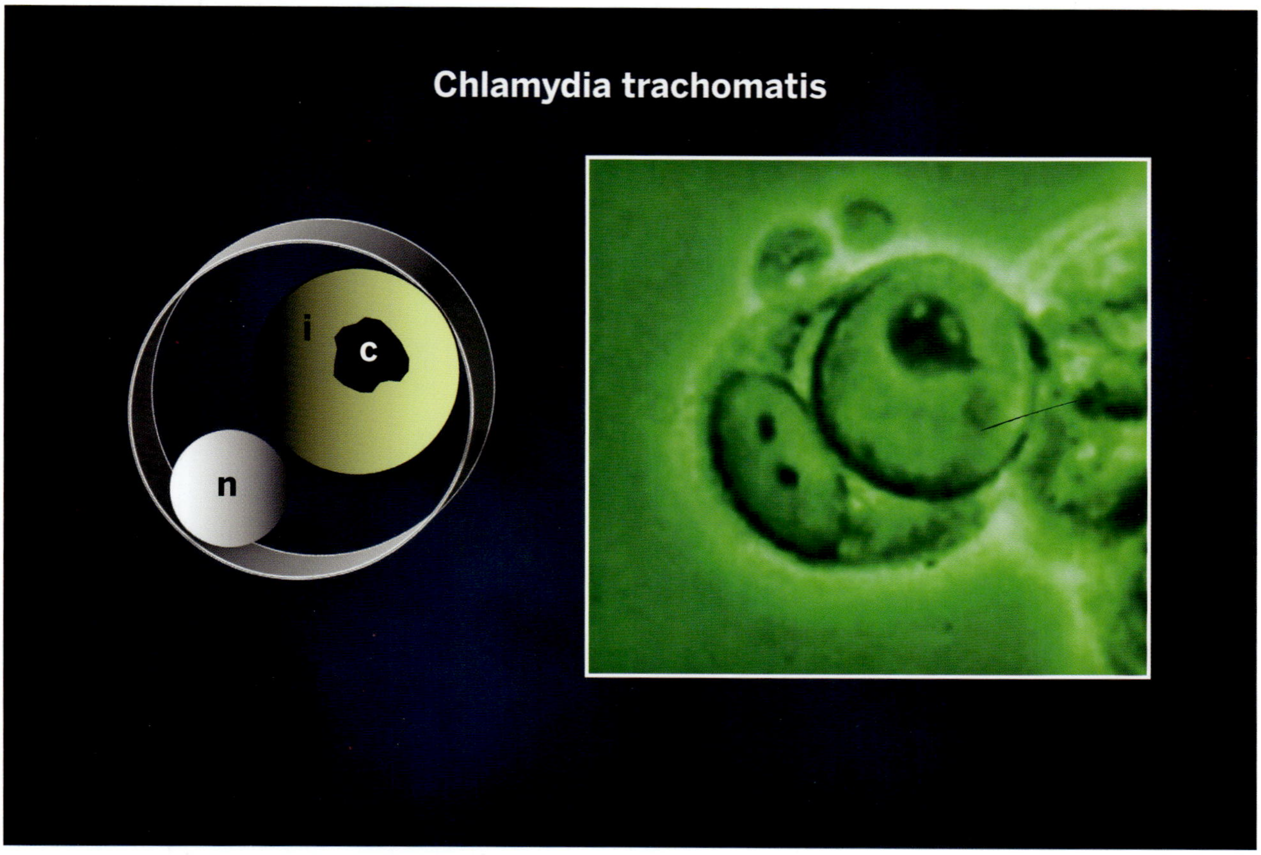

Figure 82 - Inclusion (i) containing a condensed body (c). (n) Nucleus.

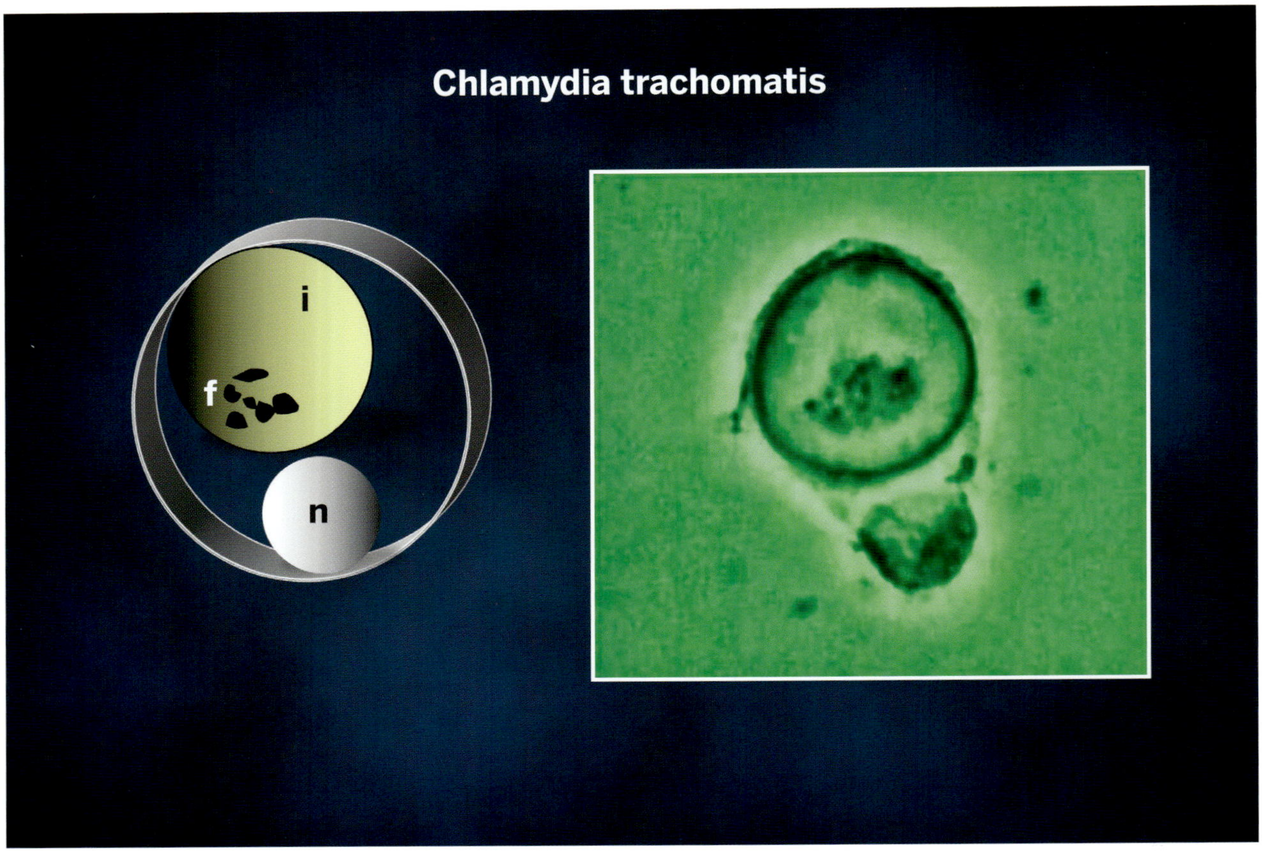

Figure 83 - Inclusion (i) containing a fragmented body (f). (n) Nucleus.

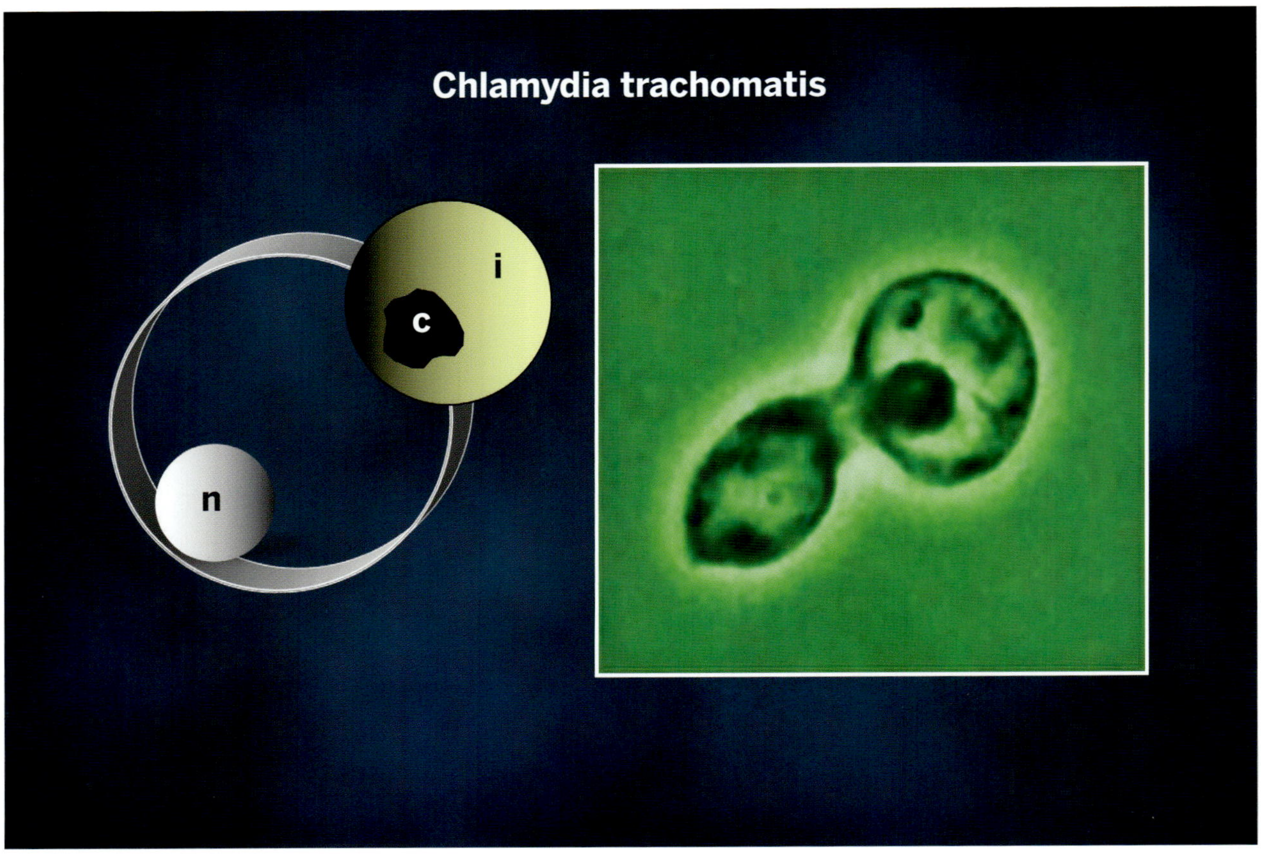

Figure 84 - Release of the inclusion (i) containing the condensed body (c). (n) Nucleus.

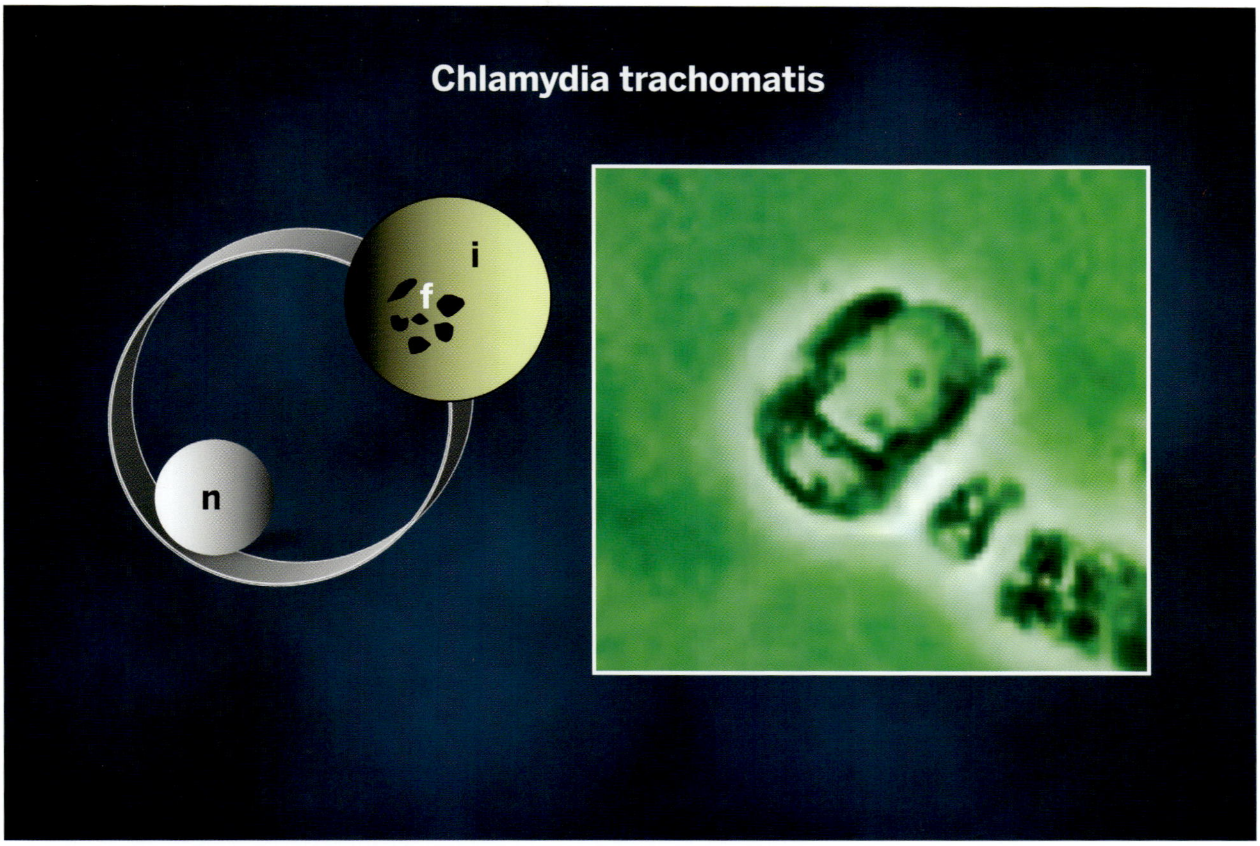

Figure 85 - Release of the inclusion (i) containing the fragmented body (f). (n) Nucleus.

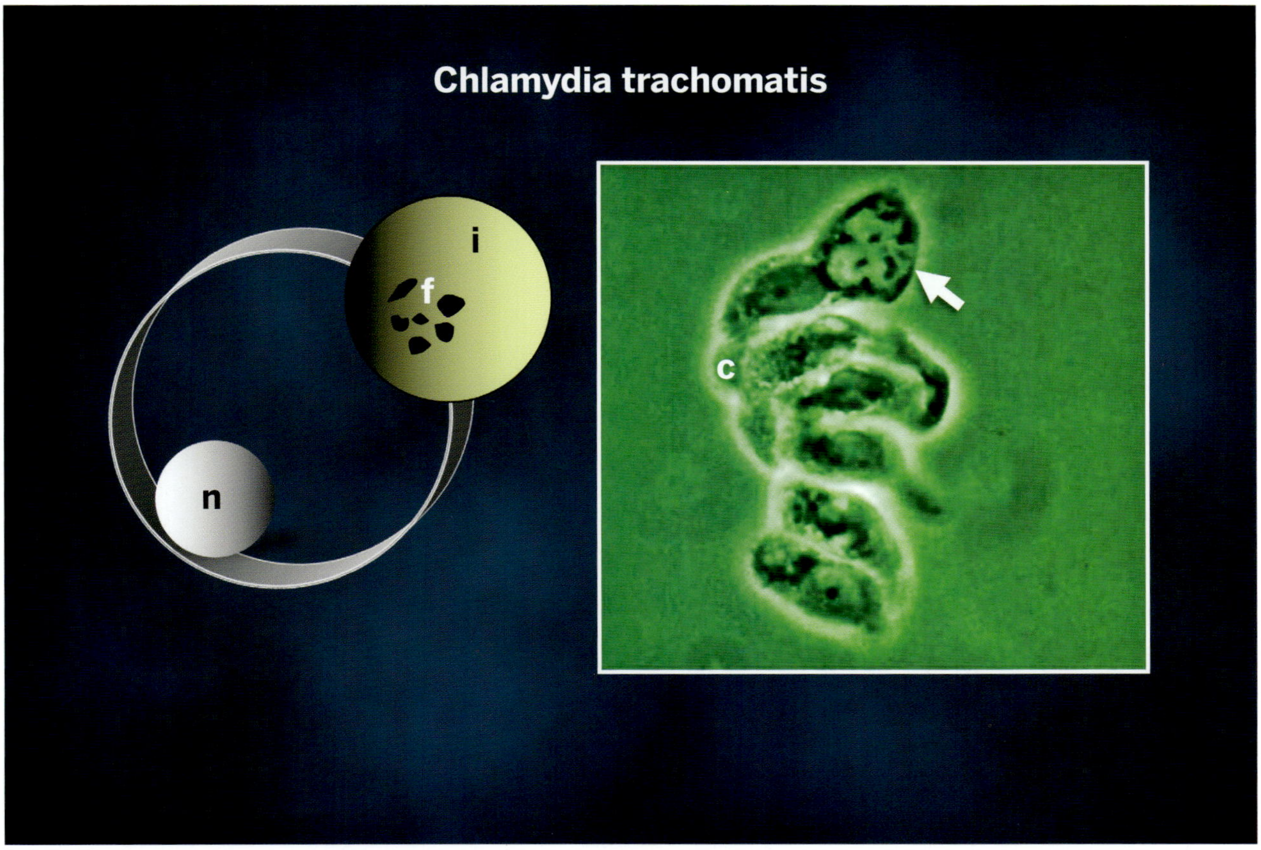

Figure 86 - Release of the inclusion (i) containing the fragmented body (f) in a columnar cell (→). (n) Nucleus, (c) columnar cells.

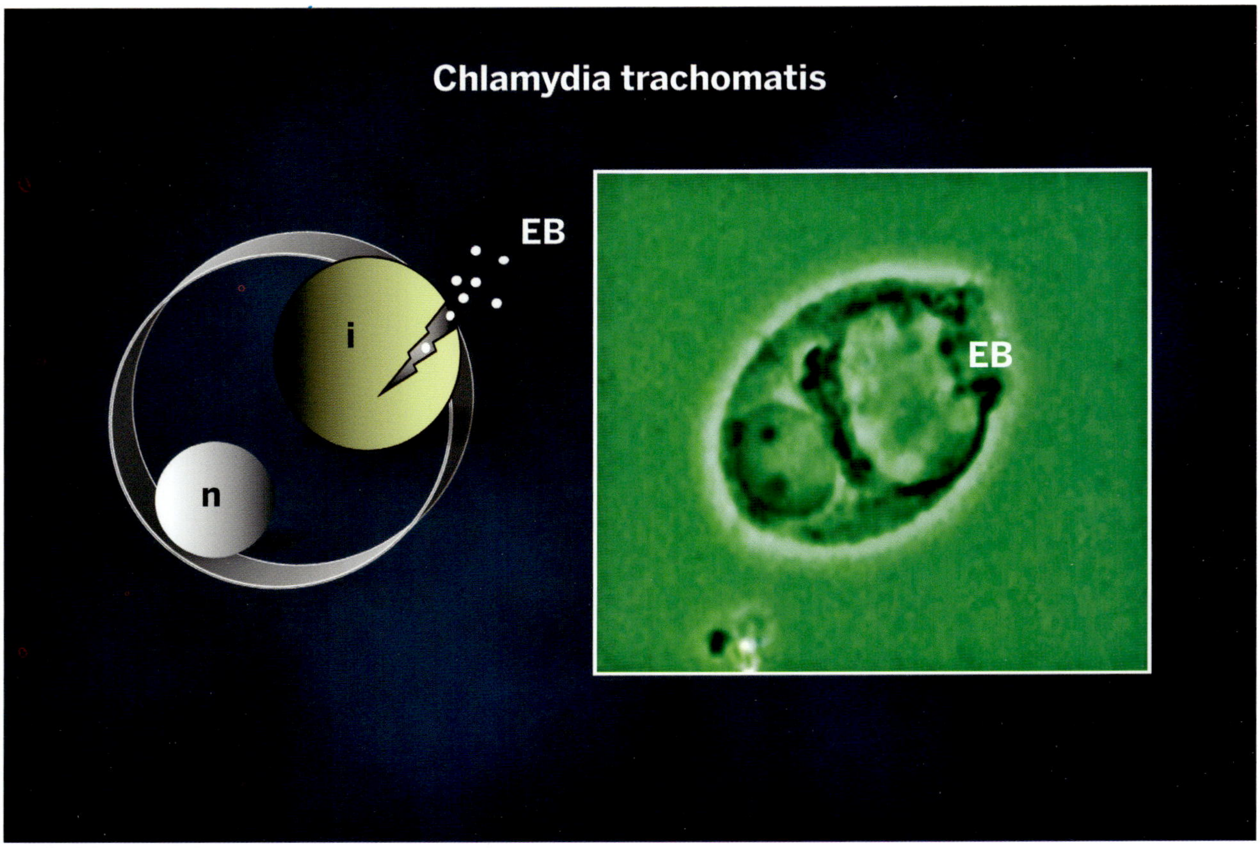

Figure 87 - Breaking of the inclusion (i) and release of elementary bodies (EB). (n) Nucleus.

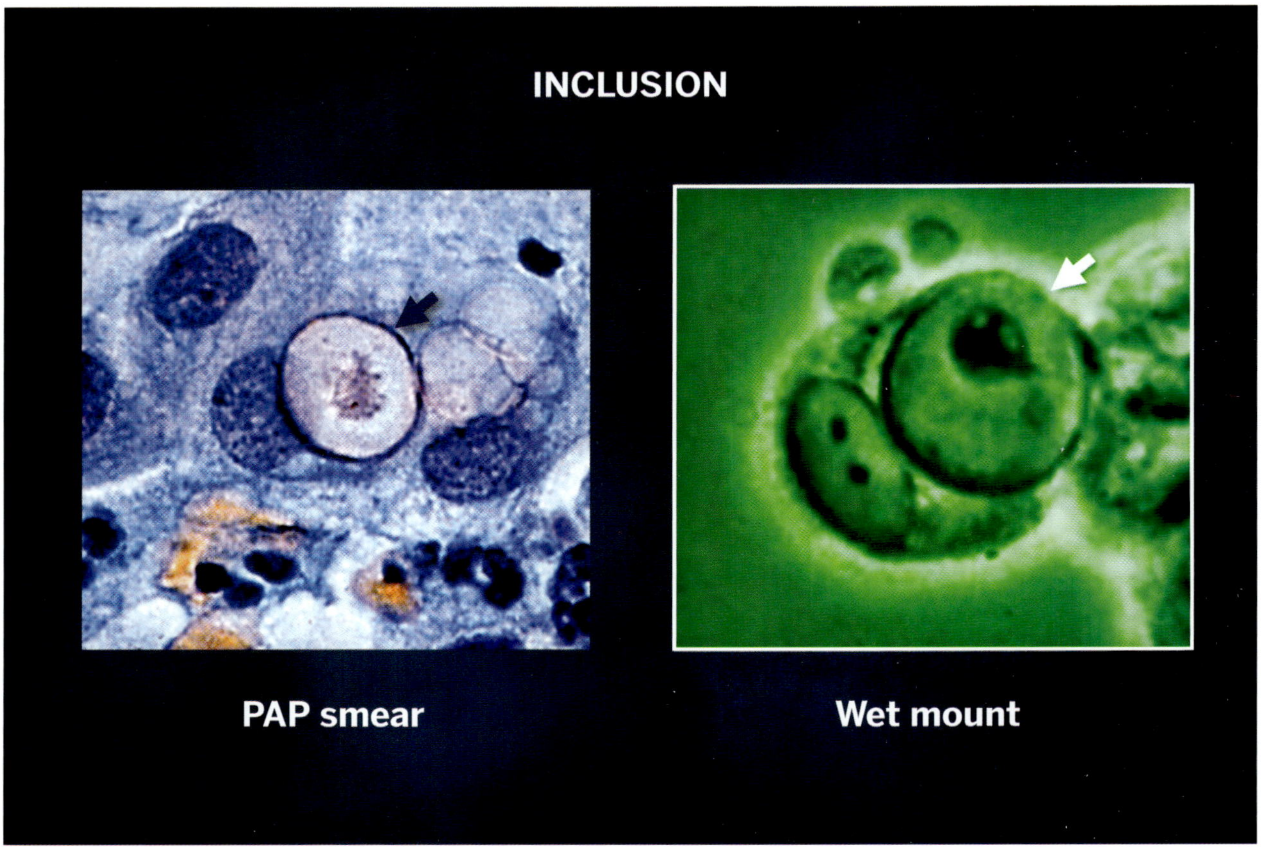

Figure 88 - Inclusion of Chlamydia trachomatis (→) observed in Pap smear and wet mount.

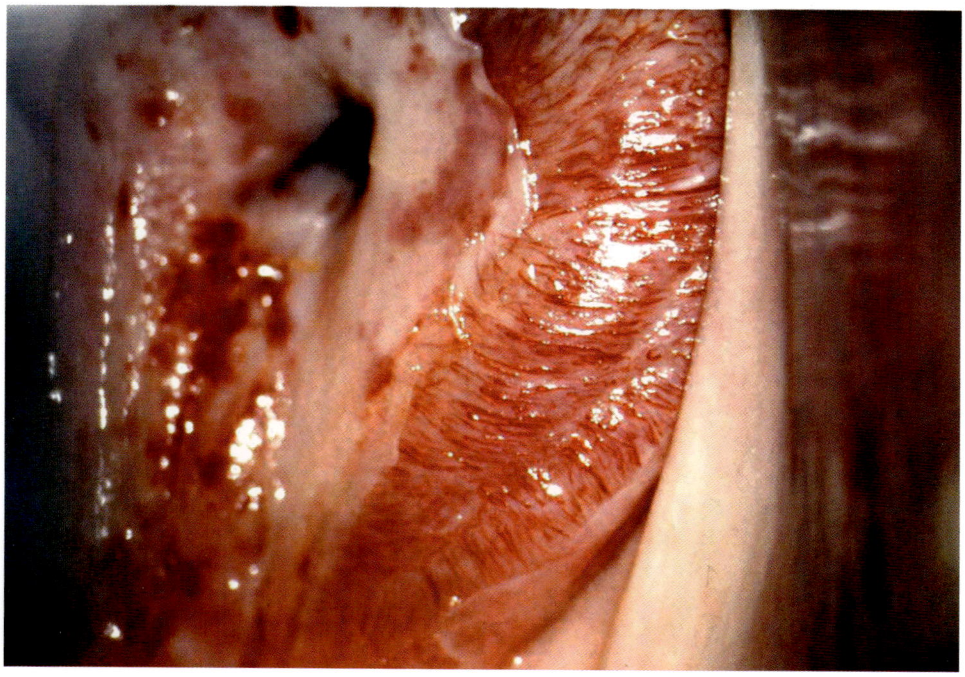

Figure 89 - Collapse of the fragile epithelium in Chlamydia trachomatis infection revealing the subepithelial capillary network.

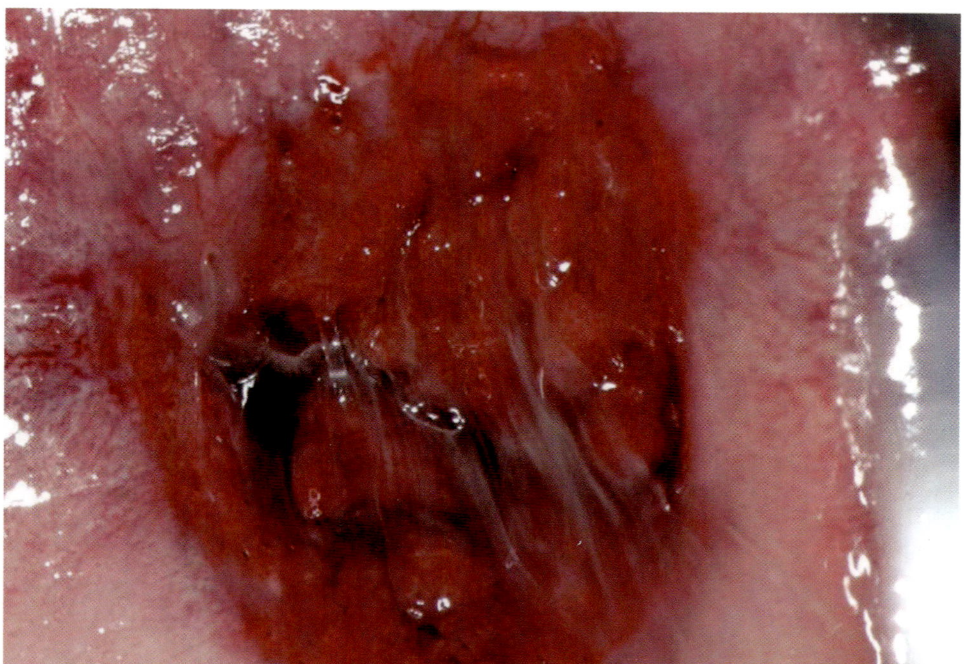

Figure 90 - Hypertrophic and congested exposed epithelium in Chlamydia trachomatis infection.

from a mother to her child during birth. Gonococci appear in pairs, as typical intracellular diplococci on microscopic examination of endocervical secretions from women, in the shape of coffee beans (Figure 92).

Women may experience a burning sensation on urination, vaginal mucopurulent discharge (Figure 93), vaginal bleeding between periods, or pelvic pain. One of the complications of this sexually transmitted infection is pelvic inflammatory disease, which can lead to serious sequelae such as infertility, ectopic pregnancy, and chronic pelvic pain. Occasionally, untreated gonococcal infection can become invasive, leading to disseminated gonococcal infections, which may result in gonococcal arthritis-dermatitis syndrome, suppurative arthritis, endocarditis with heart valves damage, and meningitis.

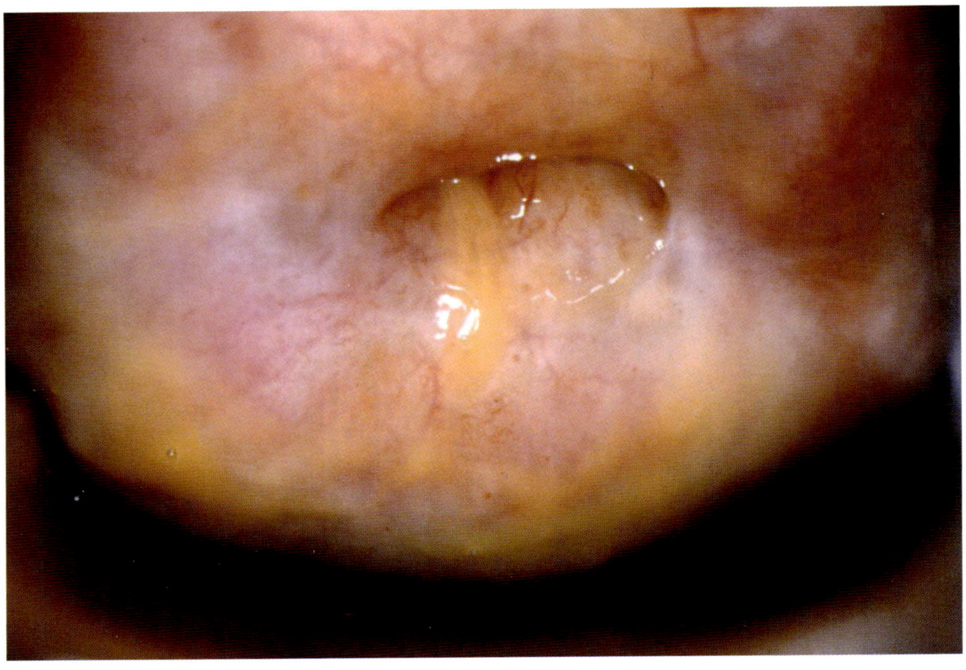

Figure 91 - Mucopurulent discharge at the os in Chlamydia trachomatis infection.

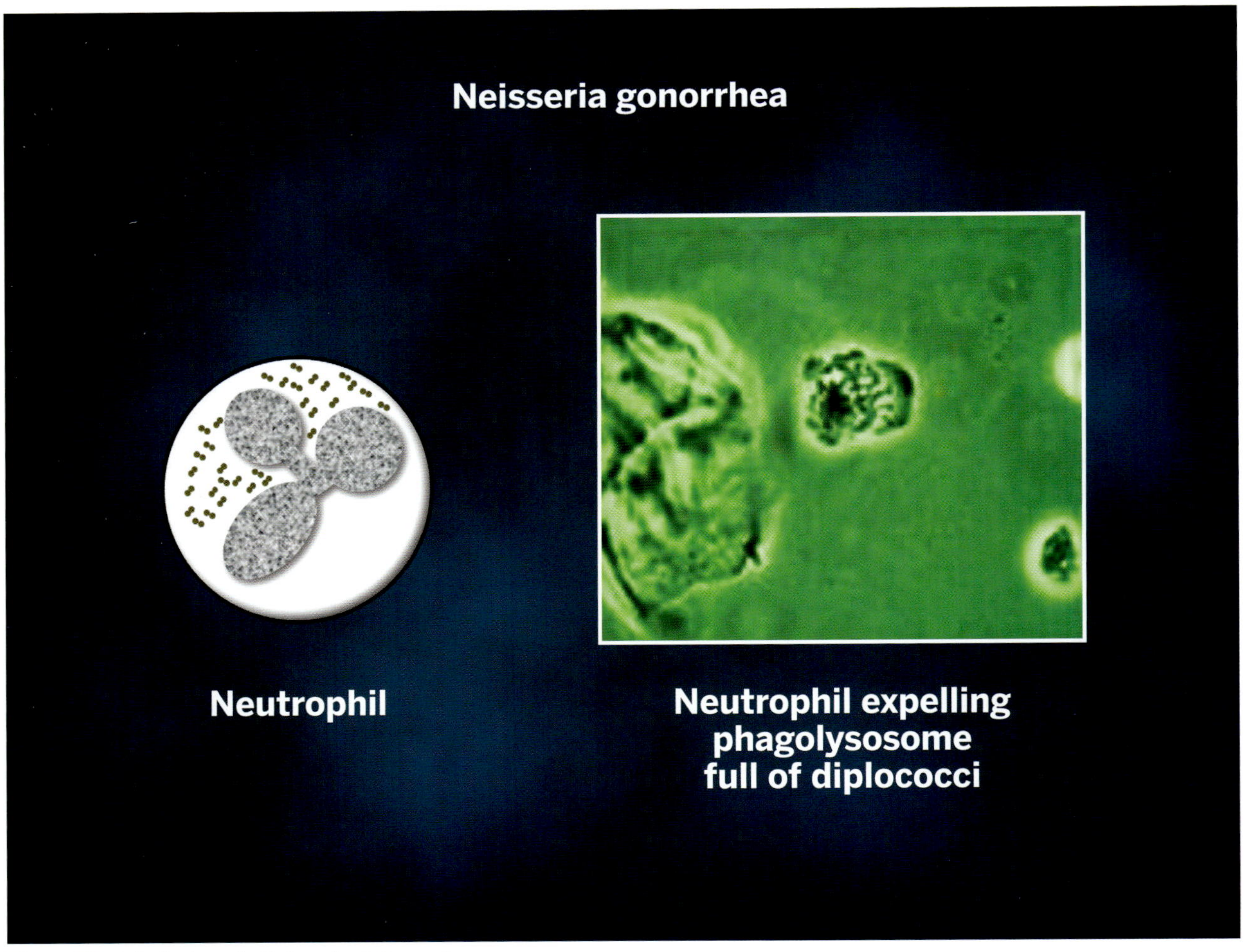

Figure 92 - Intraleukocytic Neisseria diplococci.

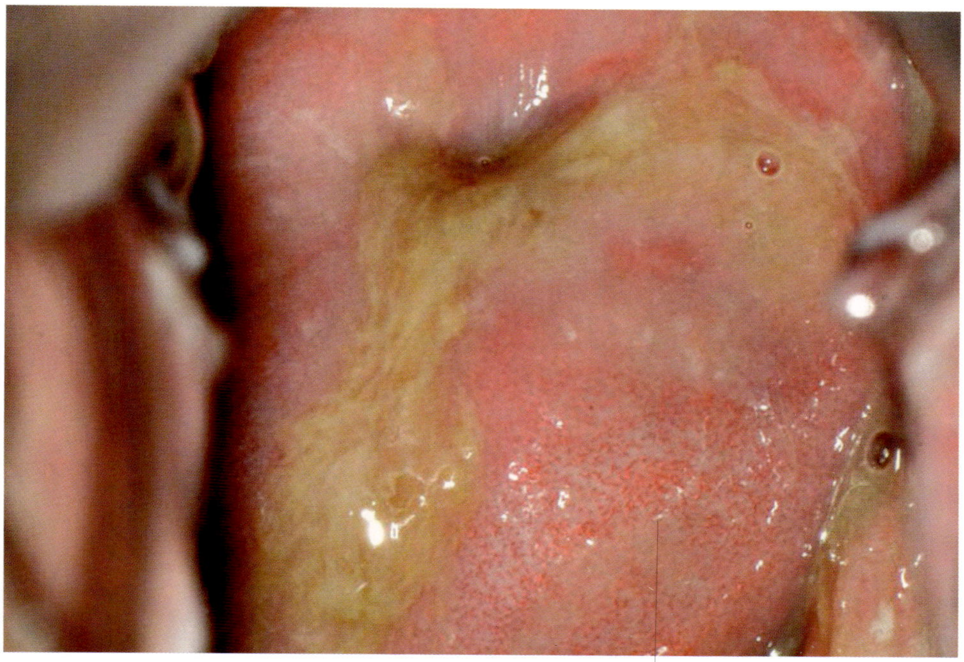
Figure 93 - Mucopurulent discharge from the cervical canal in gonorrhea.

Candidiasis

Candida and the many other microorganisms that normally live in the vaginal environment keep each other in balance. However, sometimes the amount of Candida increases, leading to a yeast infection. Vaginal yeast infections, also known as *candidiasis*, are a common female condition.

In recent years a change in epidemiological trends of vaginal fungal infections has been recorded, both regarding asymptomatic colonization and colpitis. Candida species, in fact, may be isolated from vaginal discharge in approximately 20% of healthy symptom-free women during their childbearing age. On the other hand, if we consider the symptomatic infection, candidal vulvovaginitis (CVV) shows an increase in incidence; in fact, it has been estimated that some 75% of women will complain a first CVV in their life span and that approximately half of these subjects will develop a second symptomatic event.

DNA makeup permitted to classify approximately 150 Candida species, belonging to genus 4 in blastomycetes. *C. albicans* is by far the most common etiologic agent of fungal genital infections, being responsible for 80-90% of all cases of vaginal candidiasis. *Torulopsis* or *Candida glabrata* is the second most common species (5-15%), followed by *C. tropicalis* (5%), *C. krusei* and *C. pseudotropicalis*. Other species, such as *C. guilliermondi* and *C. parapsilosis* are rarely isolated by culture.

Incidence of recurrent CCV is mistaken due to different time intervals for defining recurrence. If considering four or more mycologically-diagnosed episodes during a year as time interval, it has been estimated that some 5% of patients who experienced symptomatic vaginal candidiasis will suffer a recurrence with great psychological impact when refractory episodes are complained.

The term "yeast" is not always strictly defined, but it is generally used for single-cell fungi. Candidiasis is the second most common cause of vaginal inflammation after BV, accounting for 20 to 25 percent of cases.

The clinical pathogen Candida albicans is a budding yeast that is capable of forming a range of different vegetative structures (Figure 94):

- spore (yeast)
- blastospore (blastoconidium)
- pseudohypha
- hypha.

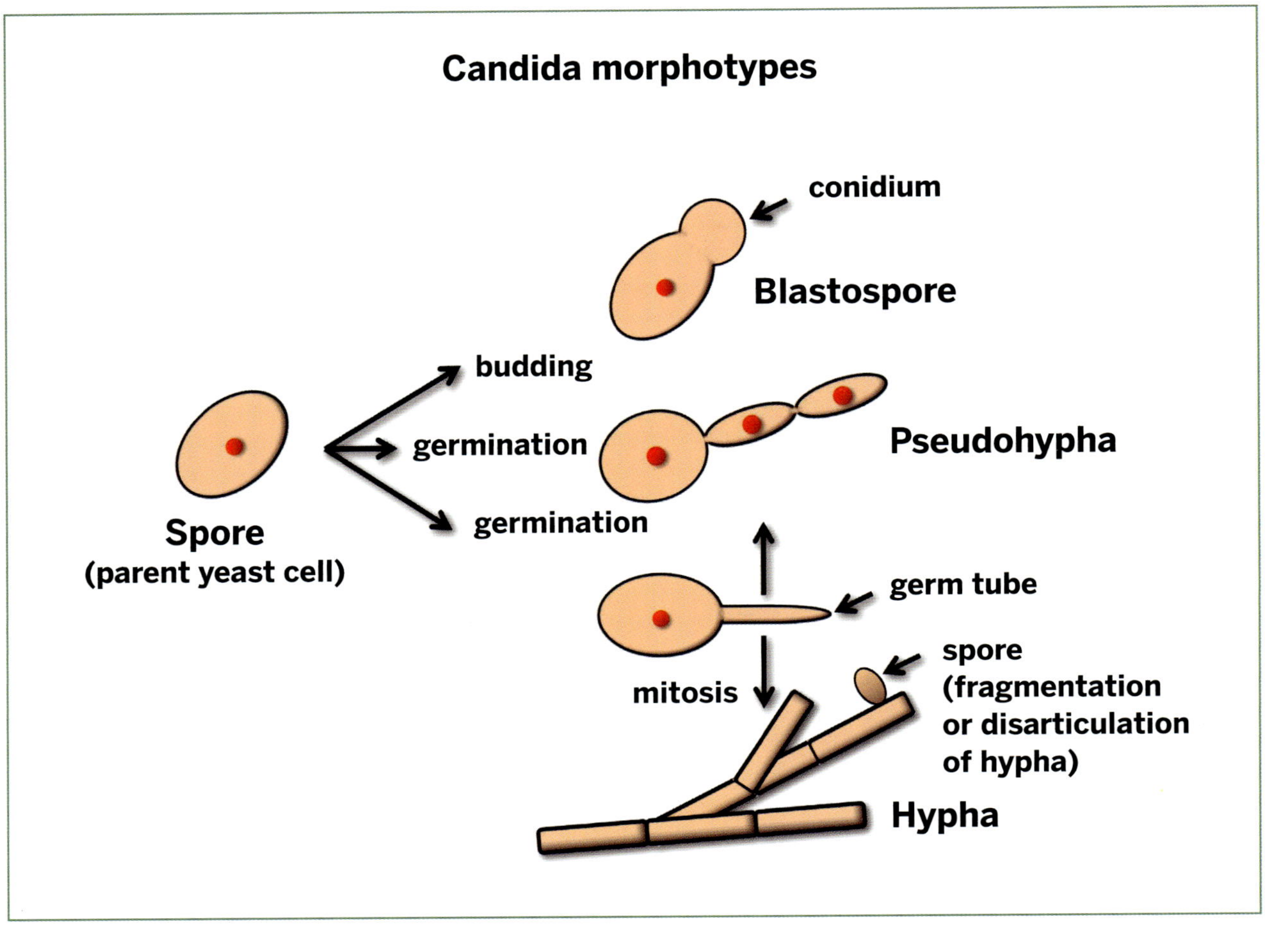

Figure 94 - Diagrammatic representation of Candida morphotypes.

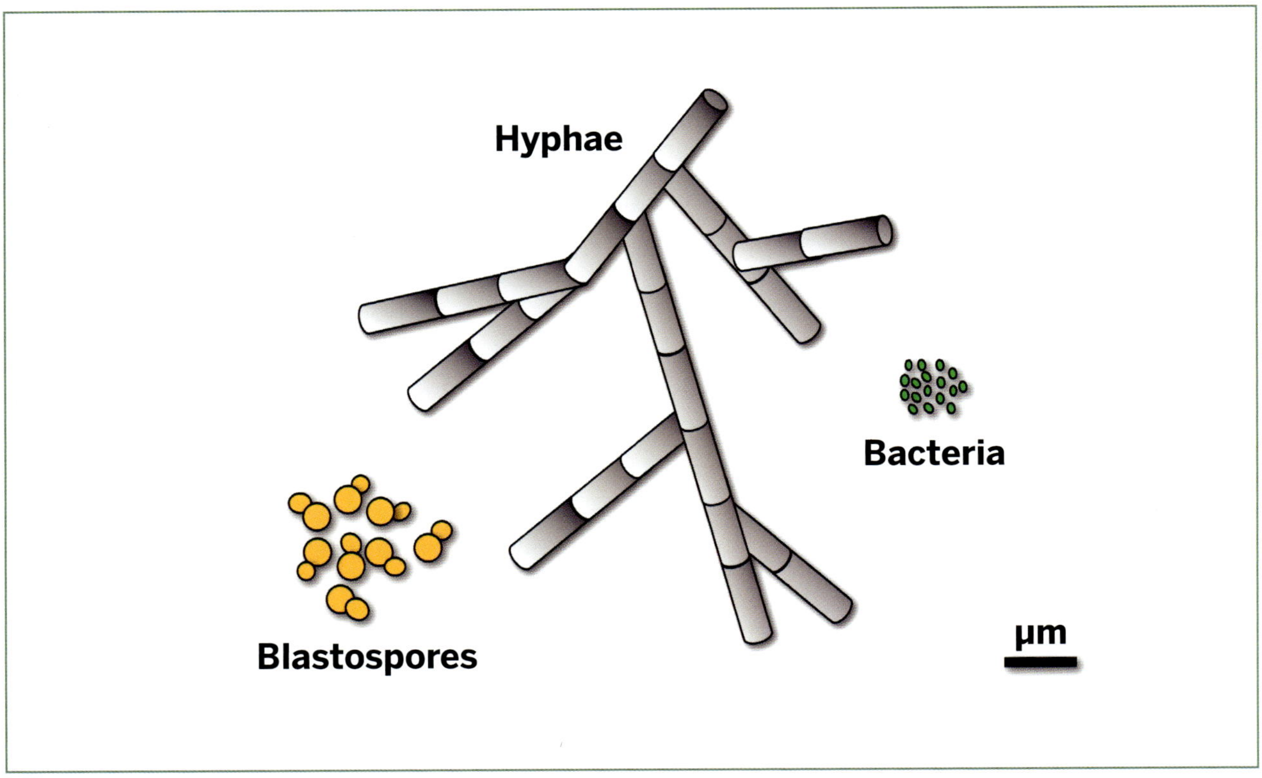

Figure 95 - Comparison of sizes among different microorganisms.

Spores are unicellular, appear round to oval, are larger than bacteria (Figure 95) and multiply by germination, generating budded cells known as *blastospores*. The formation of blastospores (Figure 94) involves three basic steps: bud emergence from the parent spore (conidium), bud growth, and conidium separation. Blastospore is a synonym of blastoconidium (blasto + conidium).

When the production of blastospores continues without separation of the conidia from each other, a *pseudohypha* consisting of a filament of attached blastospores is formed by germination.

Pseudohyphae are a type of filament that form pseudomycelia mostly in polymorphic fungi like Candida. Pseudohyphae are composed of ellipsoidal and elongated yeast- like cells. These cells remain connected as a chain with constrictions at the site where septa are found. Pseudohyphae form during the cell division and newly divided cells remain adhered as chains and branches through the budding process. Some scientists consider pseudohyphae as an intermediate state between yeast-like cells and true hyphae.

In addition to budding yeast cells and pseudohyphae, yeasts such as Candida albicans may form true *hyphae*. A *germ tube* is an outgrowth produced by spores of spore-releasing fungi during germination. The germ tube differentiates, grows, and develops by mitosis to create true hyphae.

Hyphae are defined as elongated, tubular and branching filaments that form the mycelium of a fungus. The mycelium is the vegetative part of a fungus consisting of numerous filaments.

A single hypha consists of one or more elongated tubular cells. Multicellular hyphae are internally divided by cross walls, defined as septa, displaying a chain of closely packed cells. Fragmentation or disarticulation of existing hyphae is a common mechanism of spore formation.

Both hyphae and pseudohyphae are two types of filaments that compose vegetative structures found in fungi, linked to each other as a chain.

Hyphae and pseudohyphae show some differences:

- hyphae may or may not contain septa, whereas pseudohyphae always contain septa
- there is no constriction at the site where septa are found in hyphae, whereas it is present in pseudohyphae
- hyphae can be coenocytic (single celled, multinuclear) or multicellular, but pseudohyphae are always multicellular
- hyphae do not show budding whereas pseudohyphae do show budding through which they grow continuously
- hyphae are always stationary, whereas pseudohyphae show some kind of mobility.

Several fungal forms can be observed in wet mount preparations; most of them show characteristic shape and size which define the morphotype (Figure 96).

It must be pointed out that a definitive diagnosis of fungal species rests upon isolating microorganisms on appropriate culture media; nevertheless, the detection of their morphotype may provide the key features for a presumptive diagnosis and thus for a prompt antimycotical therapy.

Candida species usually produces both blastospores and hyphae.

Torulopsis glabrata is also known as Candida glabrata or C. nana because it does not produce hyphae (glabrata=hairless) and has small sized fungal cells (nana=dwarf).

Saccharomyces is usually saprophytic in vagina. *Saccharomyces cerevisiae* (also known as "baker's yeast" or "brewer's yeast") is mostly considered to be an occasional digestive commensal. Saccharomyces can be morphologically distinguished from C. albicans because it does not develop hyphae and its characteristic blastospores appear larger, slightly dysmorphic and with a blurred outline. Furthermore, the scar at the point of detachment on the parent yeast cell is often evident.

Candidal vulvovaginitis is an estrogen-dependent disease and this explains its variable occurrence observed in different ages of life.

The pathogenetic mechanism of Candida epithelial invasion is necessary for the comprehension of such hormone-dependence. Blastospores cause the asymptomatic colonization and contagion, but are not able to penetrate into the vaginal epithelium and develop colpitis, as opposed to hyphae, which are responsible for the symptomatic infection. This process includes a three-stage pathogenetic mechanism (Figure 97):

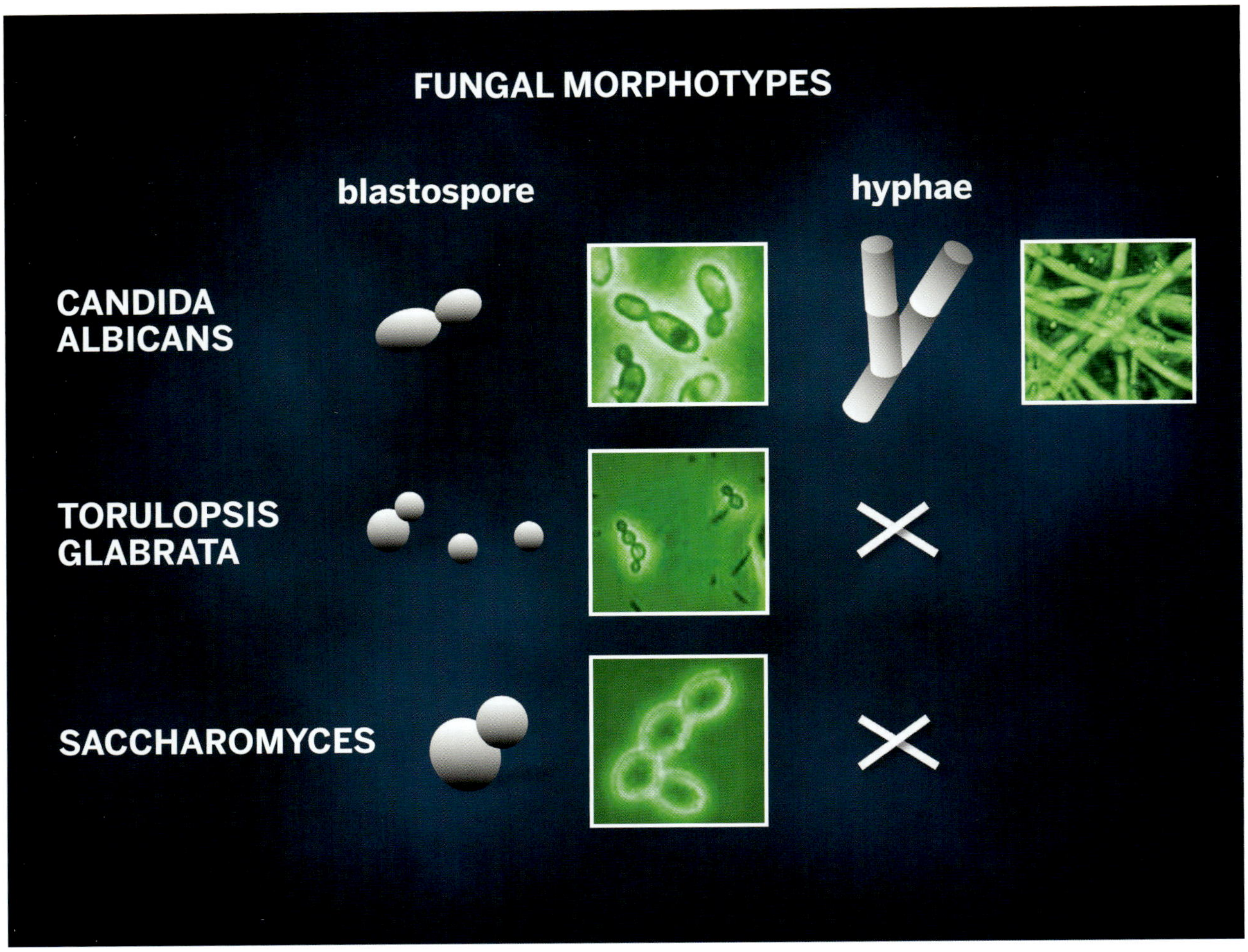

Figure 96 - Candida morphotypes.

- blastospore adhesion to the vaginal cells
- spore germination with hyphae development
- epithelial cell penetration and tissue invasion.

Estrogen impregnation in vaginal epithelium promotes blastospore adhesion and hyphae development by Candida species. This may explain the uncommon prevalence of CVV during hypoestrogenic periods such as childhood and postmenopause; on the other hand, an enhanced estrogen stimulation during pregnancy justifies a higher symptomatic infection rate.
In a cross-selectional study (Eckert et al. 1998) of 774 randomly selected women, a clinical algorithm based on symptoms, signs and selective use of wet mounts and cultures provided prompt treatment to 150 of 167 (90%) women with vulvovaginal candidiasis while minimizing the number of cultures performed.
More and more frequently, despite causing symptoms consistent with candidal vaginitis, fungal yeast cells and hyphae are not visible under direct microscopic observation and cultures may yield false negative results. Too often, vaginal specimens are inappropriately submitted for bacterial cultures that inevitably reveal bacteria which play no role in the pathogenesis of vaginitis.
This diagnostic failure depends on Candida penetration into vaginal cells by means of several proteases produced by hyphae. Hyphae may be observed while penetrating epithelium and show a characteristic diaphanous aspect when they are in the intracellular space (Figure 98). Electron microscopy studies have clearly demonstrated intracellular penetration. The electron microscopical evidence has a wet mount microscopic corresponding feature.
In 1994 the Author described a pathognomonic cell change induced by Candida during its penetration through the vaginal epithelium, defined as *Candida cytopathy* or *epithelial candidiasis*.

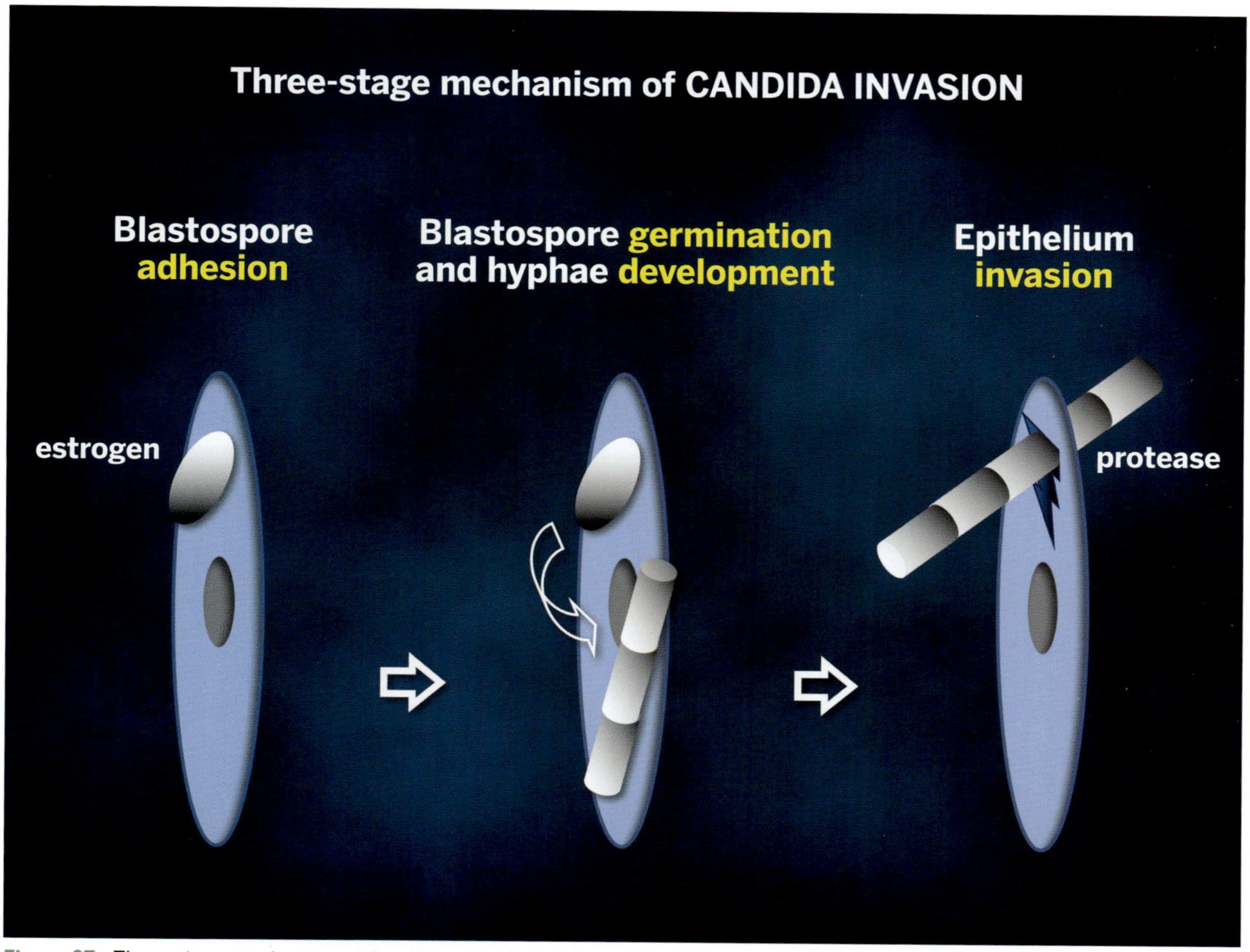

Figure 97 - Three-stage mechanism of Candida epithelial invasion.

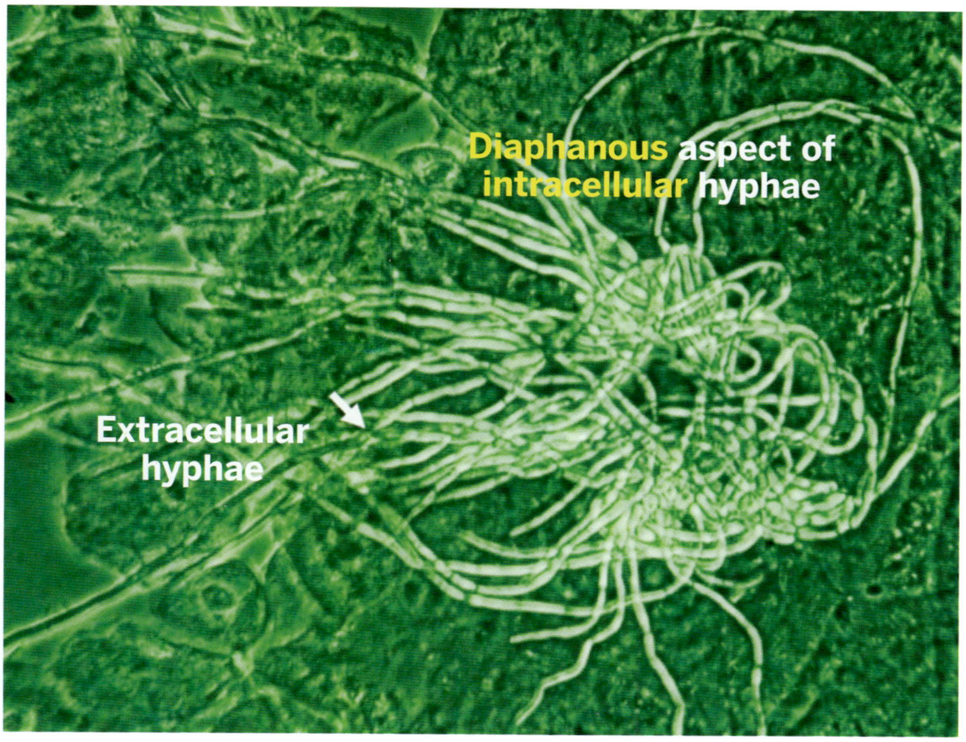

Figure 98 - Diaphanous aspect of intraepithelial hyphae. The arrow indicates the site of penetration.

This cytopathic effect can be clearly observed in different forms:

- cytoplasmic *groove*
- cytoplasmic *marginal erosion*
- cytoplasmic *hole*
- cytoplasmic *tunnel.*

When the hypha passes in parallel between two contiguous cells, it leaves a cytoplasmic groove (Figure 99). A marginal cytoplasmic erosion is formed when the hypha licks the cell surface (Figure 100). If the hypha perforates only one face of the cell, it forms a cytoplasmic hole (Figure 101). Last, when the hypha transfixes right through the cell, the cytopathic effect is represented by a cytoplasmic tunnel (Figure 102). In all its forms, Candida cytopathy is characterized by a sharply condensed border.

In presence of candidiasis, when vaginal cultures give false negative results and hyphae are not observable in vaginal smear because they are hidden inside the epithelium, the detection of Candida cytopathy by direct microscopy is the *only* diagnostic tool that provides a correct diagnosis of fungal infection. The observation of the Candida cytopathy confirmed to be a precious diagnostic tool to provide a prompt and specific treatment, above all in absence of confirmatory cultures and in recurrent episodes.

Candida cytopathy is often associated with dyskaryotic changes. In most cases, these cell changes induced by Candida infection completely regress after an appropriate therapy targeting the yeast infection. For this reason, the detection of the specific Candida cytopathy is extremely important when blastospores and pseudohyphae are not visible, in order to defer or avoid unnecessary excisional procedures on the cervix.

The detection of Candida cytopathy is essential to diagnose hidden fungal infections in several districts different from vagina, like in the lower urinary tract (Figures 16, 17), on the skin (Figure 18), in the oral cavity (Figure 19) and in the rectum (Figure 20).

Candidiasis symptoms include itching and burning of the vagina and labia, painful intercourse and burning on urination.

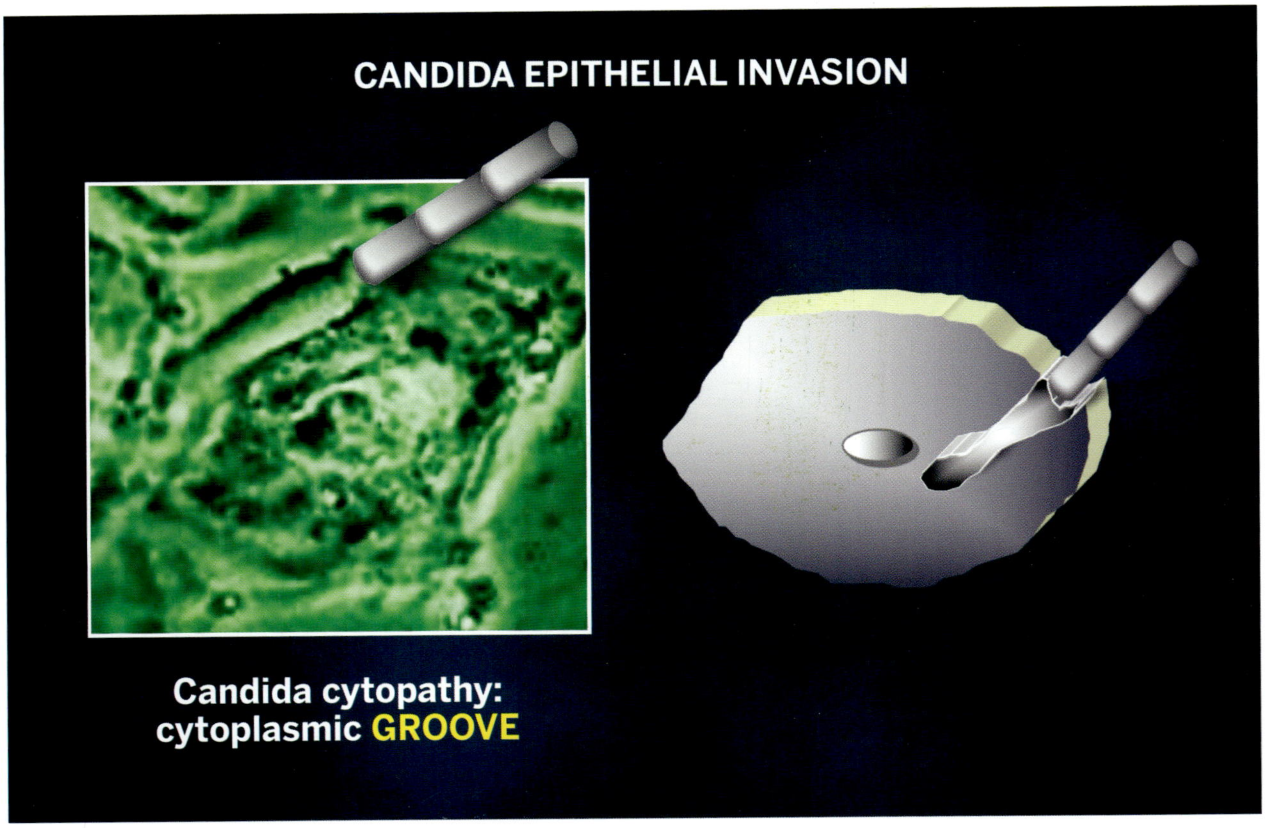

Figure 99 - Candida cytopathy: cytoplasmic groove.

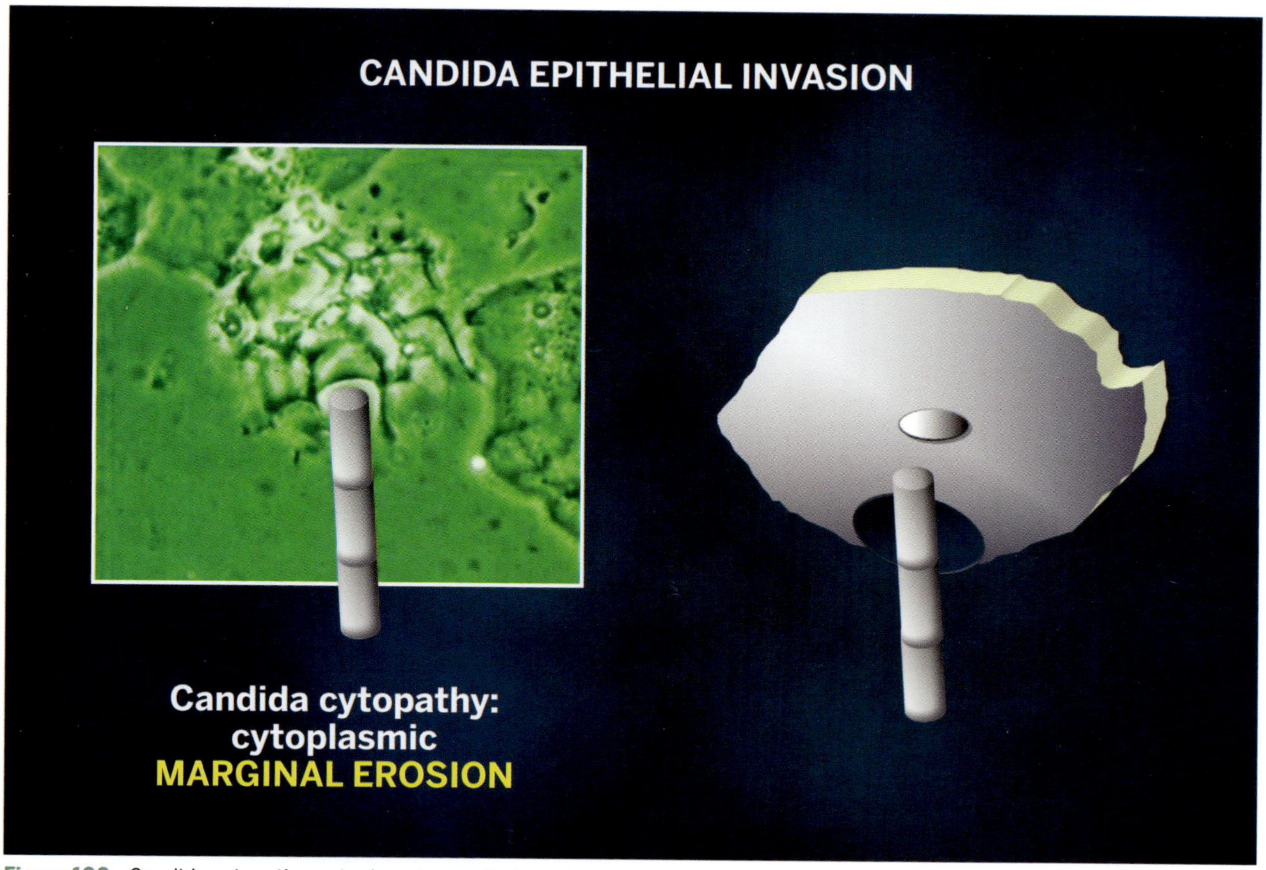

Figure 100 - Candida cytopathy: cytoplasmic marginal erosion.

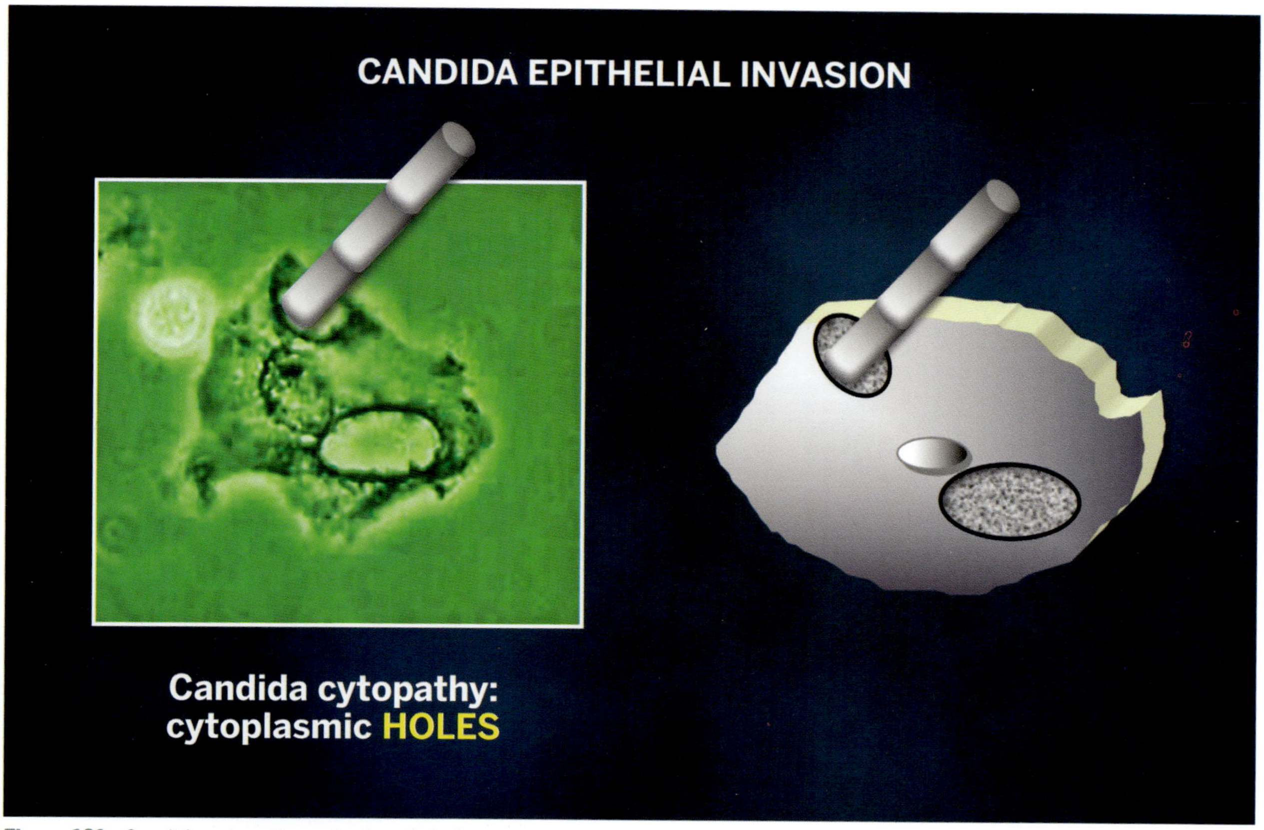

Figure 101 - Candida cytopathy: cytoplasmic holes.

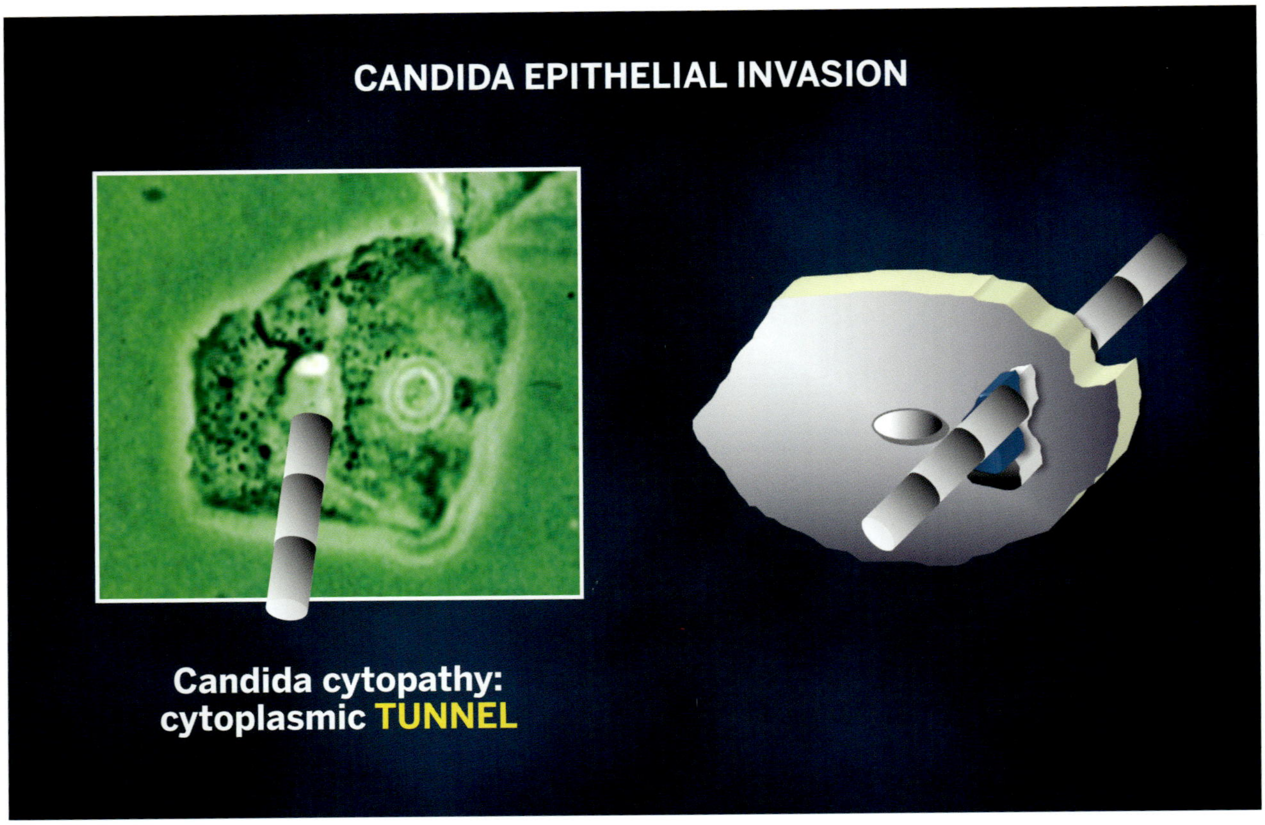

Figure 102 - Candida cytopathy: cytoplasmic tunnel.

Yeast infection in the vagina and on the cervix may cause different objective signs and colposcopic features:

- discharge can range from slightly watery, white discharge to thick, white, lumpy discharge that looks like cottage cheese (Figure 103)
- redness of cervix and vagina
- diffuse erithematous macules (Figure 104), usually larger than subepithelial punctate petechiae that characterize strawberry appearance in trichomoniasis
- cervical and vaginal centrally depressed erithematous papules (Figure 105)
- white punctation (Figure 106), distinguishable from the same colposcopic finding induced by Human Papillomavirus infection or the one observed in metaplasia as fungal white punctation is often seen associated with centrally depressed erithematous papules (white dots colpitis).

All these colposcopic features disappear after an appropriate treatment for candidiasis.

The signs of vulvar inflammation include:

- erythema (redness) (Figure 107)
- edema due to swelling from fluid build-up (Figure 108)
- fissuring (cracked skin) (Figure 109) which may involve the perianal area (Figure 110).

Sometimes the evaluator may find some fungal forms such as Alternaria and arthroconidia, usually having no pathogenetic role but representing only a contamination of the wet mount (Figure 111).

Alternaria

Alternaria has a worldwide distribution, with many species being common saprophytes in soil, air and a variety of other habitats. However, it can also cause several different types of human infections, such as bronchial asthma, hypersensitivity pneumonitis, allergic paranasal sinusitis and rhinitis, ocular infections, onychomycosis, cutaneous and subcutaneous infections.

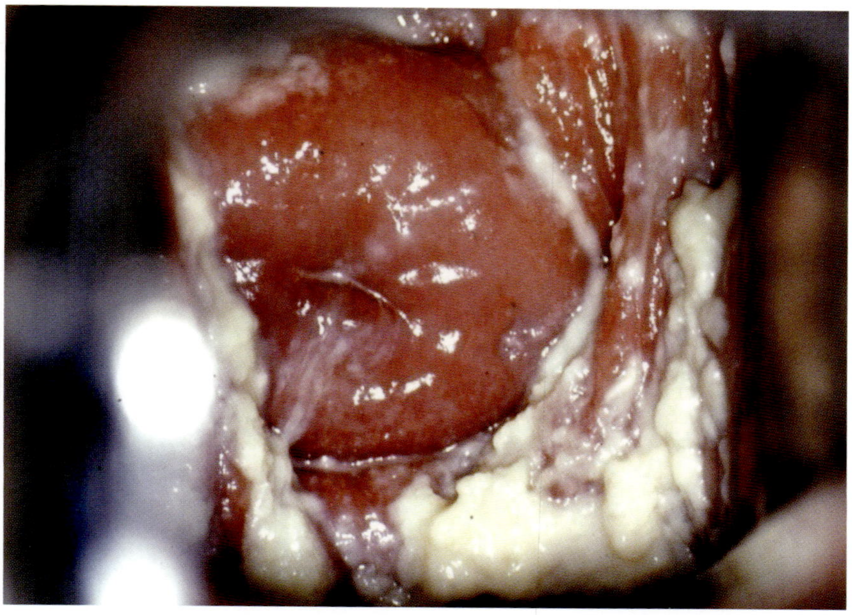

Figure 103 - White and clumpy discharge in candidiasis.

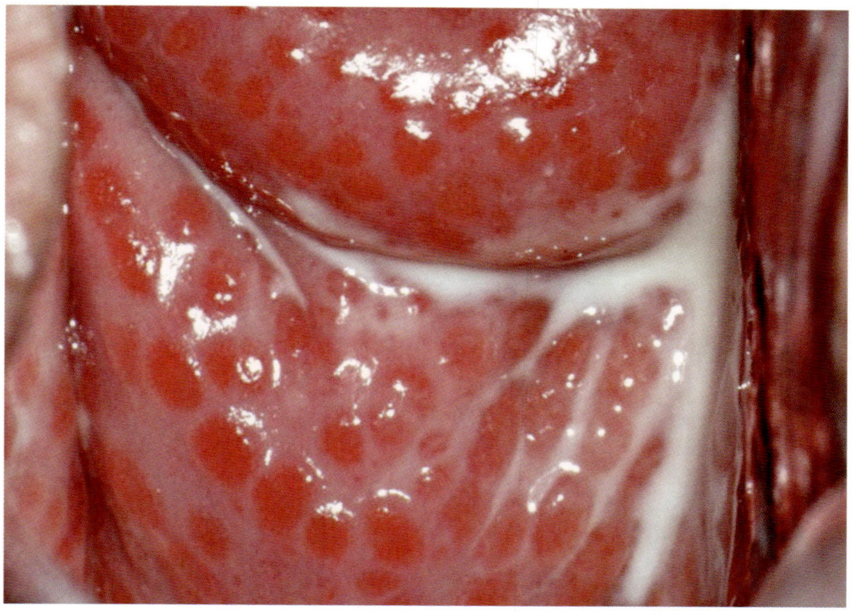

Figure 104 - Fungal macular vaginitis.

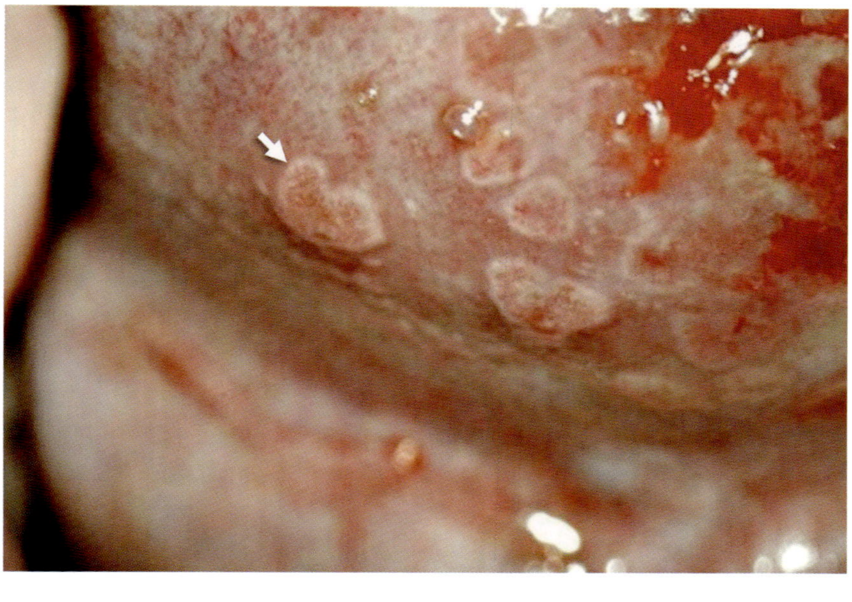

Figure 105 - Fungal erithematous papules, centrally depressed.

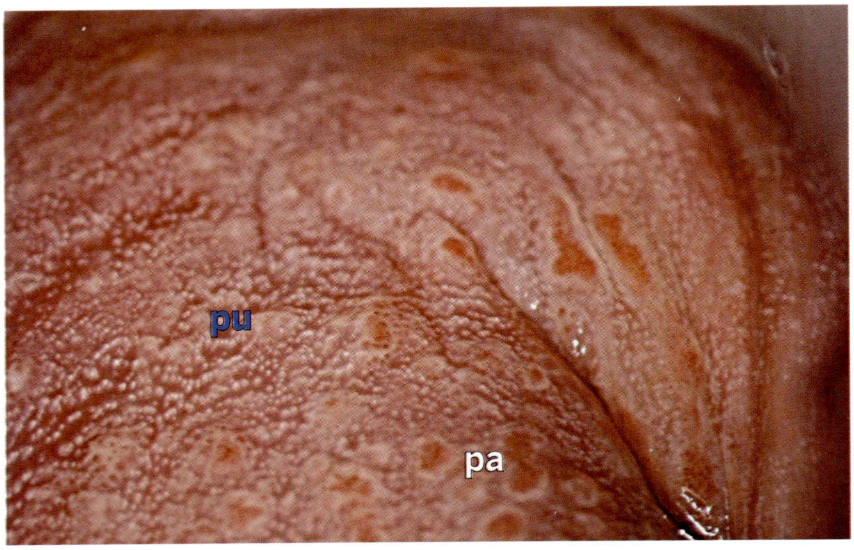

Figure 106 - Fungal white punctation (pu) associated with erithematous papules (pa) (white dots colpitis).

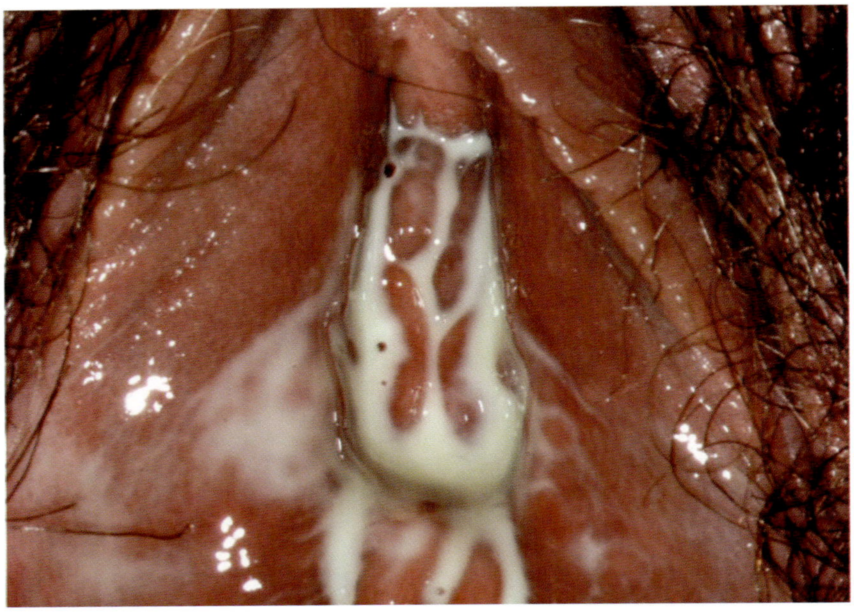

Figure 107 - Vulvar erythema and milky discharge in candidiasis.

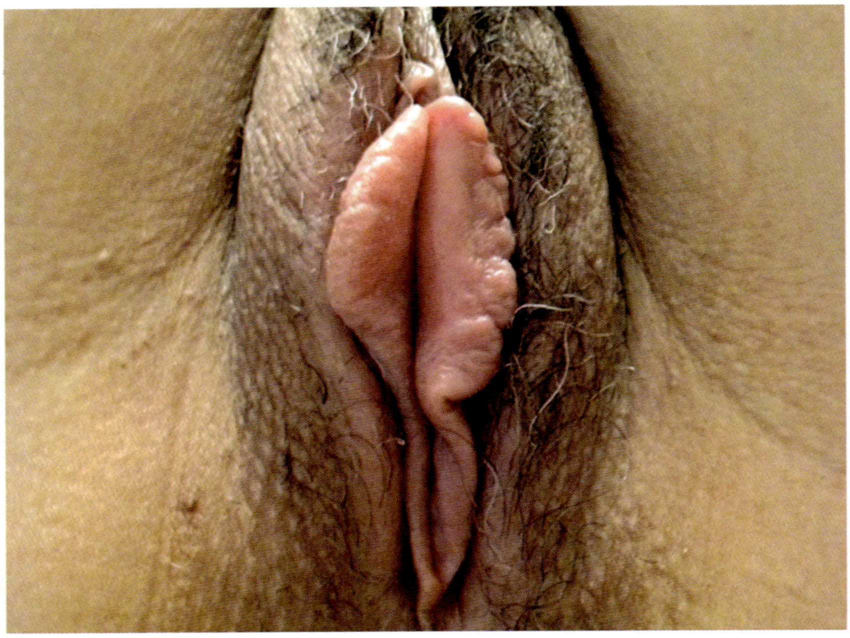

Figure 108 - Vulvar edema in candidiasis.

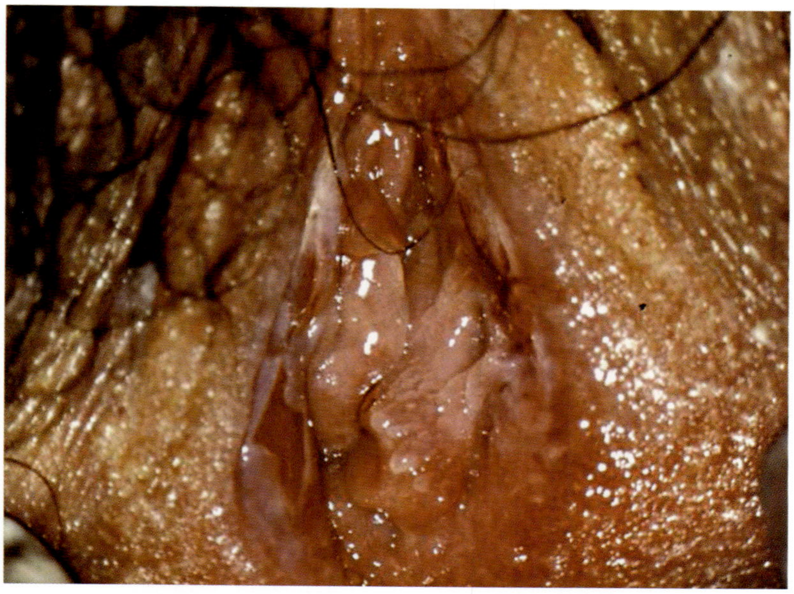

Figure 109 - Vestibular fissuring in candidiasis.

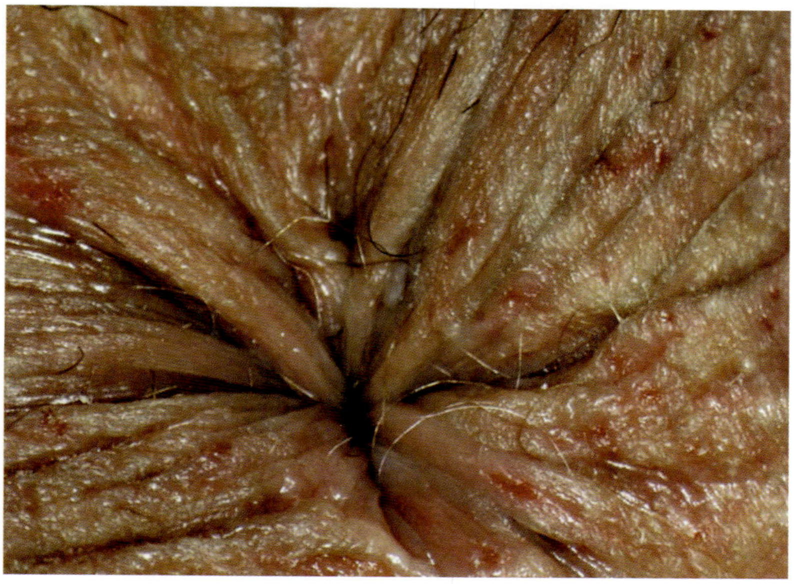

Figure 110 - Perianal fissuring in candidiasis.

Occasionally, *Alternaria* has been reported as a contaminant of soft contact lenses.

Microscopically multicelled, obclavate to obpyriform conidia with short conical beaks can be observed. Blastoconidia of Alternaria may be observed solitary or much more often in branching acropetal chains (Figure 112).

Alternaria is not a vaginal pathogen and its presence in a wet mount is always a sign of contamination.

Dermatophytosis

Dermatophytosis (tinea or ringworm) of the scalp, glabrous skin, and nails is caused by a closely related group of fungi known as dermatophytes having the ability to utilise keratin as a nutrient source, i.e. they have a unique enzymatic capacity (keratinase). Dermatophytes can survive solely on outer cornified layers of the skin.

Natural infection is acquired by the deposition of viable arthroconidia (arthrospores) (Figure 111) or hyphae on the surface of the susceptible individual. After the inoculation in the host skin, suitable conditions favour the infection to progress through the stages of adherence and penetration. Under certain predisposing conditions, dermatophytes produce arthroconidia.

Arthroconidium formation, characteristic of der-

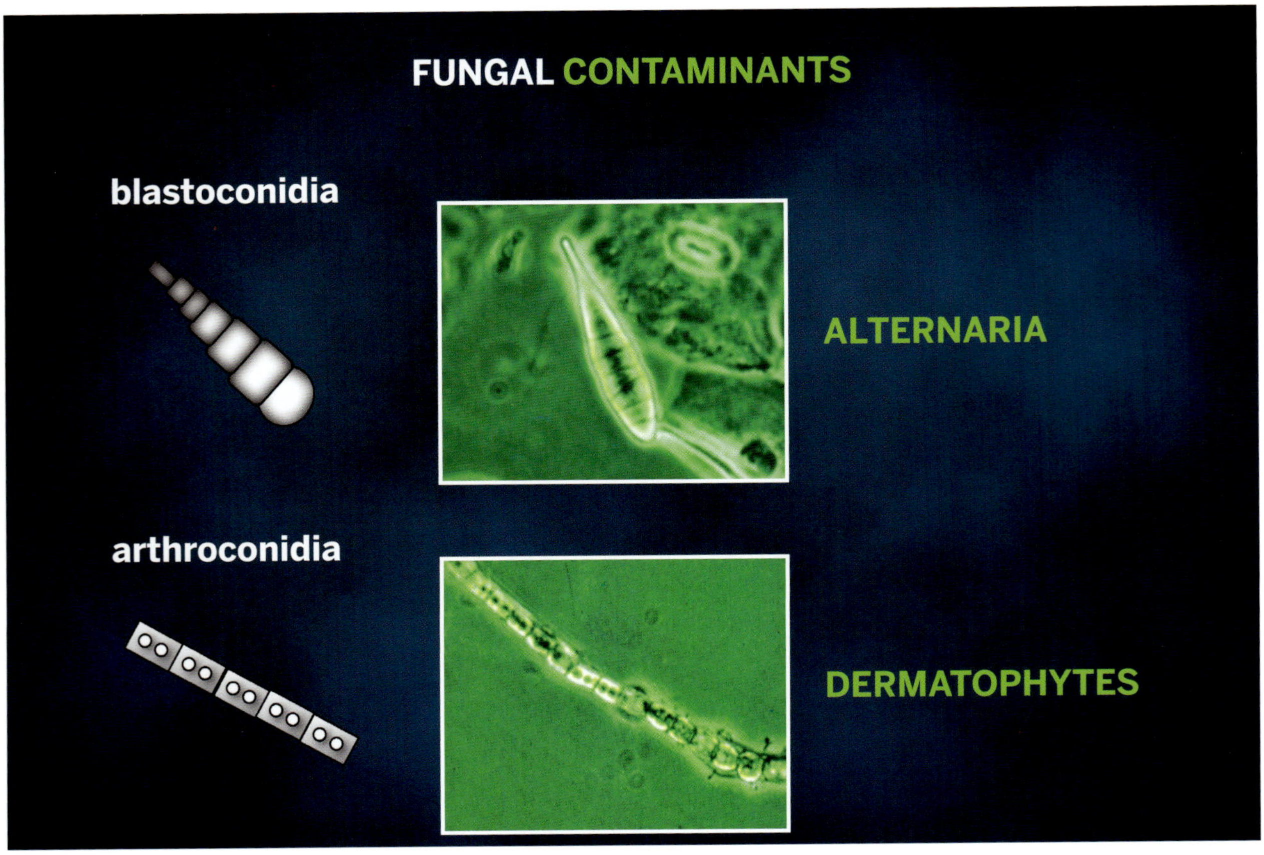

Figure 111 - Fungal contaminants.

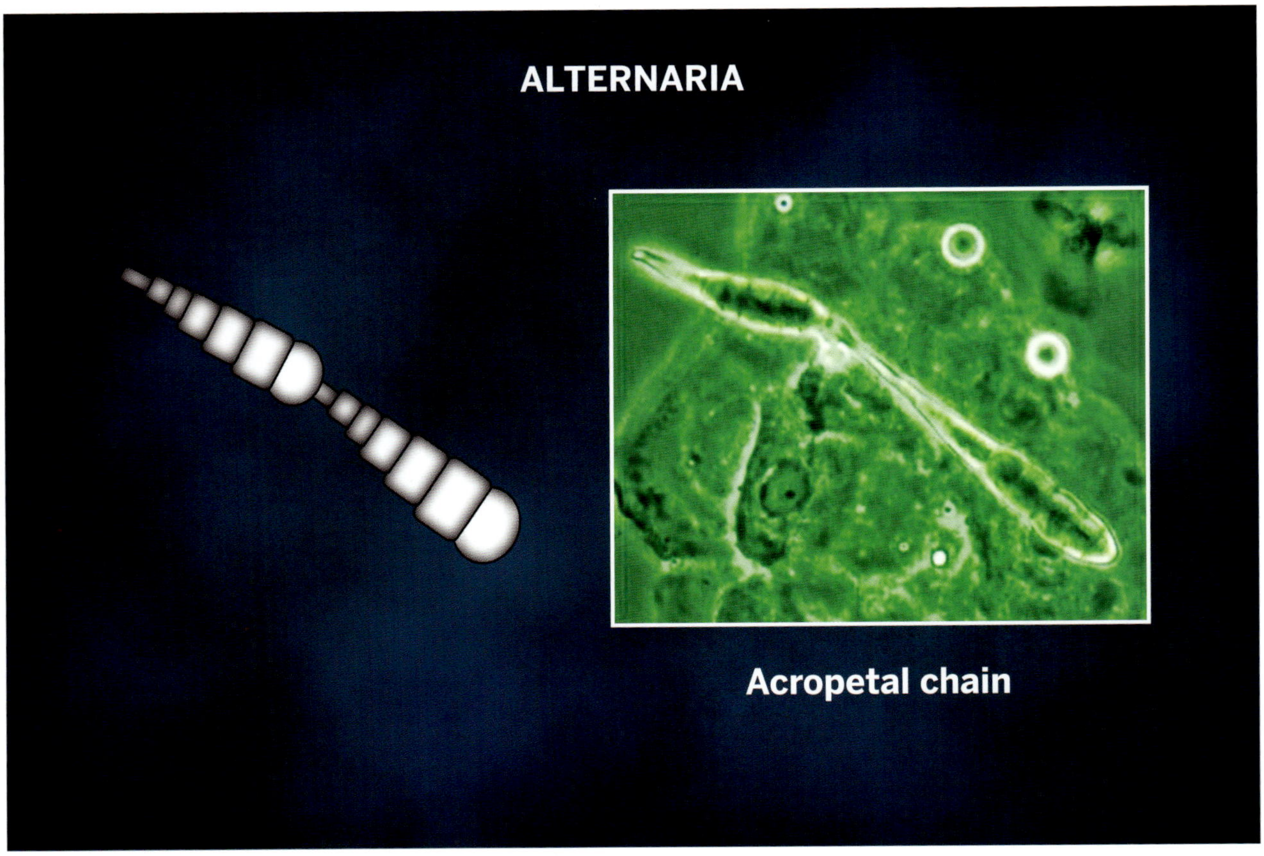

Figure 112 - Acropetal chain of Alternaria.

matophyte infection of skin, hair or nails, results from the fragmentation of a hypha following multiple septum formation. Growth in the stratum corneum of skin, nails and hair occurs in the form of hyphae, which may then form arthroconidia. It has been suggested that arthroconidia are more commonly found in wet skin lesions and nails. Arthroconidia are seen, for example, within nail-bed infections caused by Trichophyton rubrum, within nail-plate infections caused by Trichophyton mentagrophytes interdigitale, and in infections of scalp hair.
Microscopy shows typical single-celled, rectangular to barrel-shaped alternate arthroconidia, separated from each other by a disjunctor cell.
Arthroconidium presence in the vagina often depends on contamination from nail infections or vulvar wet skin infections.

Actinomycetes

Actinomycetes are a specific group of bacteria, acting as fungi, but being actual bacteria. They are discussed in this session as morphologically they resemble fungi because of their elongated cells that branch into filaments or hyphae. We prefer the term filaments to avoid confusion with fungal hyphae.
Wet mounts can show both thick and thin filaments (Figure 113) that tend to form palisades and V-shaped pairs. Thick filaments (Figure 114) may appear zebrine or homogeneous and must not be confused with fungal hyphae which show a characteristic bamboo cane aspect (Figure 115).
Thick zebrine filaments in some species may undergo fragmentation, form a beaded filament (Figure 116) and finally give rise to coccoid-shaped forms (coccoid fragments) (Figure 117). Coccoid fragments can arise diagnostic doubts because they look similar to budding blastospores of Torulopsis glabrata. For a differential diagnosis (Figure 118), it is useful to point out that coccoid fragments exhibit the same size because they are generated by fragmentation, whereas the small blastospores of Torulopsis glabrata have progressively smaller sizes during budding.
Thick homogeneous filaments in some species assume a wave shape (Figure 119) before undergoing snapping fission to generate rod-shaped bacteria called diphteroid fragments. Such fragments are commonly referred to as "diphtheroids", due to their

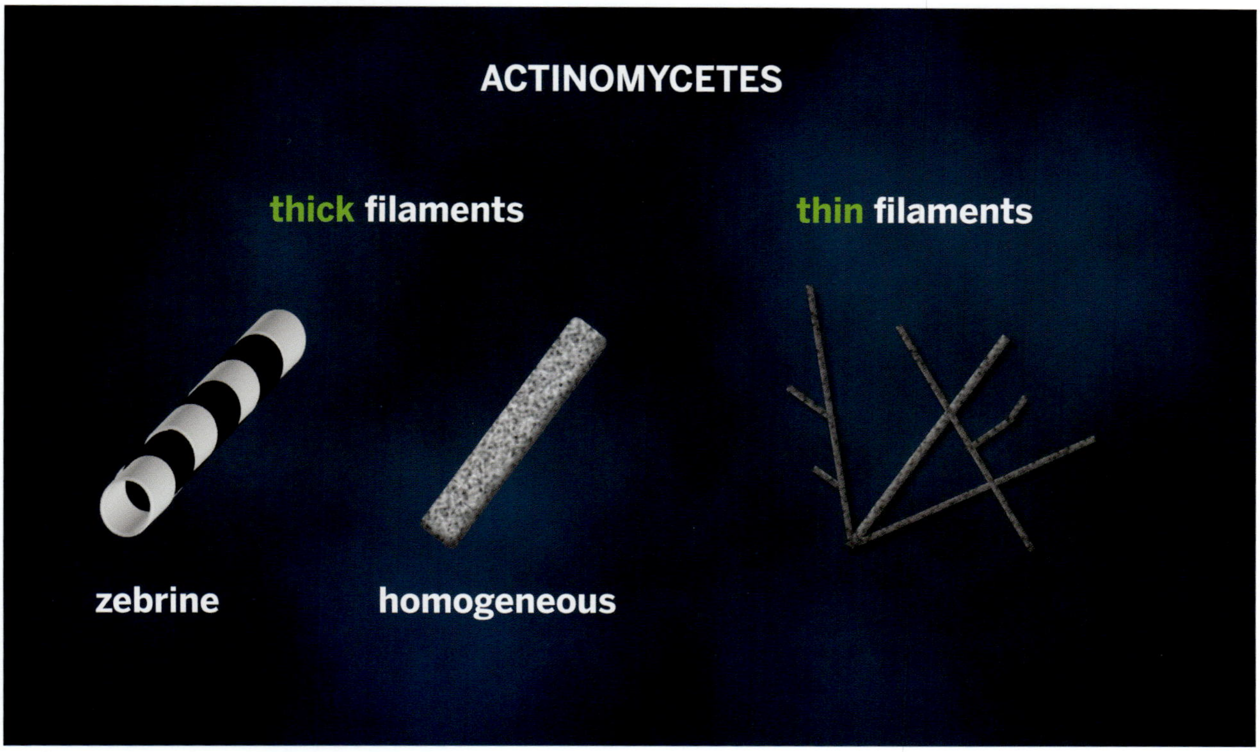

Figure 113 - Different filaments of Actinomycetes.

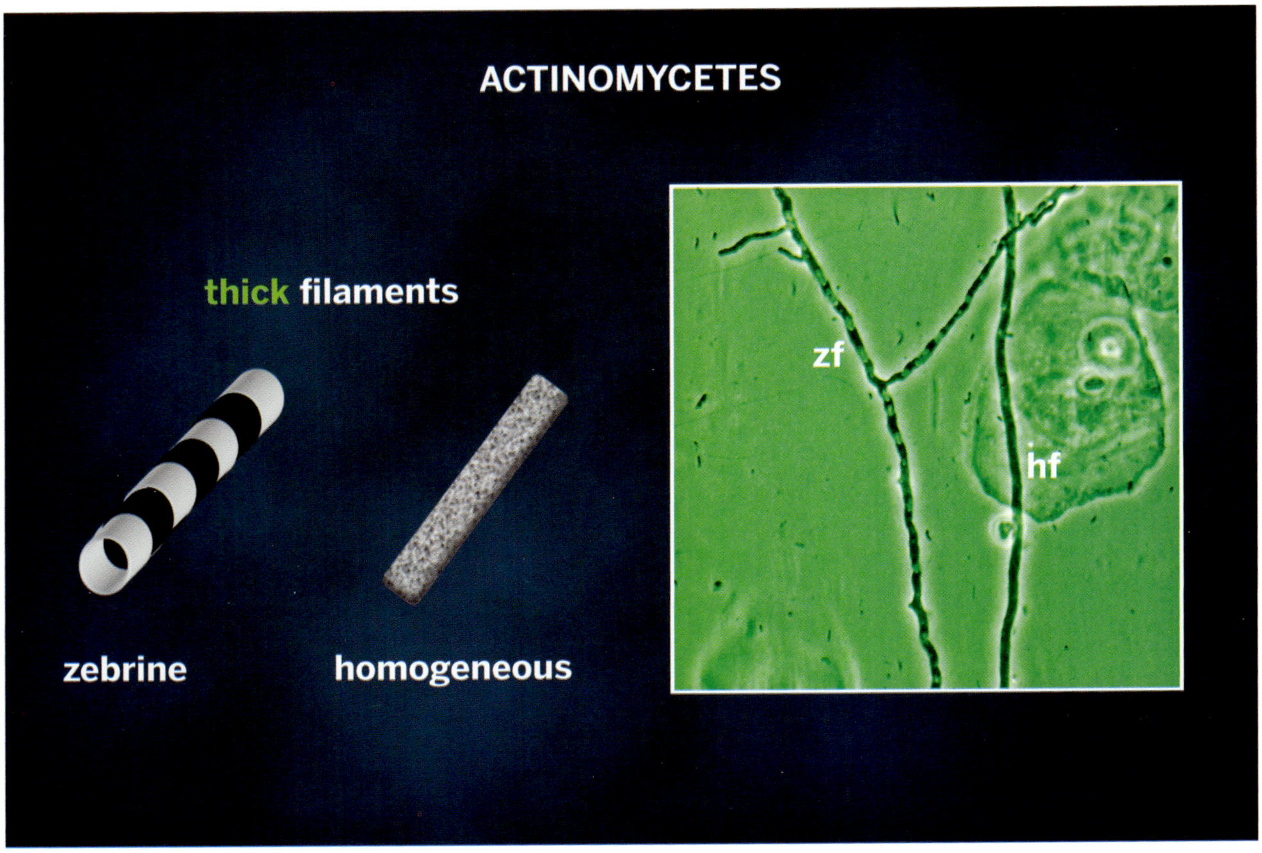

Figure 114 - Thick filaments of Actinomycetes.

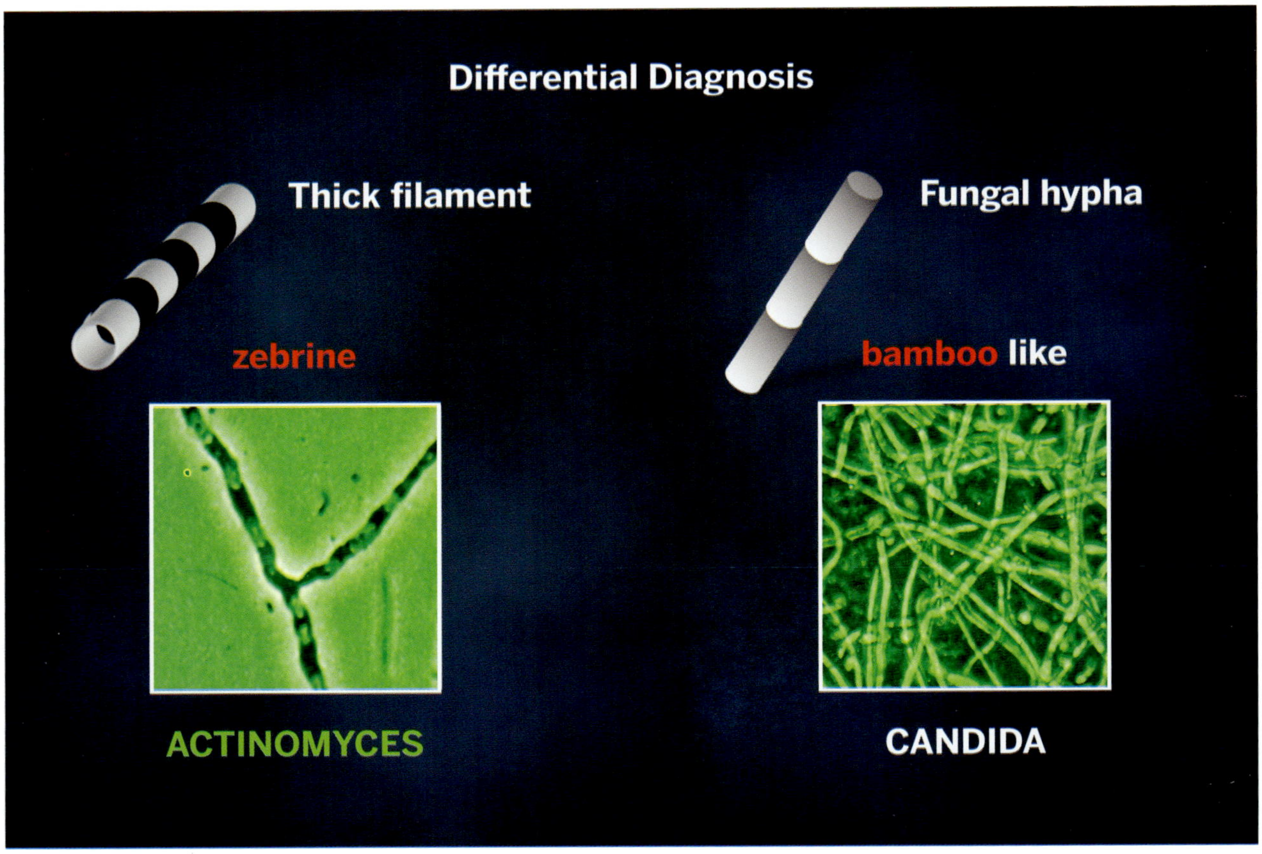

Figure 115 - Differential diagnosis between zebrine thick filaments of Actinomycetes and Candida hyphae.

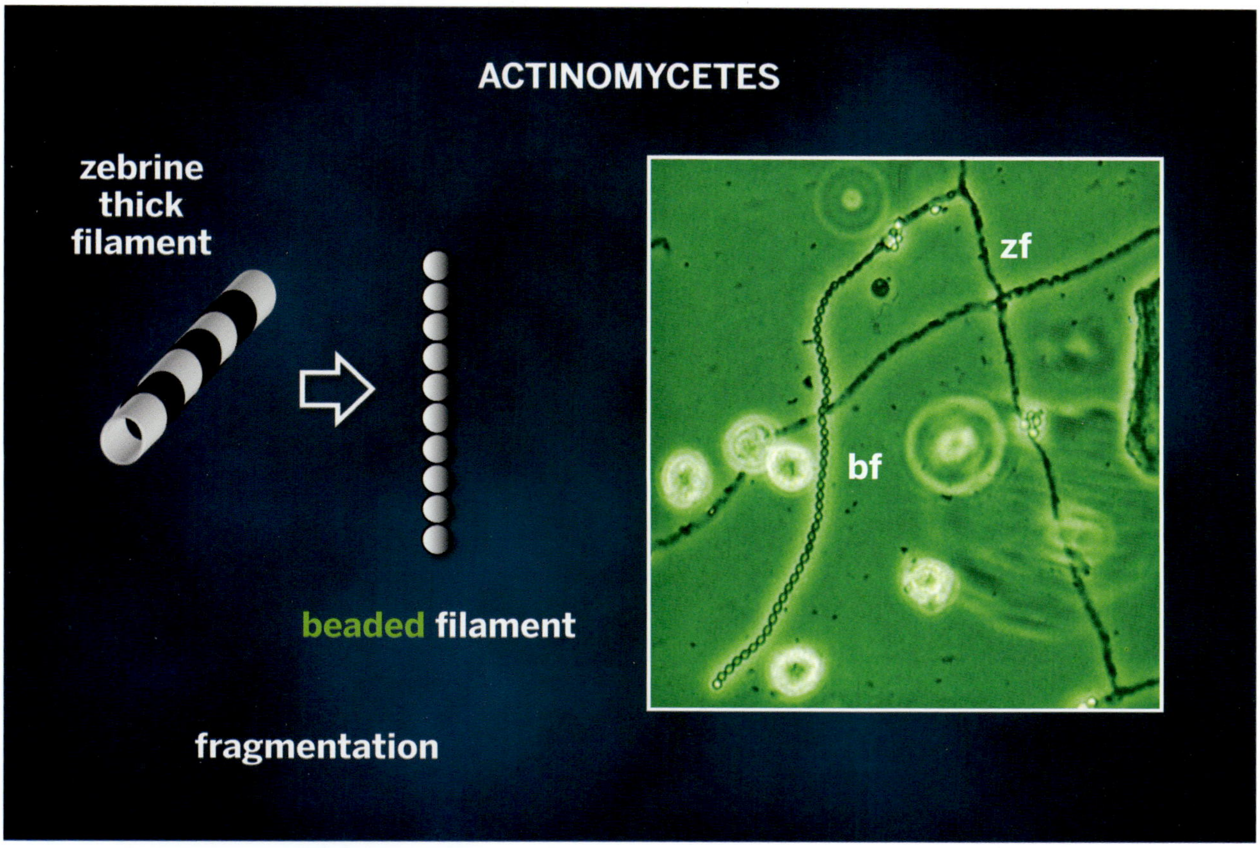

Figure 116 - Formation of beaded filaments of Actinomycetes.

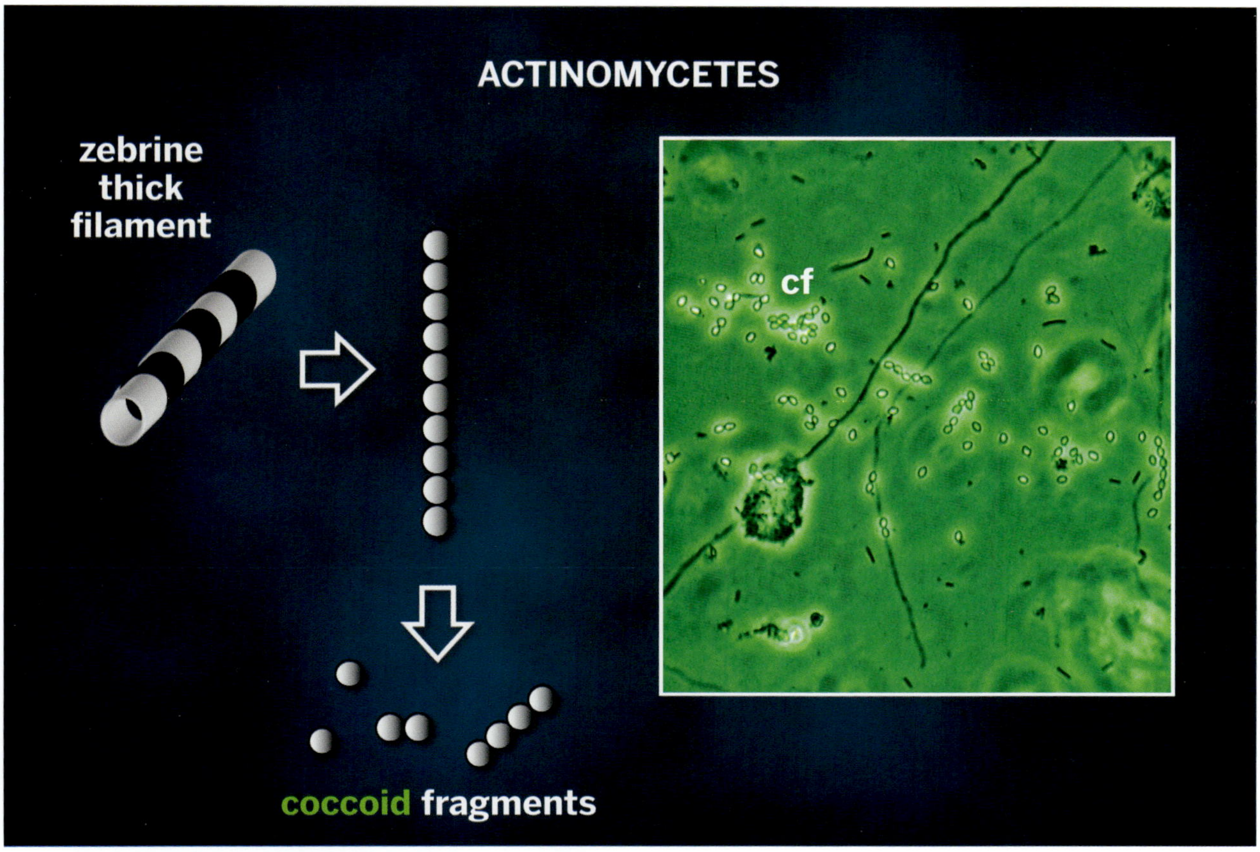

Figure 117 - Formation of coccoid fragments of Actinomycetes.

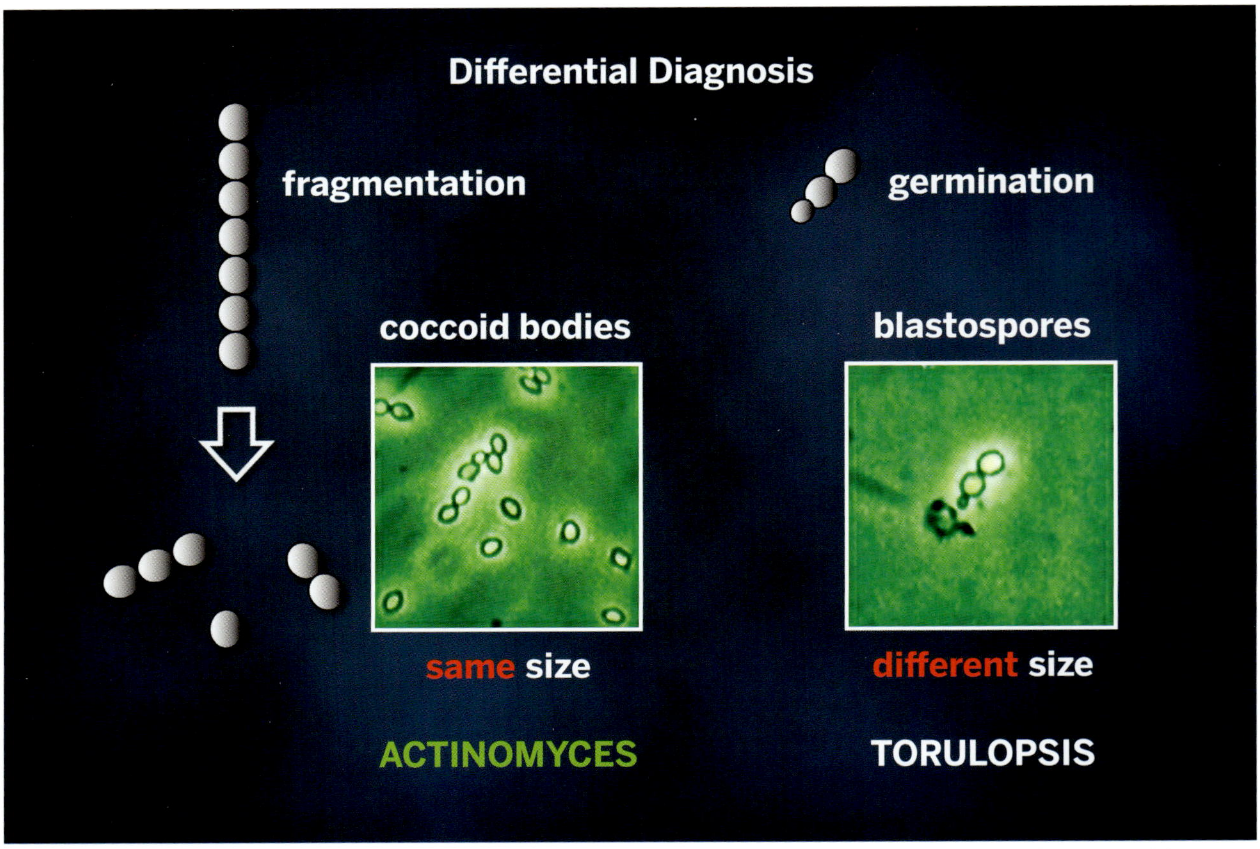

Figure 118 - Differential diagnosis between coccoid fragments of Actinomycetes and budding blastospores of Torulopsis glabrata.

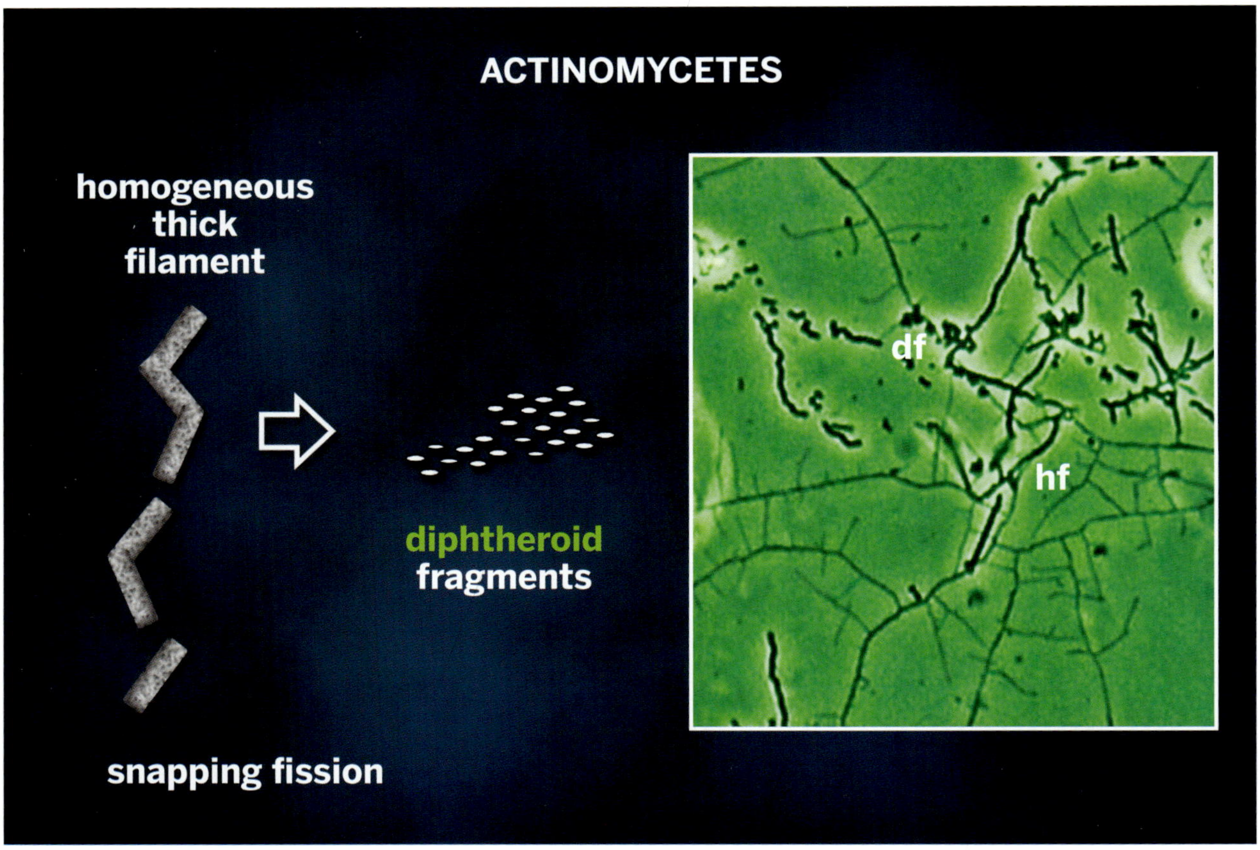

Figure 119 - Formation of diphteroid fragments of Actinomycetes.

morphological resemblance to Corynebacterium diphtheriae, the agent of diphtheria. Diphteroid fragments may be confused with pleomorphic (diphtheroid) bacteria in Bacterial vaginosis. For a diagnostic support, it is useful to consider that diphteroid fragments are always found close to Actinomycetes (Figure 120). Thick filaments generate thin and brighter filaments (Figure 121). Finally, Actinomycetes can develop arthrospore-like aerial units; their presence close to filaments facilitates the diagnosis (Figure 122).

Some actinomycetes are found to be responsible for allergic symptoms in the respiratory tract. Pelvic actinomycotic disease occurs infrequently in women and is indistinguishable from other forms of pelvic inflammatory disease.

Evidence suggests that there is a cause-effect relationship between IUD use and pelvic actinomycosis. Actinomyces israelii, a branching bacterium, infects 1.6-11.6% of IUD users worldwide. It appears that A. israelii infection is more common in women with plastic IUDs than in those with copper IUDs and in women who have had an IUD for more than 4 years. In patients with an intrauterine device, actinomycetes should be considered in differential diagnosis of pelvic infections. As culture techniques tend to be inadequate, many health professionals use a microscope to identify A. israelii and often confirm the microscopy findings with direct immunofluorescent techniques. Preoperative diagnosis is of the utmost importance in order to prevent morbidity of this infiltrative infection.

Nocardia is a genus (family Actinomycetes) that includes fungus-like bacteria. *Nocardia* species are found worldwide in soil rich in dead decaying organic matter, water, dust and on vegetation. In addition, this Actinomyces can be part of the oral microflora in healthy gingiva and periodontal pockets. The presence of Nocardia in vagina is assumed to be the consequence of contamination from the oral cavity of the male sexual partner during cunnilingus. Most *Nocardia* infections are acquired by inhalation of the bacteria or through traumatic introduction. Nocardiosis is a chronic bacterial disease

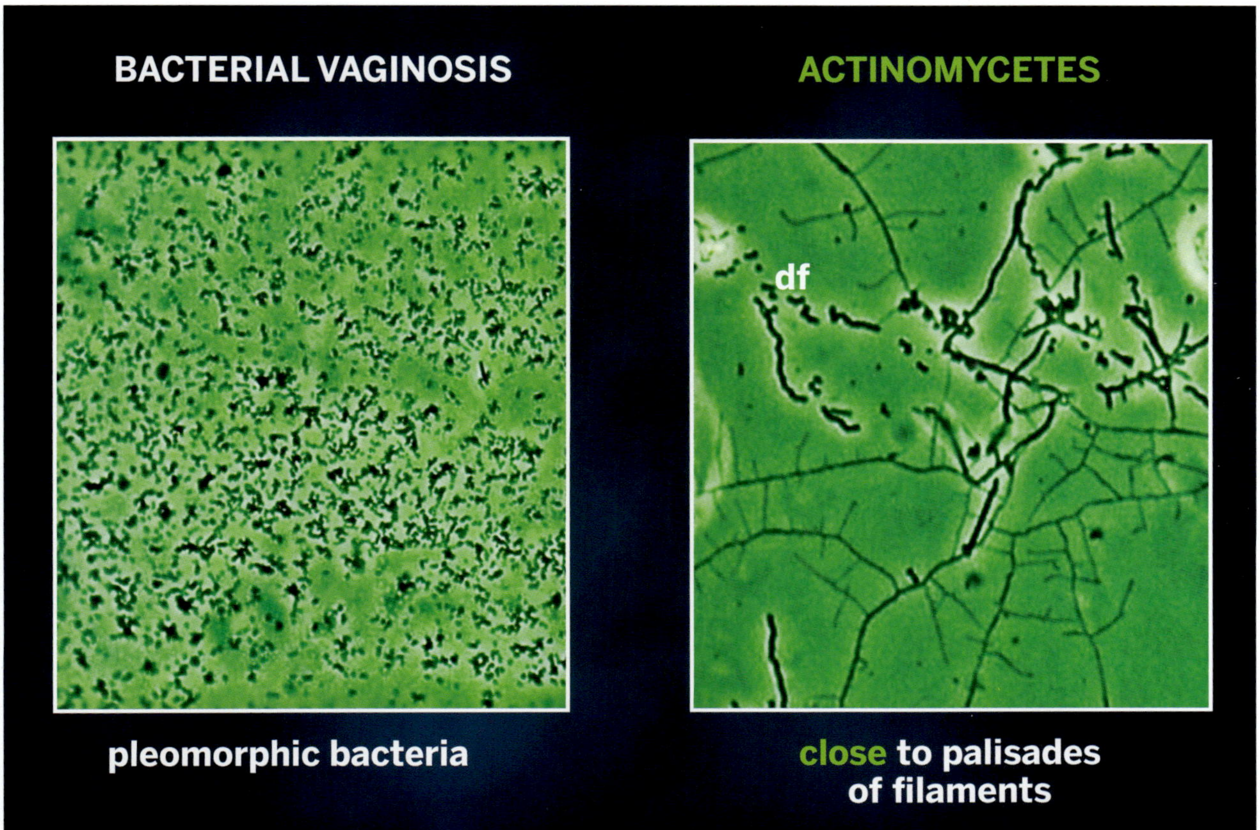

Figure 120 - Differential diagnosis between pleomorphic bacteria of Bacterial vaginosis and diphteroid fragments (df) of Actinomycetes.

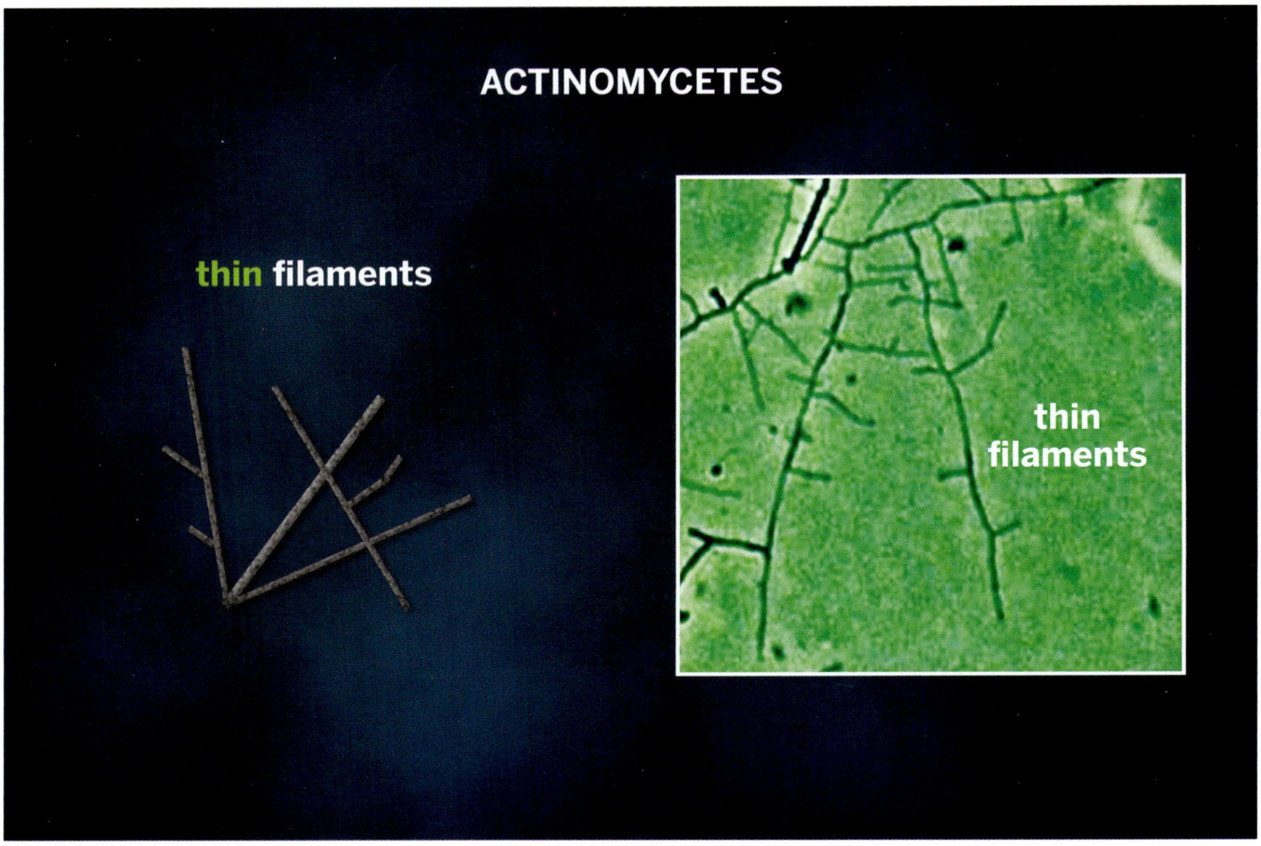

Figure 121 - Thin filaments of Actinomycetes.

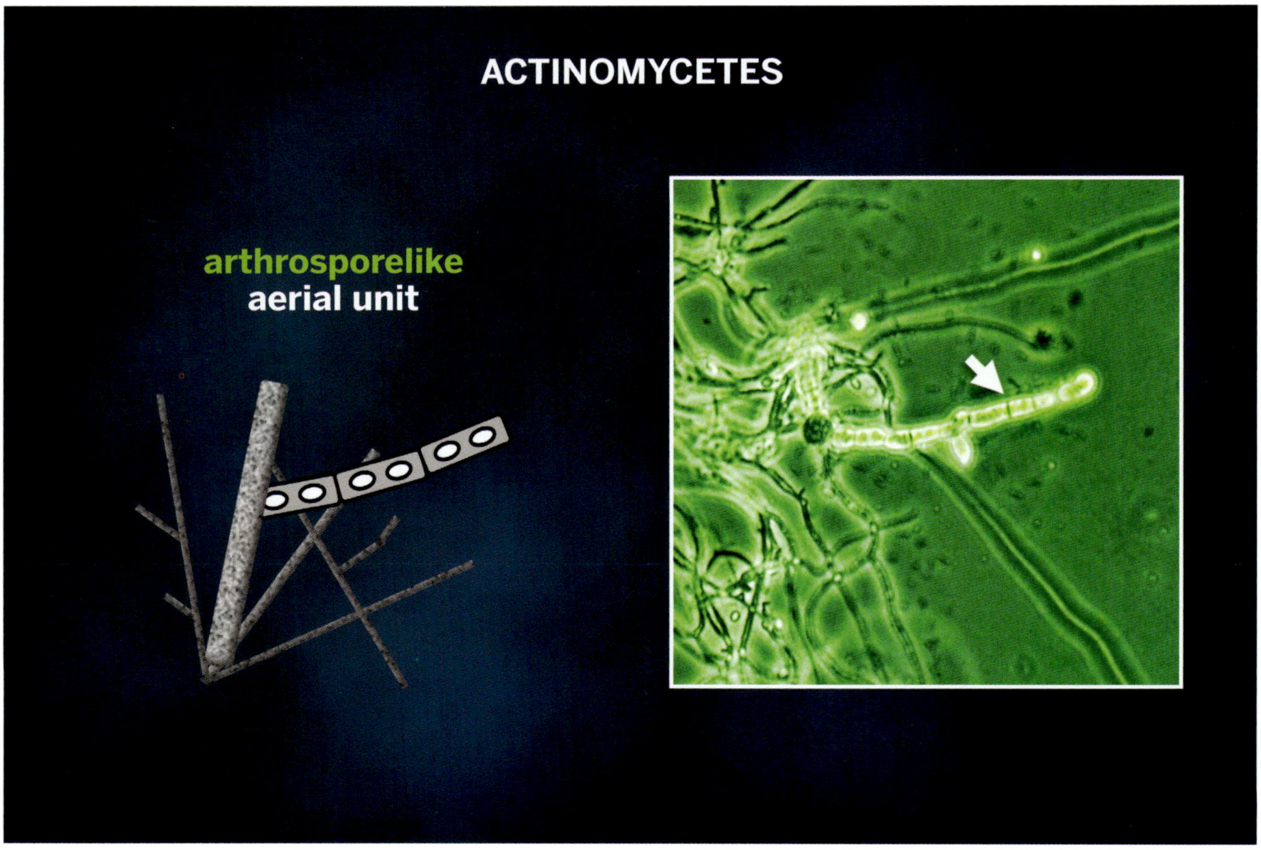

Figure 122 - Arthrospore-like aerial unit (→) of Actinomycetes.

of humans originating in the respiratory tract and disseminated through blood supply to other organs. The majority of infections occur in people with weakened immune systems, such as subjects who have received bone-marrow transplantations and are on immunosuppressive therapy, subjects with HIV/AIDS or with malignancies.

The observation of Actinomycetes in vaginal wet mount generally indicates a contamination of the microscopic glass during storage or processing.

Trichomoniasis

Trichomoniasis ("trich") is the most common non-viral sexually transmitted infection caused by the one-celled protozoan organism *Trichomonas vaginalis* (TV), which is most often spread through vaginal, oral, or anal sex. The WHO has estimated that more than 160 million people worldwide are annually infected.

About 70% of infected women and men do not experience any symptoms. Symptoms can include itching in the genital area, a bad smelling, thin and frothy vaginal discharge, burning on urination, and pain during sexual intercourse. Trichomoniasis increases the risk of getting HIV/AIDS. It may also cause PID and complications during pregnancy.

Trichomonas vaginalis (Figure 123) is a flagellated protozoan possessing five flagella, four of which protrude from its front end (Figure 124). The fifth flagellum extends rearward and is incorporated within the undulating membrane of the parasite supported by a slender noncontractile costa. The parasite propels itself using the four whip-like flagella. The undulating membrane gives T. vaginalis a characteristic quivering motility. The functionality of the fifth flagellum is not known. A barb-like axostyle (Figures 125, 126) projects opposite the four-flagella bundle, as a posterior prolongation of cyto-skeleton. The axostyle supposedly participates in locomotion, attachment to tissue and host cell damage, but also in mitosis during cell division (Figure 127). The direct observation of parasite replication is rare.

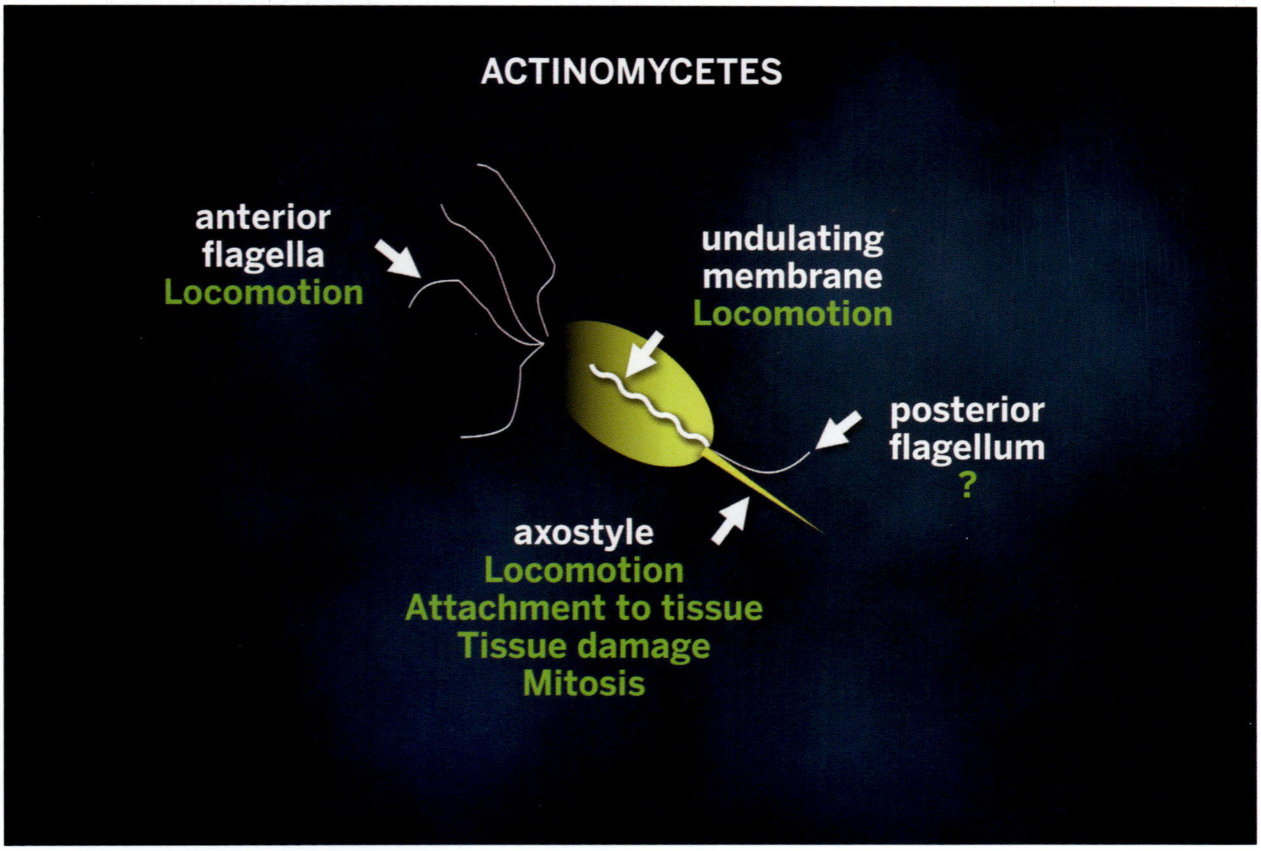

Figure 123 - Diagrammatic representation of Trichomonas vaginalis.

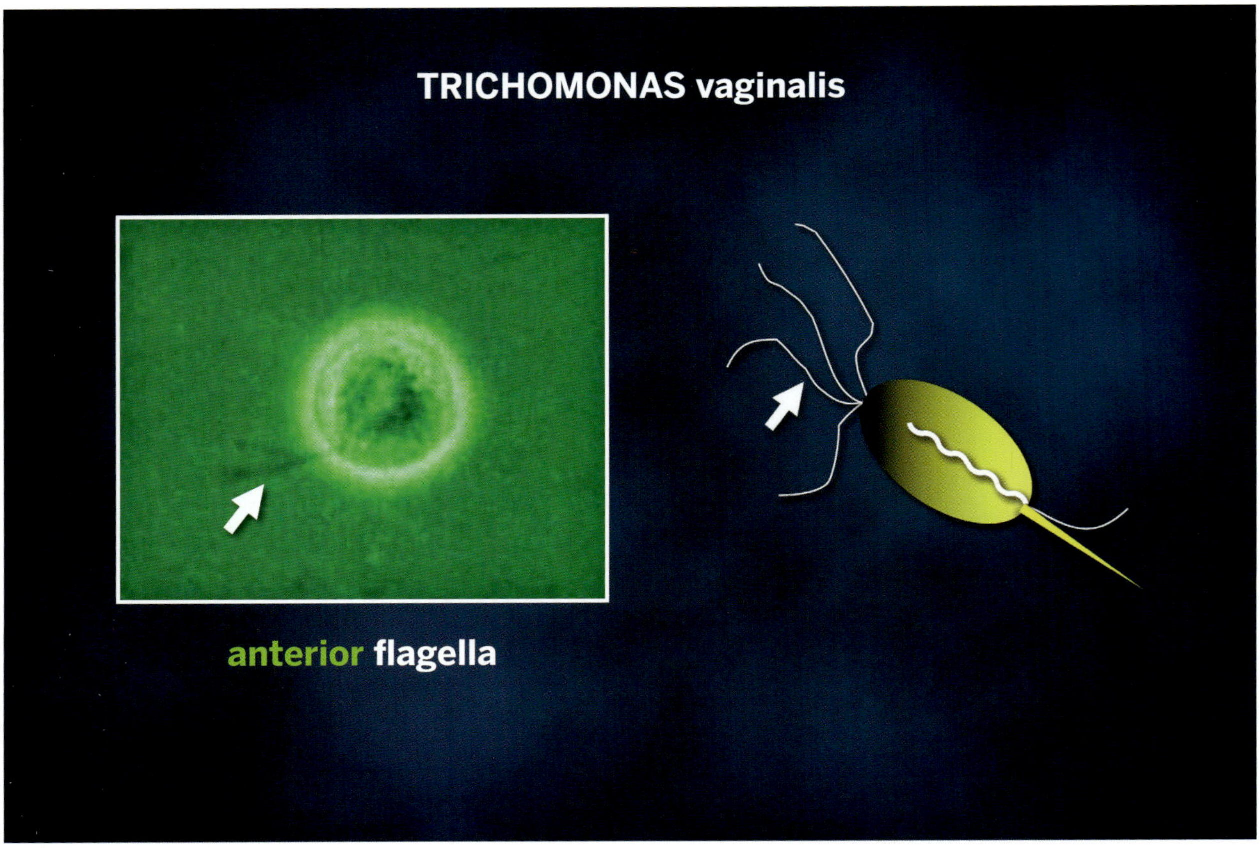

Figure 124 - Anterior flagella of Trichomonas vaginalis.

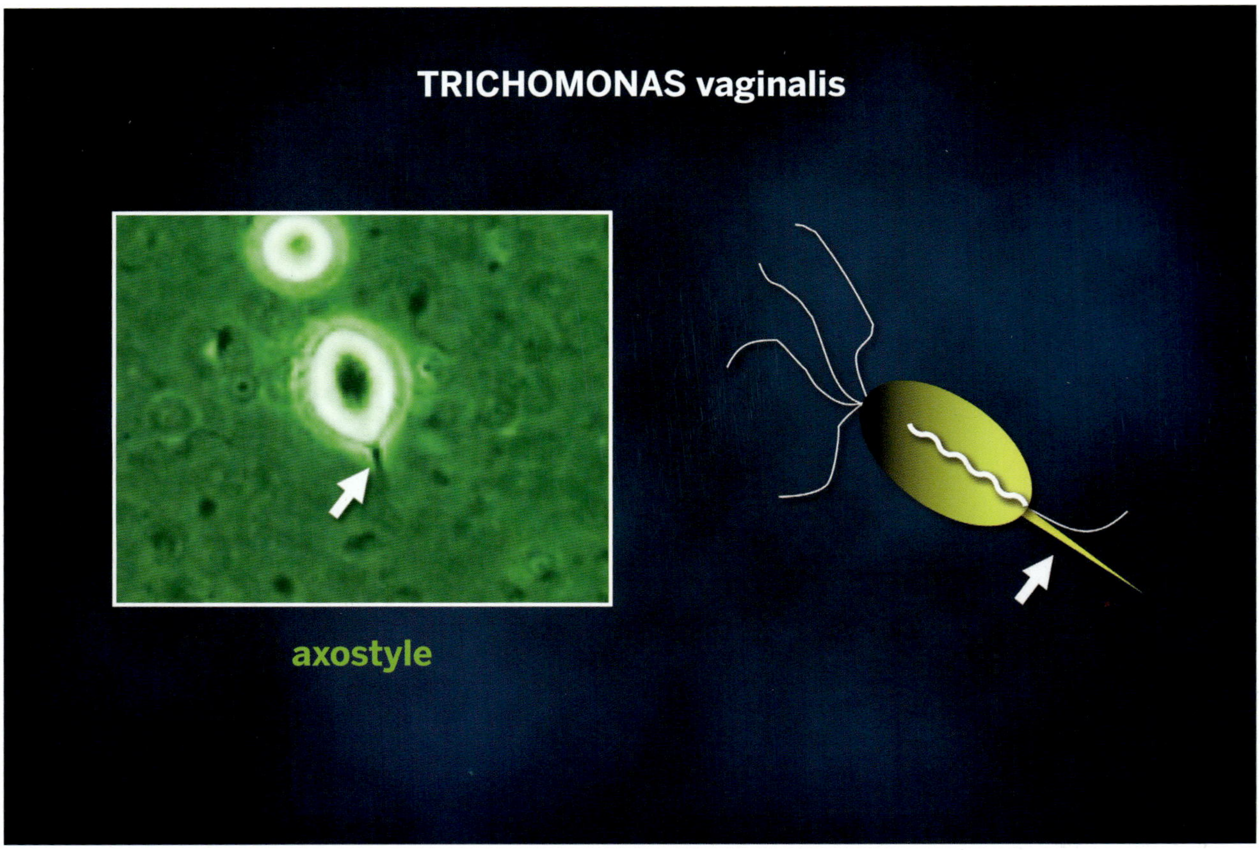

Figure 125 - Axostyle in Trichomonas vaginalis.

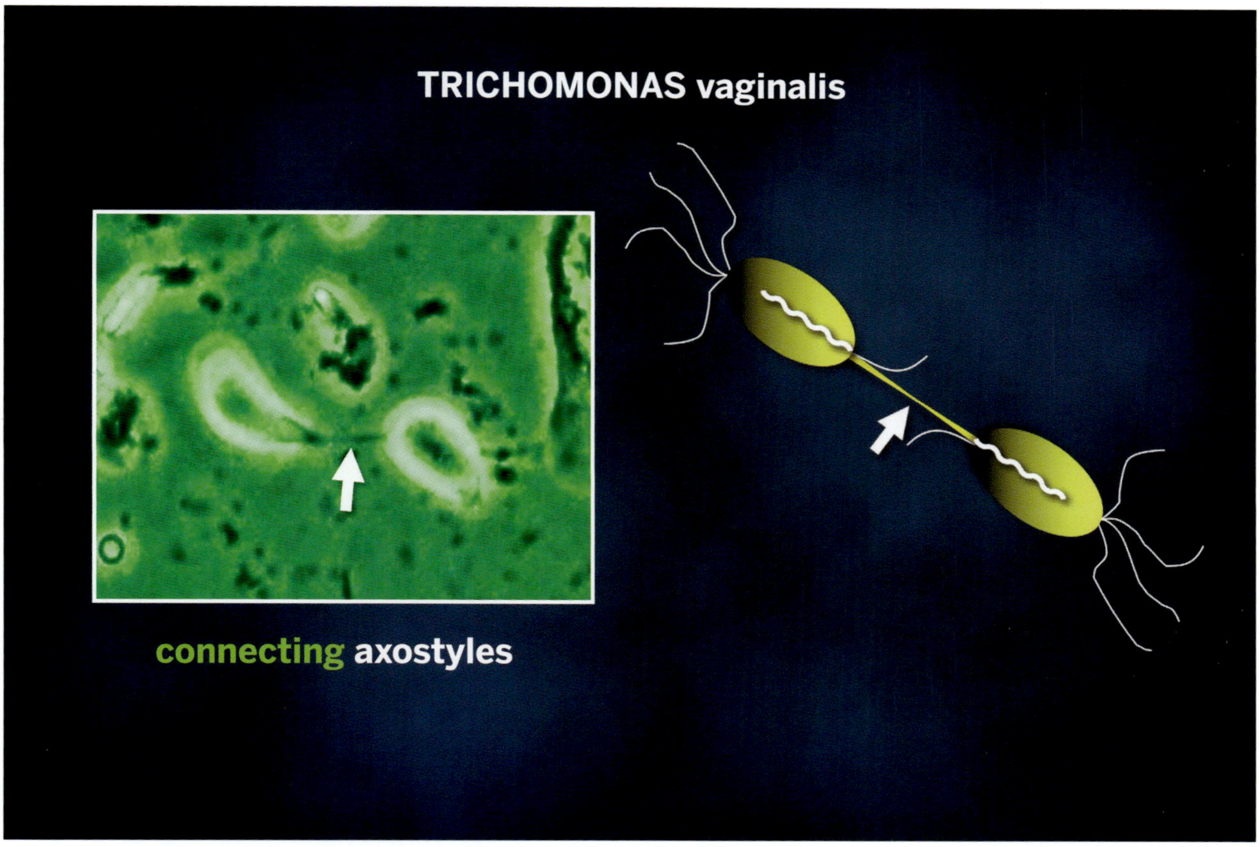

Figure 126 - Connecting axostyles between two trichomonads.

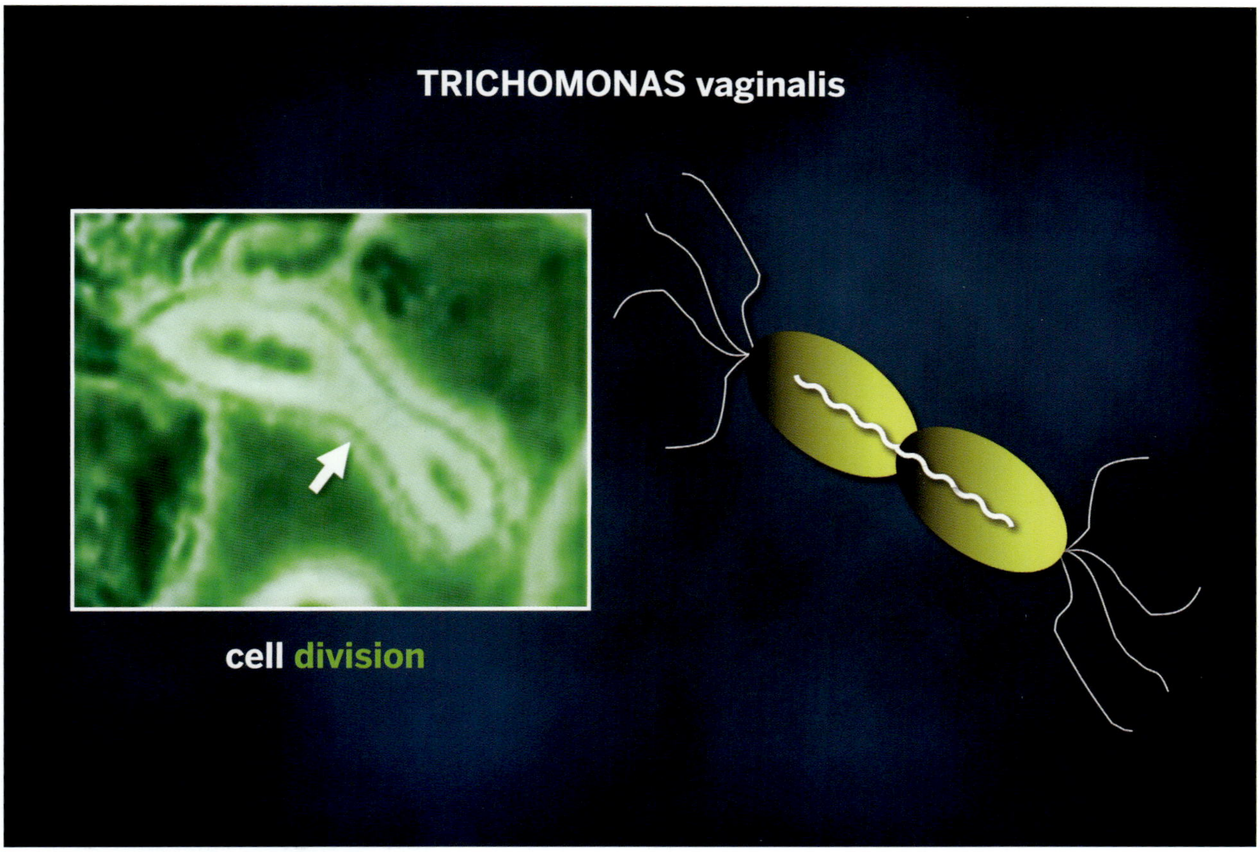

Figure 127 - Cell division of a trichomonad.

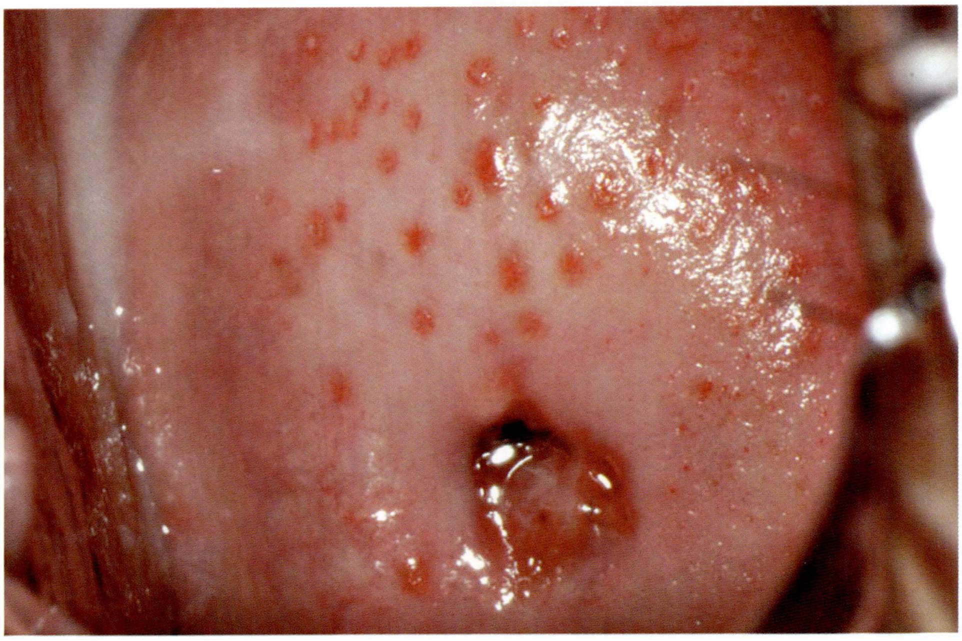

Figure 128 - Colpitis macularis in trichomoniasis ("strawberry cervix").

Currently, wet prep is a quick and easy test that can be done in real time and is commonly used to diagnose TV, that can be easily recognized for its jerky, swaying, or tumbling motion.

On colposcopic examination, Trichomonas infection is often associated with colpitis macularis or "strawberry" cervix (Figure 128). The cervix has a punctate and papilliform appearance, resulting from microscopic, punctate haemorrhages.

Viruses are not observable under bright-field or phase contrast microscope; nevertheless, they induce specific cell changes that usually represent the only warning signal to their presence. In consideration of the crucial role played by some viruses as carcinogens or co-carcinogens in the development of cervical intraepithelial neoplasia or other malignancies of the lower female genital tract, the recognition of characteristic viral cell changes must be further investigated, making careful colposcopic examination and molecular biology methods advisable.

Human Papillomavirus

Human Papillomavirus (HPV) infection is the most common sexually transmitted infection. HPV is so common that nearly all sexually active men and women get the virus at some point in their life. Although the majority of sexually active adults will be infected with HPV at least once in their lives, the highest rates of infection are found in sexually active women under 25.

HPV is a DNA virus belonging to the papillomavirus family, of which over 150 types are known.

More than 30 to 40 types of HPV are transmitted through sexual intercourse and anal sex. Some HPV infections that result in oral or upper respiratory lesions are acquired through oral sex. Since HPV is a skin-to-skin infection in the genital region, intercourse is not necessary to acquire the infection. Human Papillomavirus is not transmitted via common objects like toilet seats. In rare cases, an infected mother can infect her baby during delivery.

HPV targets the basal cells in the stratified squamous epithelium and the metaplastic cells at the squamocolumnar junction of the cervix. Additionally, high-risk HPV may infect the glandular epithelium of the endocervix, resulting in glandular neoplasms (Figure 129), such as adenocarcinoma in situ or invasive adenocarcinoma.

Unlike many genitourinary infections, HPV infection is not usually associated with immediate symptoms such as itching, burning, and vaginal discharge. Most HPV infections are cleared by the immune system and do not result in clinical sequelae. Although the host immune system successfully

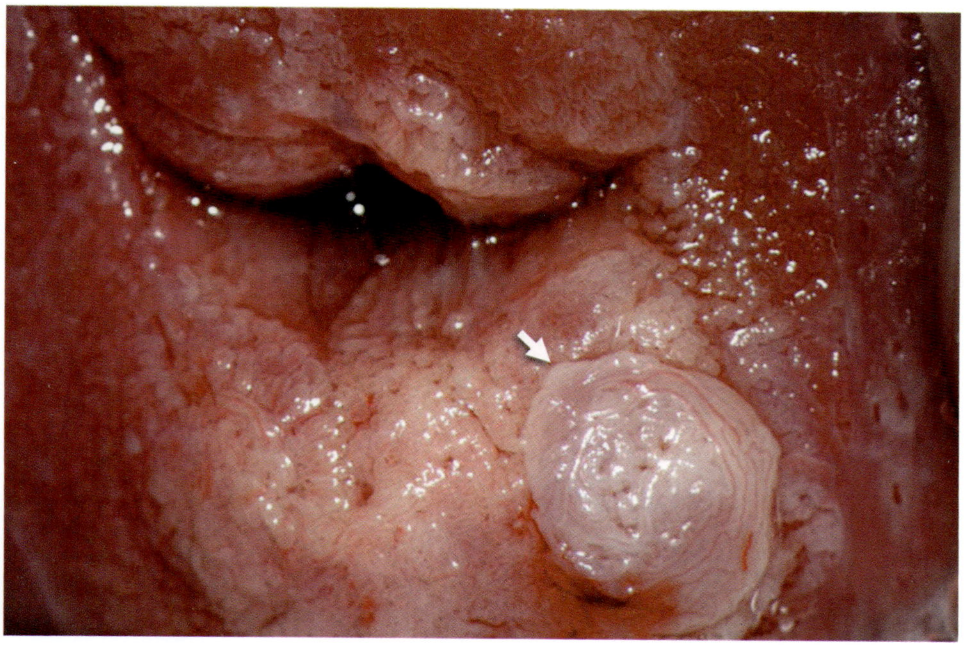
Figure 129 - Adenocarcinoma.

clears most of these infections, some women will develop disease such as genital warts, cervical dysplasia – distinguished in low-grade squamous intraepithelial lesions (L-SIL) and high-grade squamous intraepithelial lesions (H-SIL) – and invasive cervical cancer. Clinical complications in cases of low-risk HPV infection consist of genital warts, while clinical manifestations of high-risk HPV infection include dysplasia and cervical cancer. Usually, the process from initial HPV infection to the development of cancer takes years, if not decades. The strains of HPV known to cause genital warts are low-risk HPV 6 and 11, while the strains of HPV associated with dysplasia and cancer include high-risk HPV 16, 18 (which cause about 70% of cervical cancers), 31, 33, 45, 52, 58 and a few others. Human papillomavirus infection is a necessary, although not sufficient, cause of cervical cancer.
The methods to diagnose HPV infection are:

- pap smear and wet mount microscopy
- colposcopy and acetic acid test
- histology
- DNA test (PCR, Southern Blot Hybridization, In Situ Hybridization).

Human Papillomavirus can induce specific cytopathic effects that are easily detectable by microscopy (Figure 130):

- koilocyte
- dark nuclei
- multiple nuclei.

Koilocyte (Figures 130, 131) shows a characteristic wide perinuclear halo with a sharply condensed border. The nucleus may exhibit an irregular membrane contour and usually appears enlarged (two to three times the normal size) with abnormal chromatin distribution. The sharp-edged halo seen in koilocyte must be distinguished from the perinuclear halo with blurred edge of reactive cells (false koilocyte), due to coarctation of cytoplasm around the nucleus (Figure 132).
A darker than normal staining pattern in the nucleus known as *hyperchromasia* can be observed in HPV infection. As wet mount microscopy does not recur to staining, the term *dark nuclei* (Figures 130, 132) is preferred to hyperchromasia.
Multiple nuclei (Figures 130, 133, 134) derive all from one nucleus. When multinucleation is present, nuclei are dispersed in the cytoplasm or at least appear overlapping, but they are never gathered and moulded as in polykaryocyte by Herpes Simplex Virus.
Different HPV cytopathic effects may be combined in the same cell (Figures 135, 136, 137, 138, 139, 140). Cell changes induced by HPV may be associated

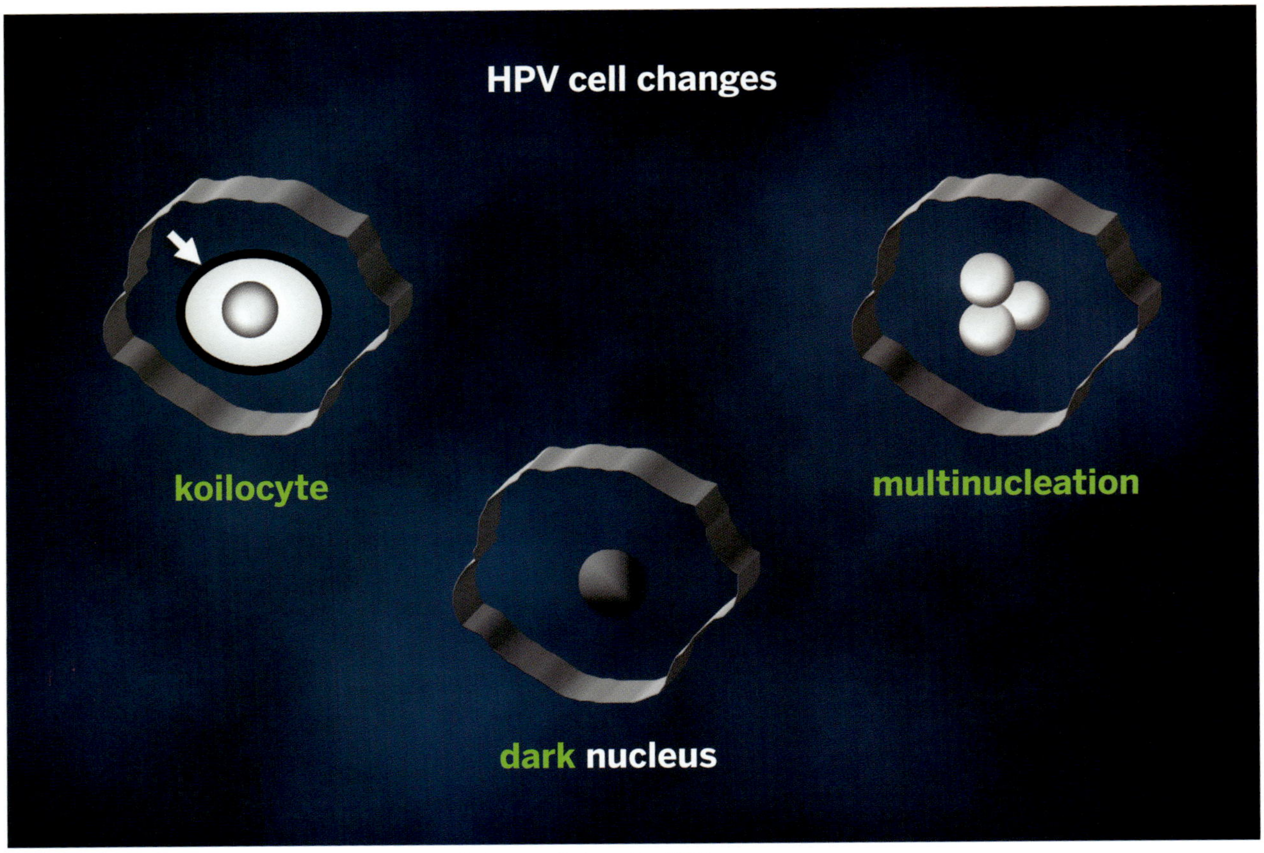

Figure 130 - Diagrammatic representation of cell changes induced by HPV.

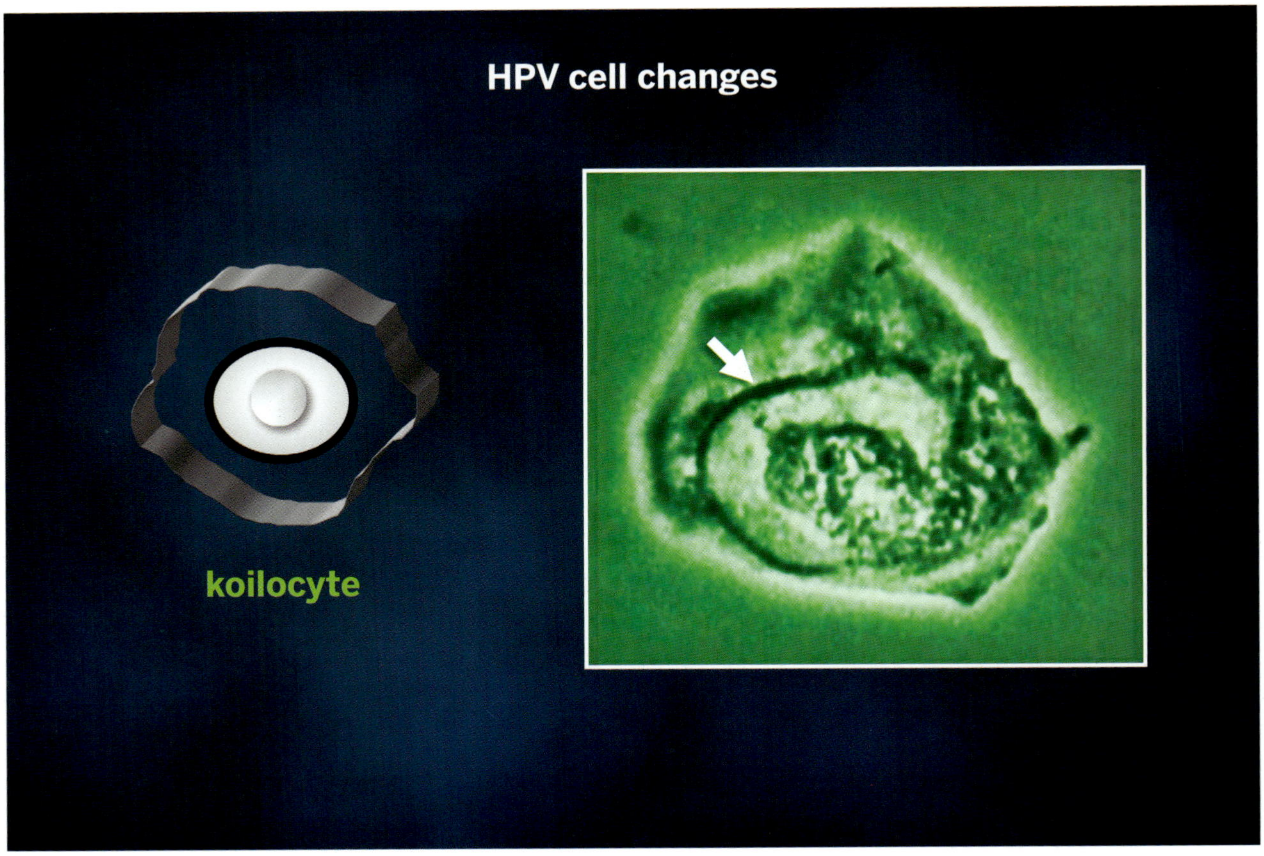

Figure 131 - Koilocyte.

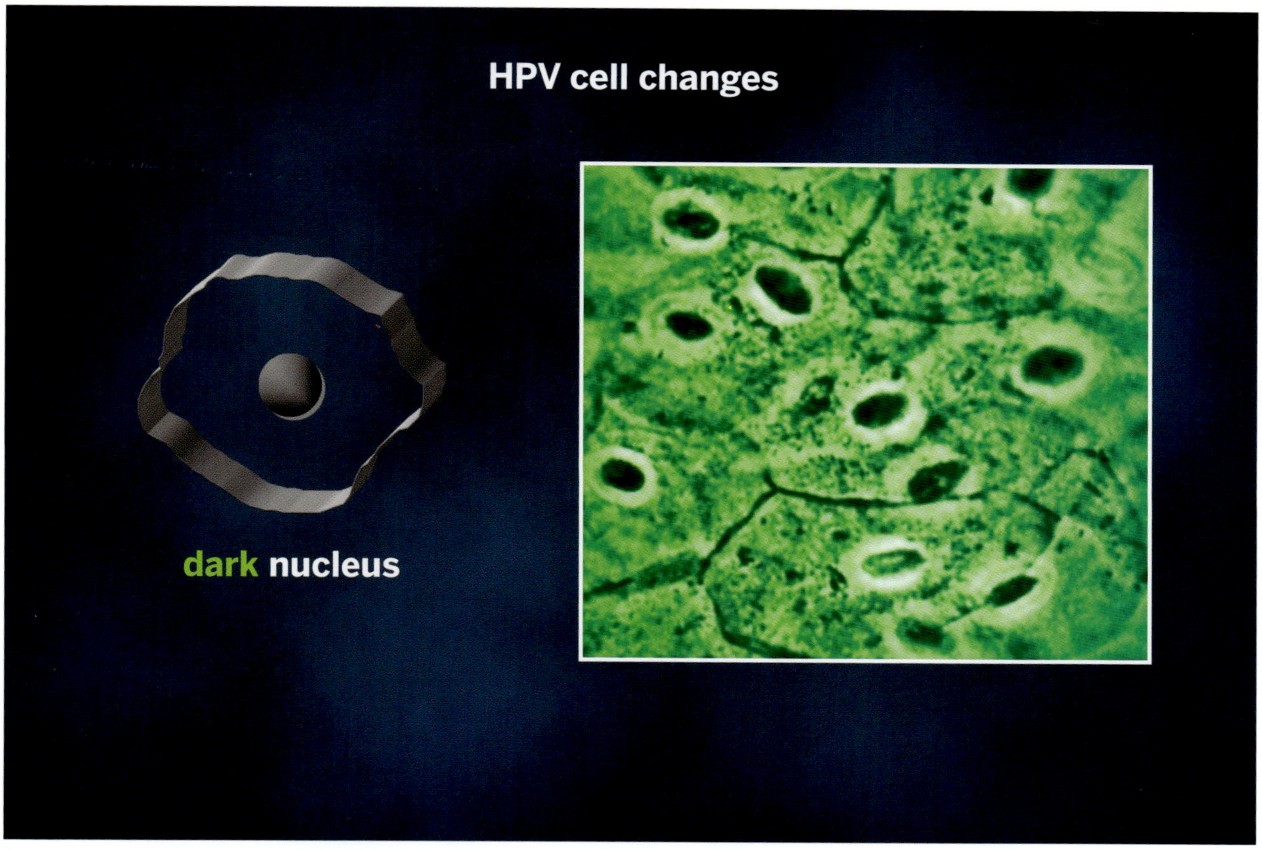

Figure 132 - Dark nuclei in HPV infection. The cells show a perinuclear halo with blurred edge (false koilocytes).

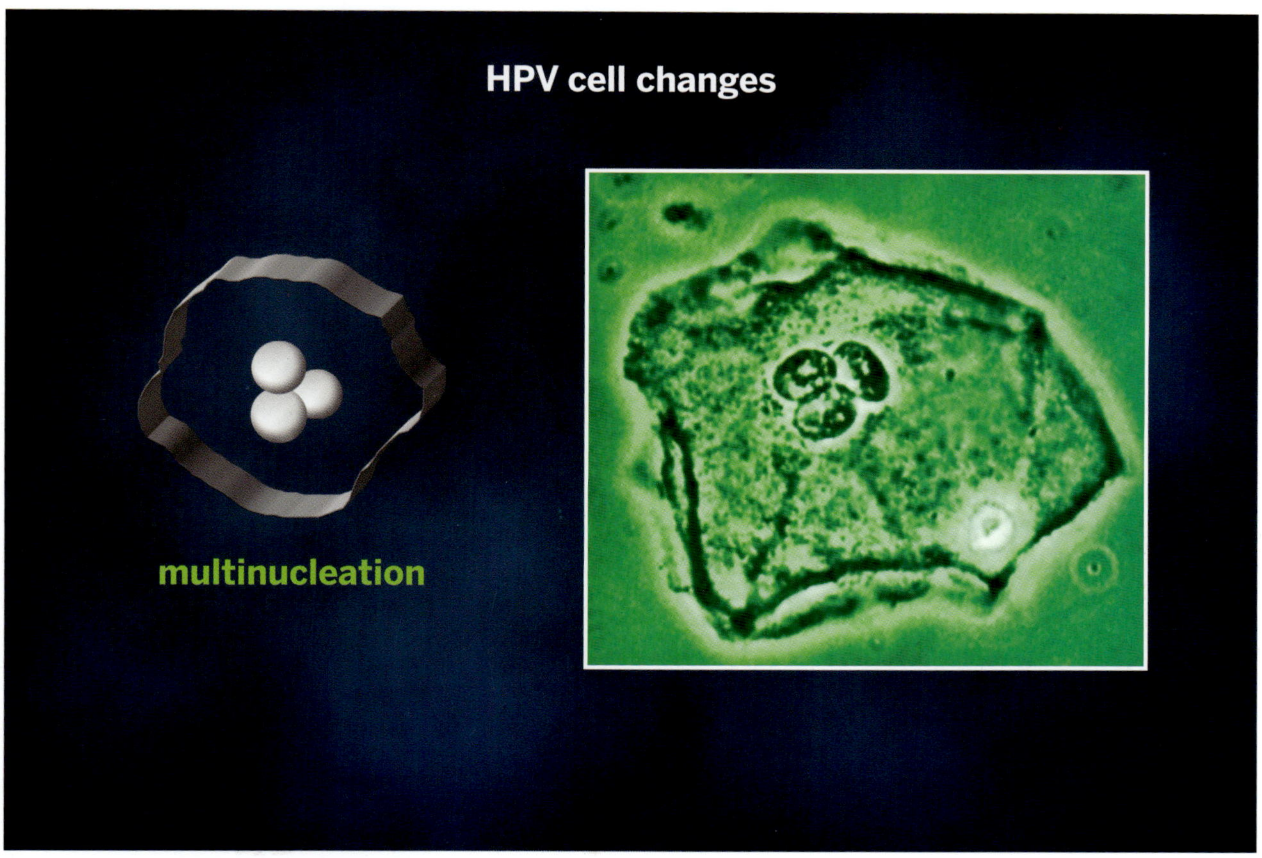

Figure 133 - Multinucleation in HPV infection.

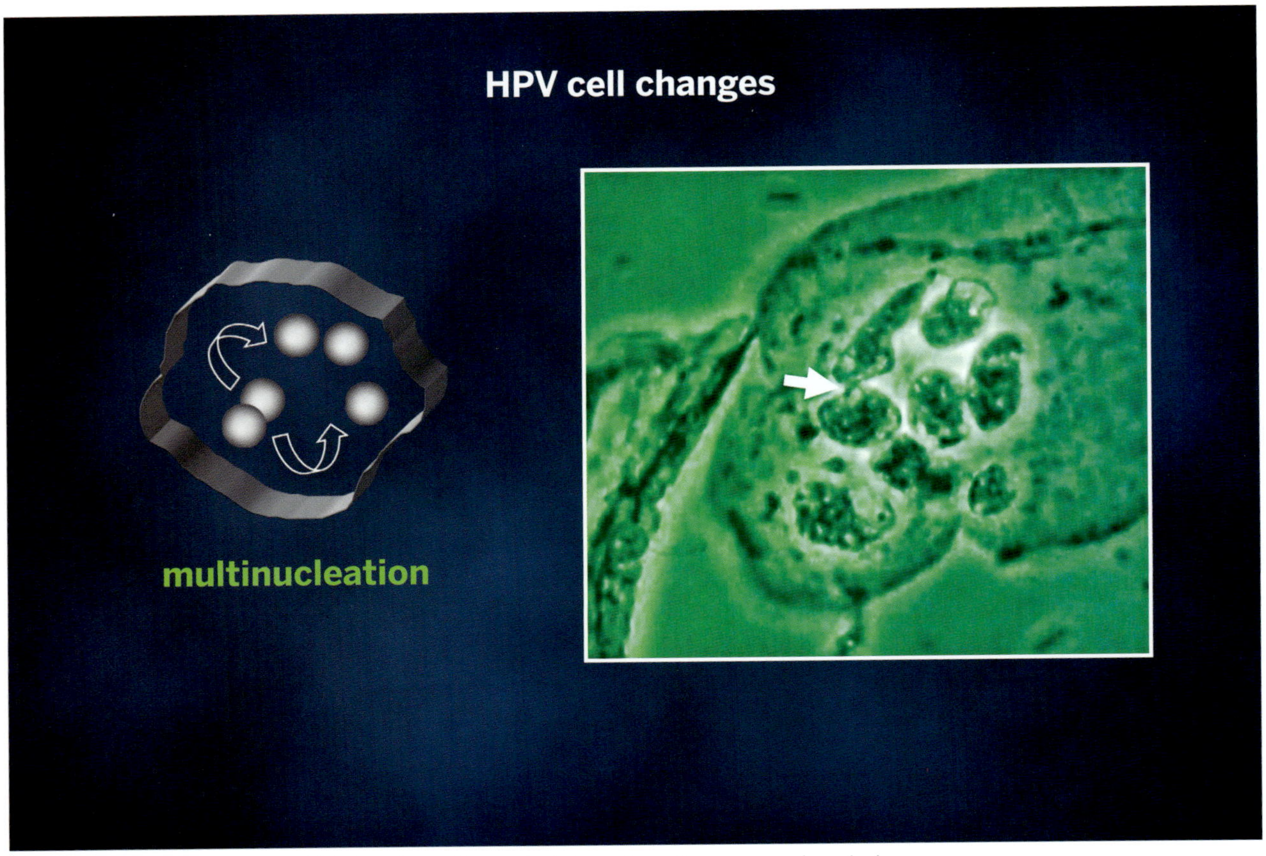

Figure 134 - Multinucleation in HPV infection. All nuclei originate from the same nucleus (→).

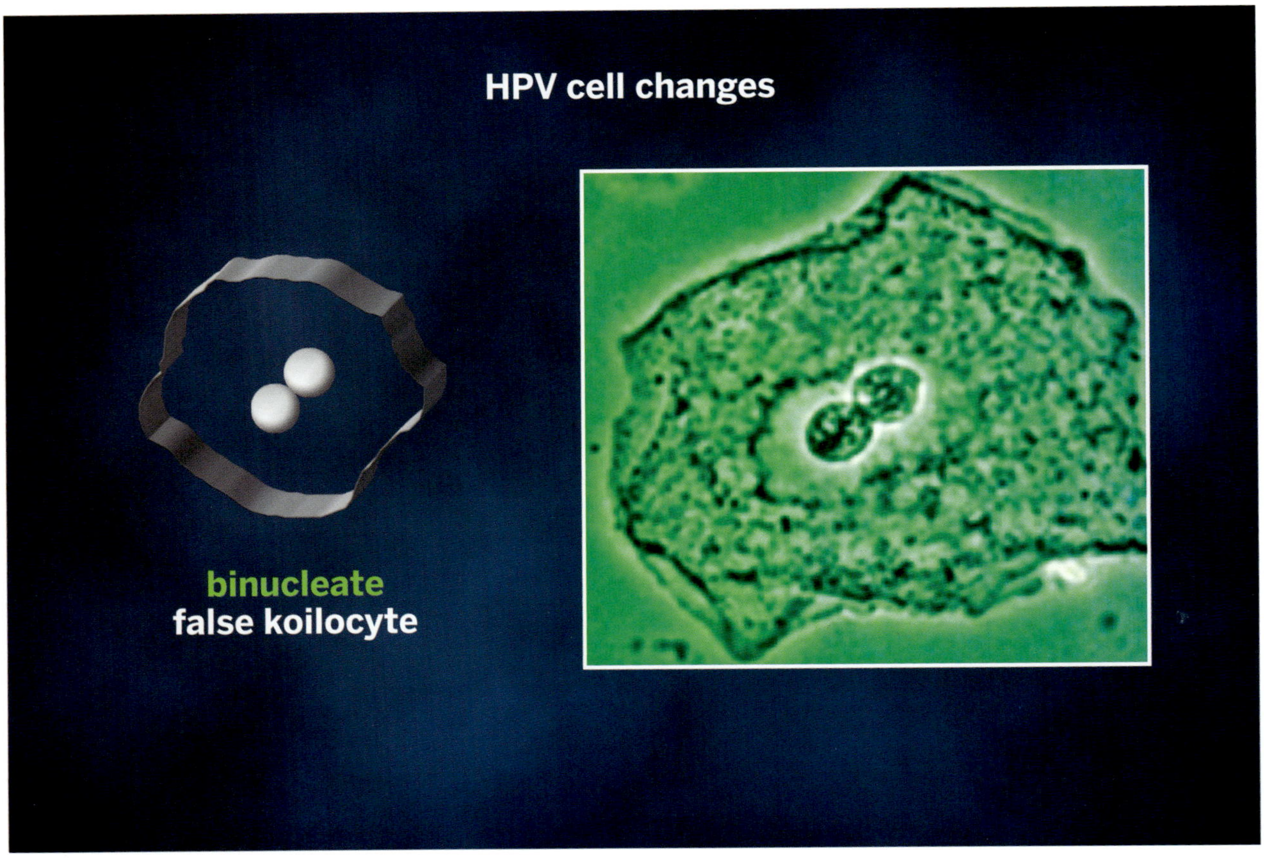

Figure 135 - Binucleate false koilocyte.

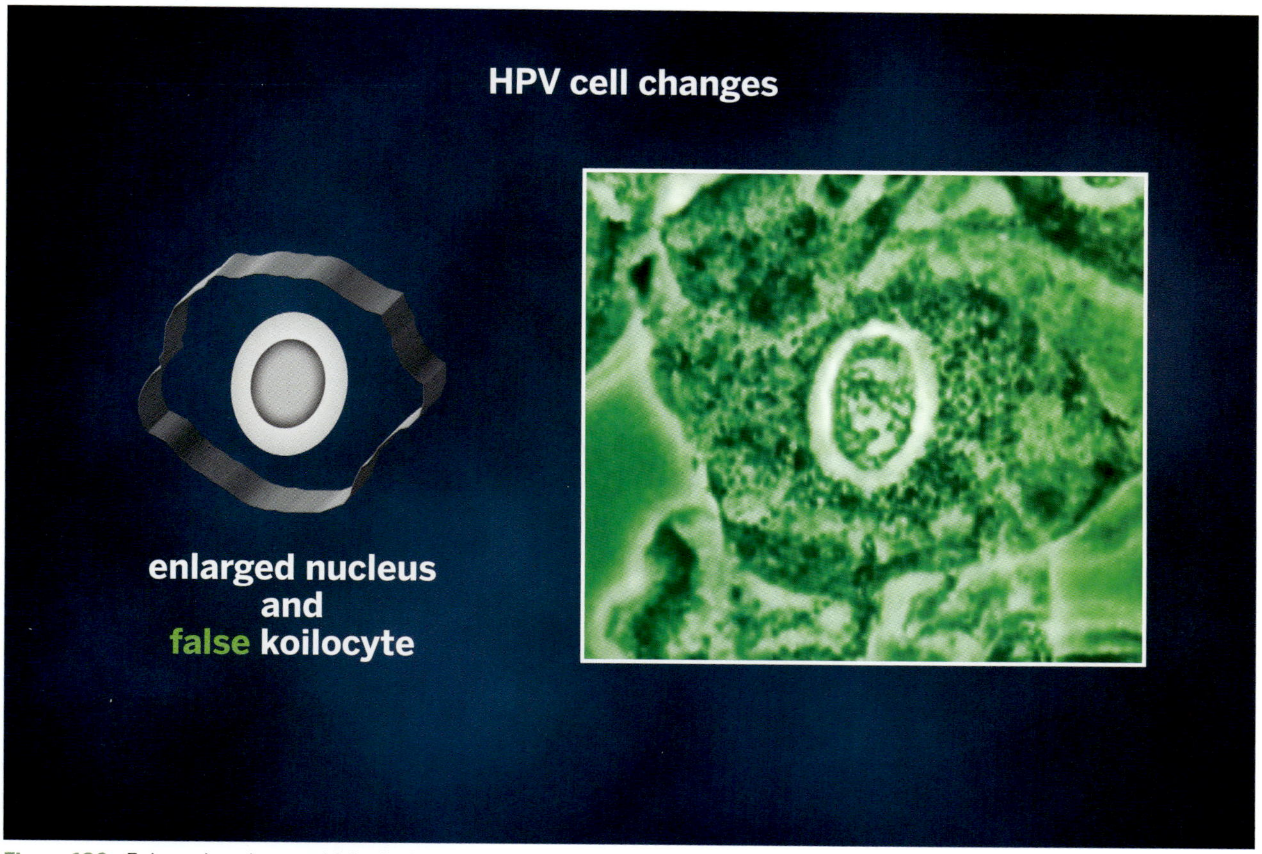

Figure 136 - Enlarged nucleus and false koilocyte.

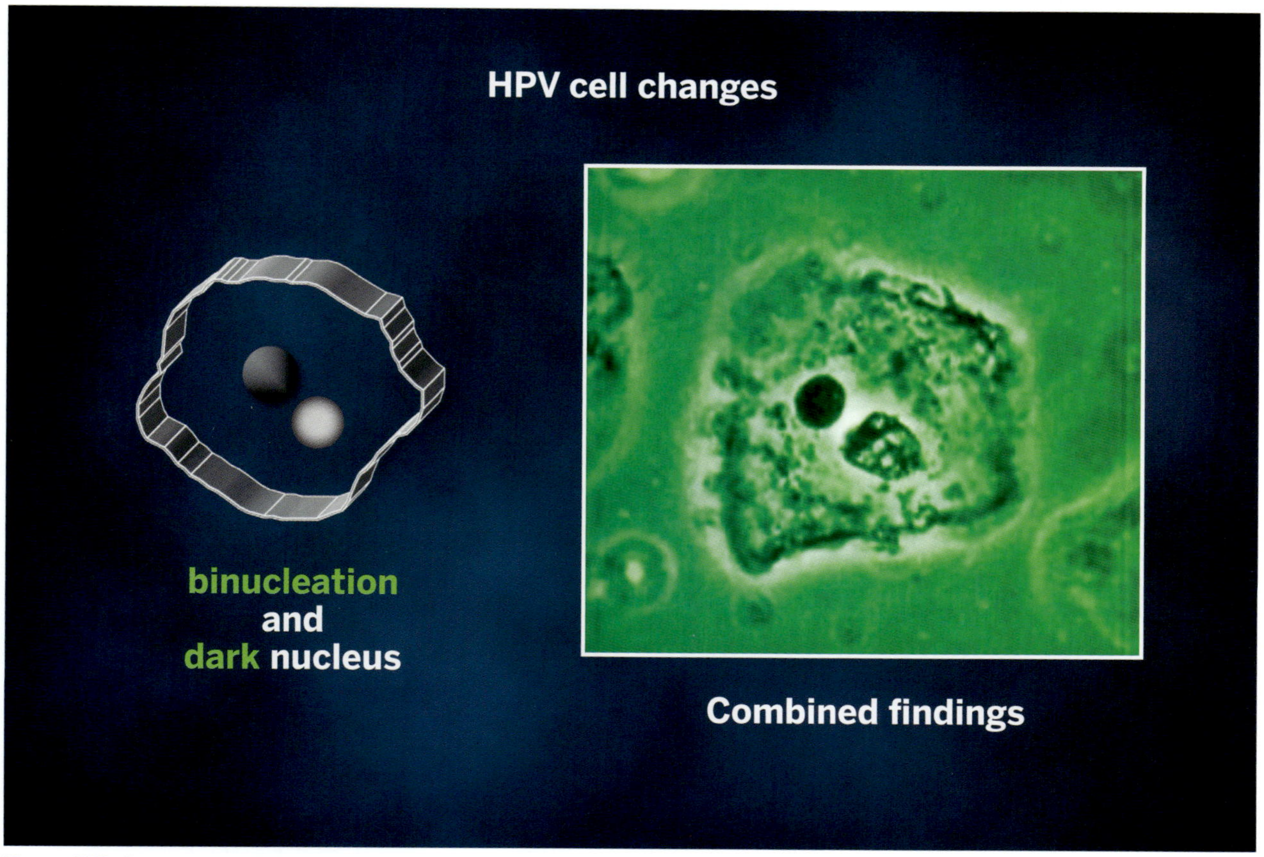

Figure 137 - Binucleation and dark nucleus.

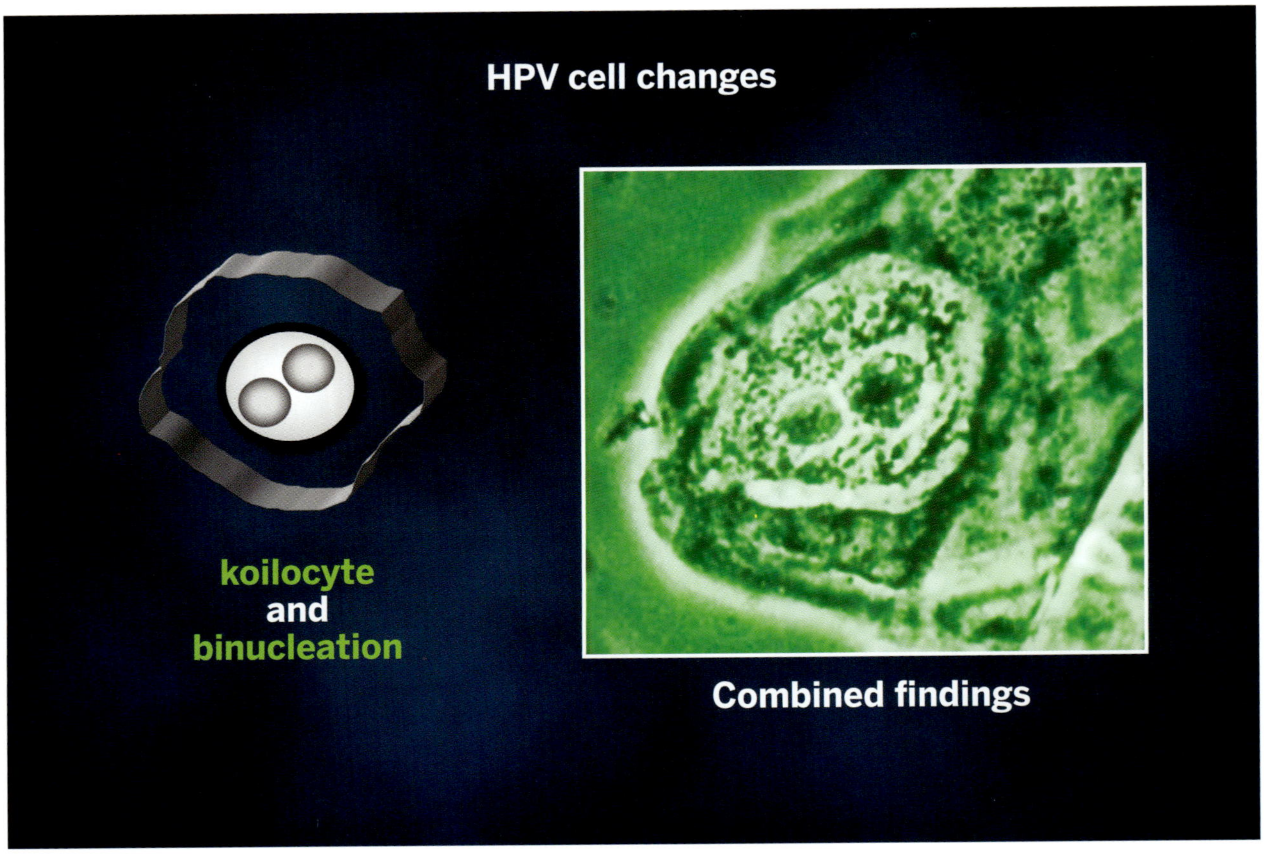

Figure 138 - Binucleate koilocyte.

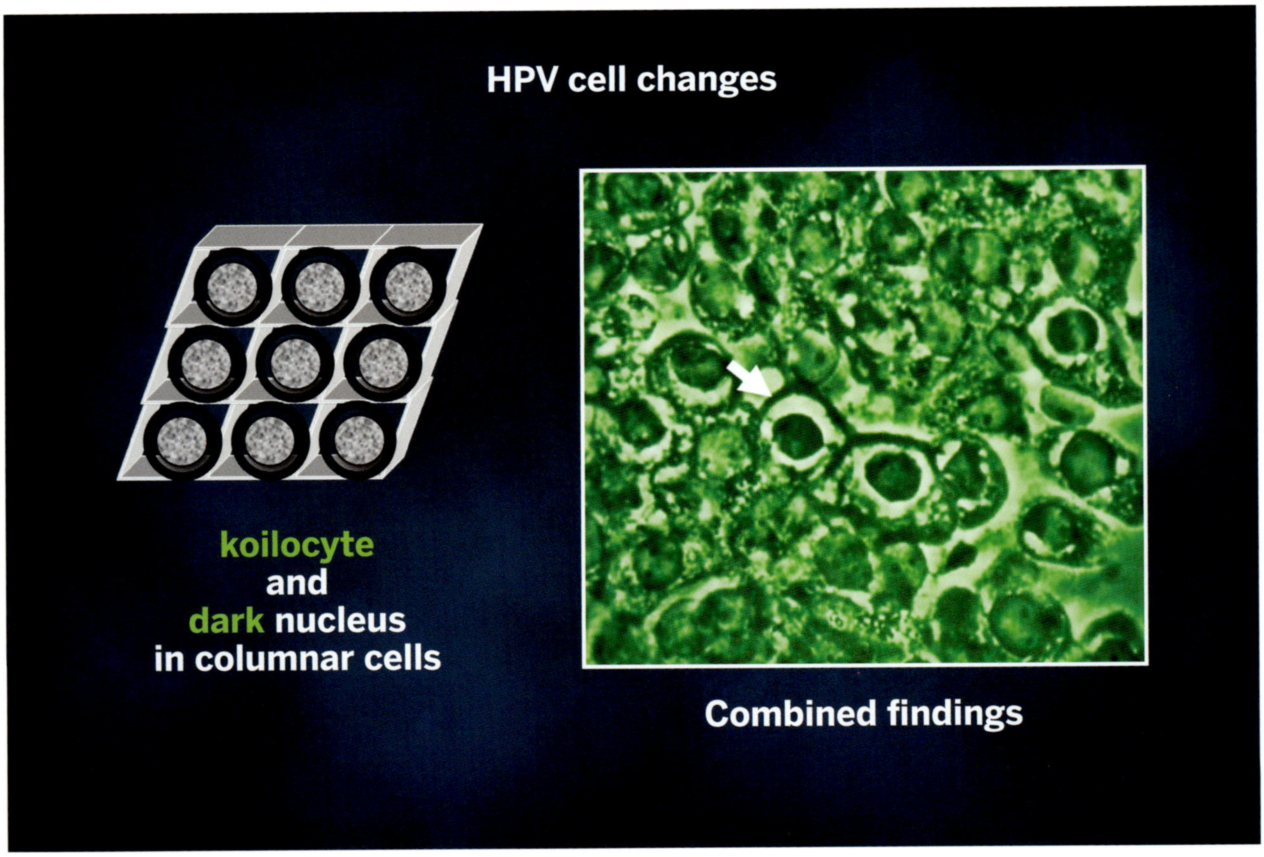

Figure 139 - Koilocytes and dark nuclei in columnar cells.

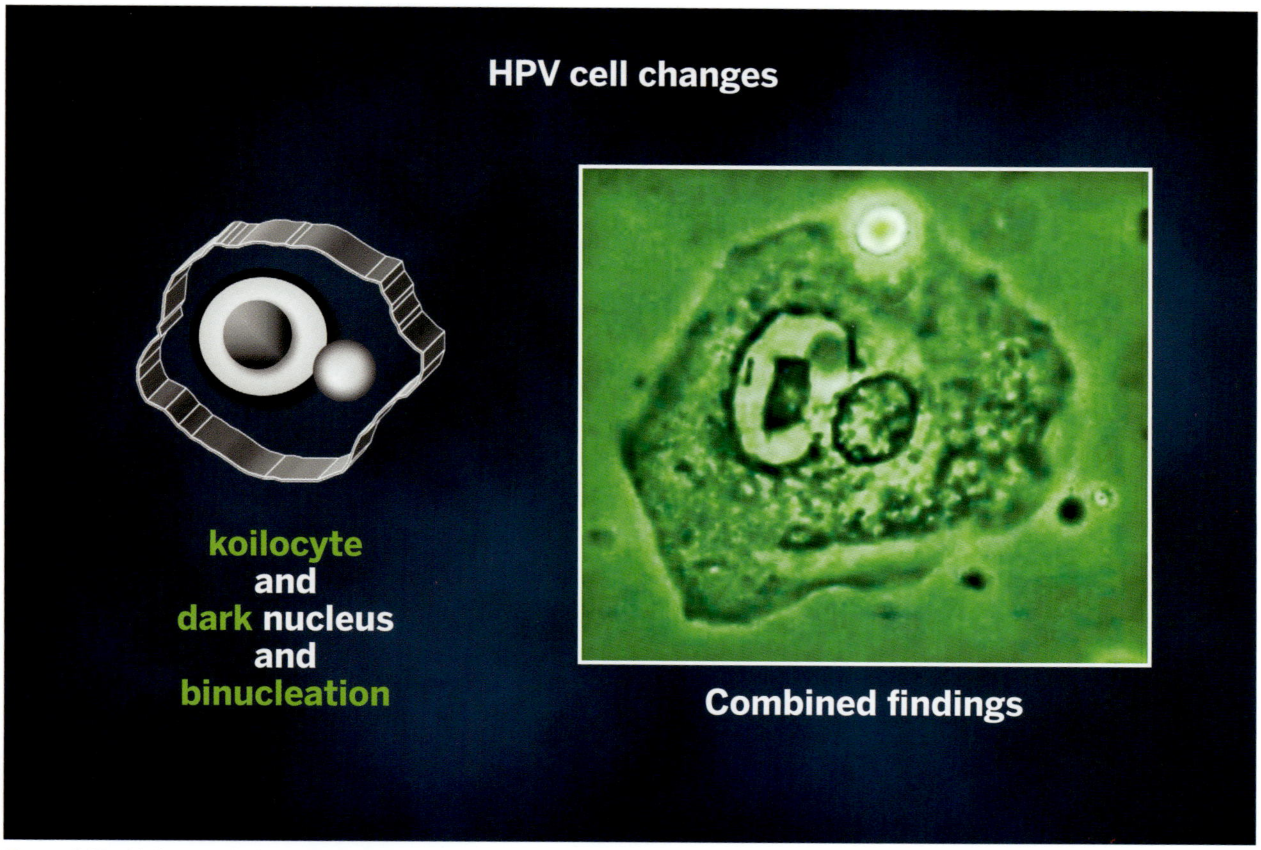

Figure 140 - Koilocyte, dark nucleus and binucleation in the same cell.

with altered cytoplasm/nucleus ratio (C/N r) in CIN 2 (Figure 141) or with inverted C/N r in CIN 3 (Figure 142).

HPV infection may exhibit no abnormal colposcopic findings or may induce extremely variable colposcopic findings which are graded according to degree of acetowhite lesion (Figure 143), surface contour, mosaic pattern (Figure 144), and punctuation (Figure 145). Greater abnormalities of these parameters are related to the degree of severity of the lesions.

Colposcopic features induced by HPV infection may be divided into two groups: exophytic or productive lesions and flat or subclinical papillomavirus infection (SPI):

- *exophytic lesions*
  - exophytic condyloma
  - micropapillary lesions
- *flat lesions* (SPI)
  - flat condyloma
  - white punctuation.

The former group includes macroscopic lesions, like exophytic condyloma and early micropapillary lesions, that are visible to the naked eye.

Exophytic condyloma may involve vulvar mucosa (Figure 146), clitoris (Figure 147), vagina (Figure 148) and cervix (Figure 149). Condyloma acuminata or warts refer to an epidermal manifestation of exophytic condyloma (Figure 150). Warts appear as small to large soft, flesh-coloured lumps. Condyloma acuminata may occur in clusters and some of these clusters have a cauliflower-like appearance. In presence of florid anal warts (Figure 151) it is advisable to inspect the lower rectum (Figure 152). Genital and anal warts can spread, even when no warts seem to be present. The incubation period after exposure ranges from three weeks to eight months.

Micropapillary lesions are not easily detected without a special examination of the skin (Figure 153), vaginal vestibule (Figure 154), vagina (Figure 155) and cervix (Figure 156). Micropapillary lesions induced by HPV must be distinguished from

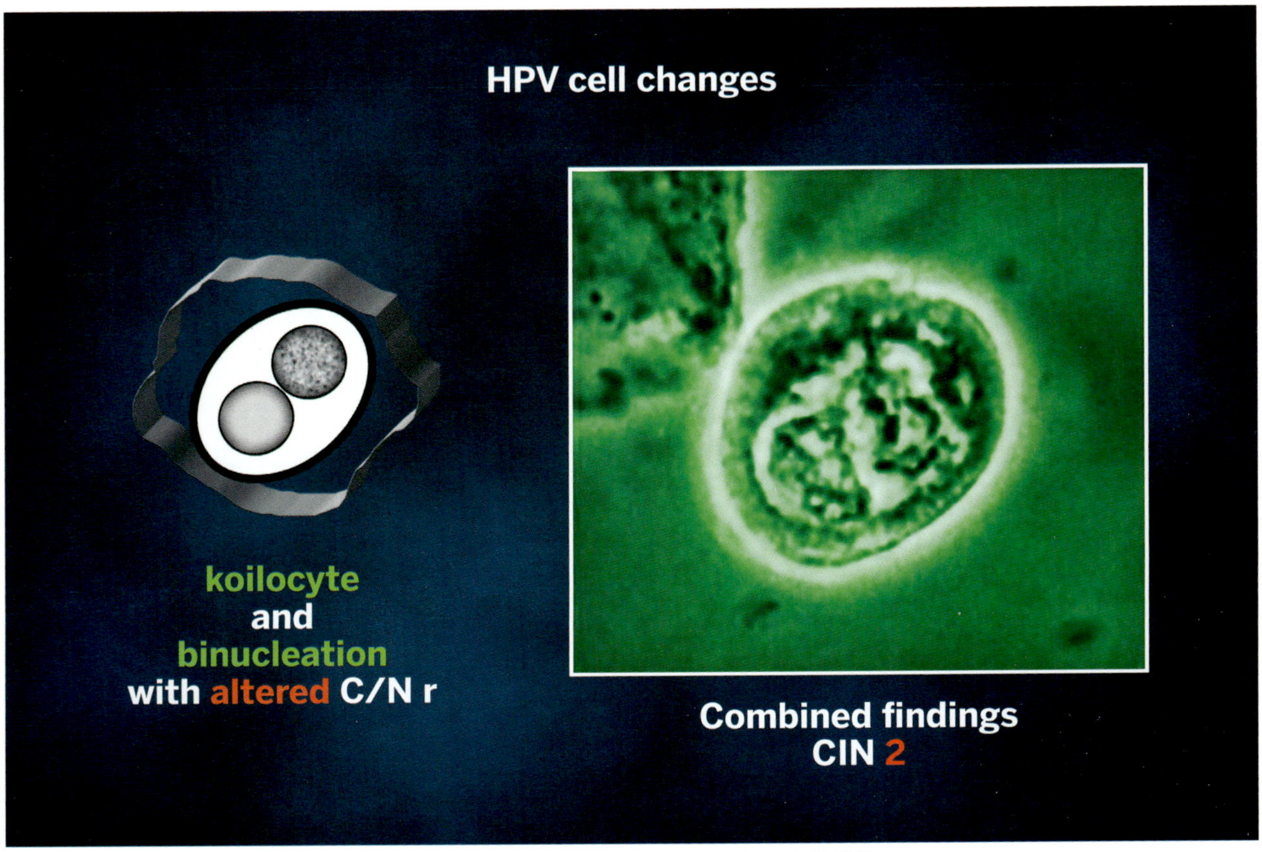

Figure 141 - Koilocyte and binucleation with altered cytoplasm/nucleus ratio (C/N r) (CIN 2).

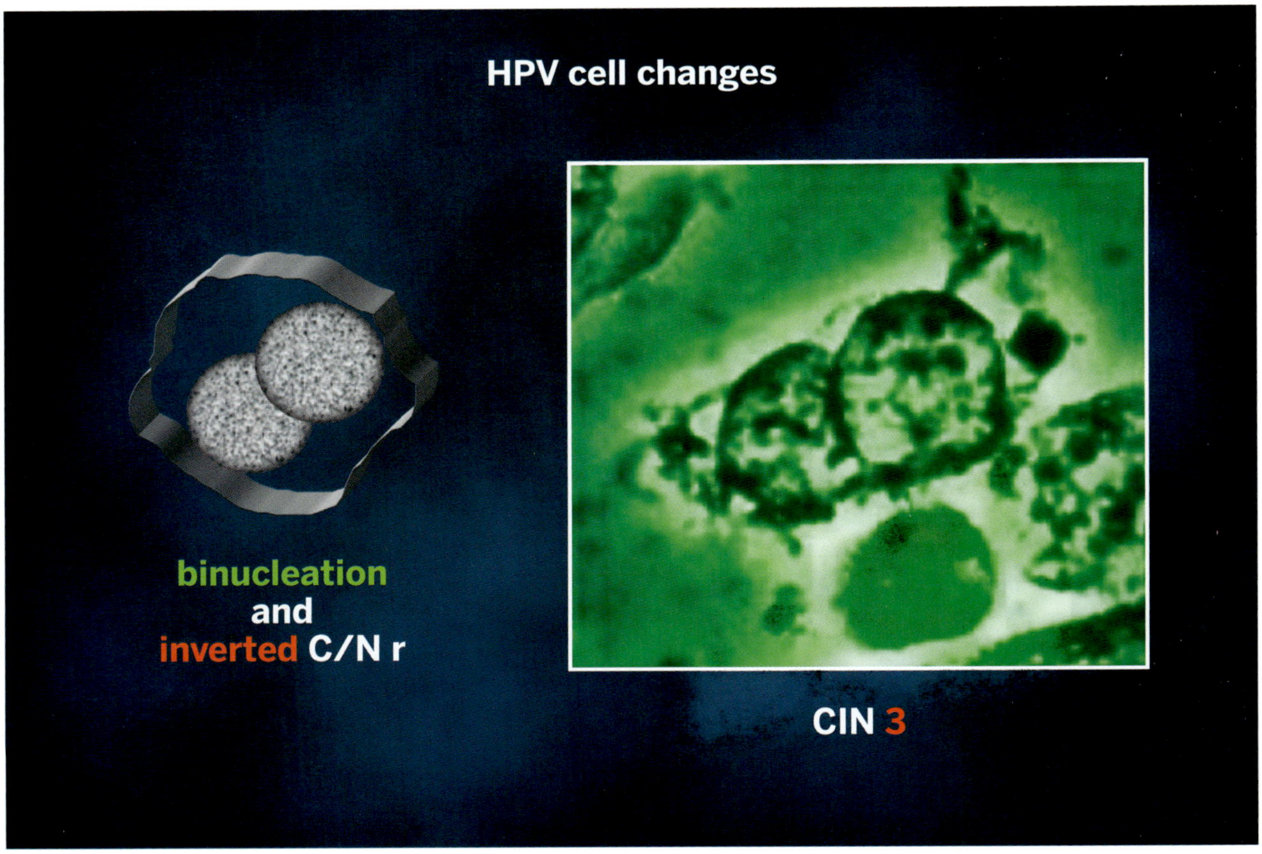

Figure 142 - Binucleation and inverted C/N r in CIN 3.

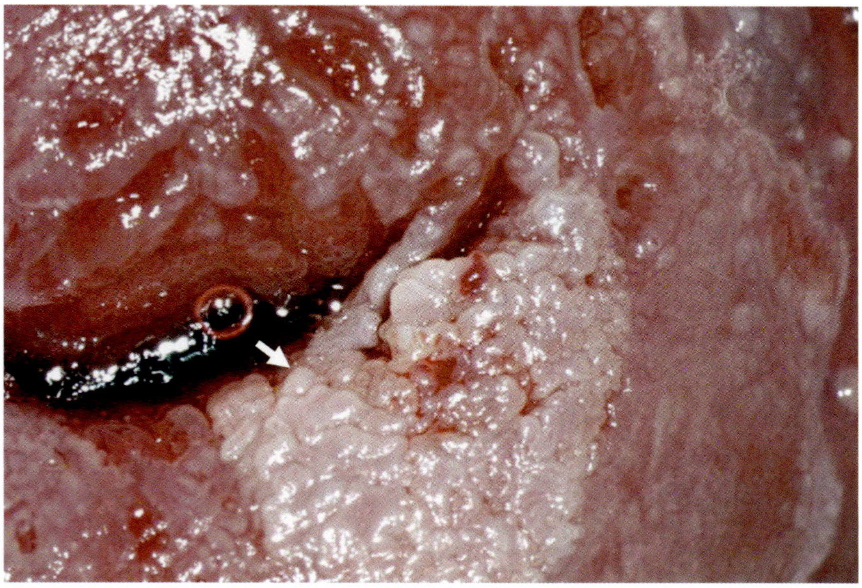

Figure 143 - Early cervical exophytic condyloma (→).

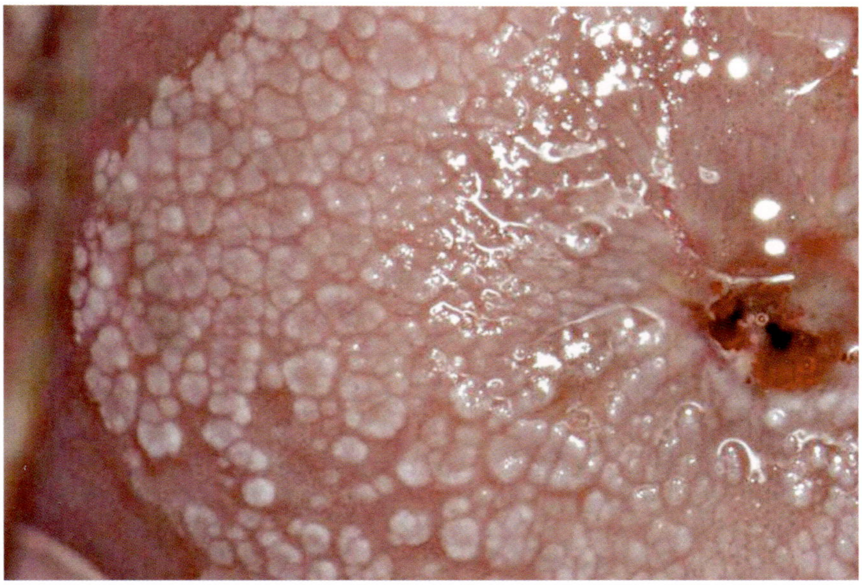

Figure 144 - Coarse mosaic pattern.

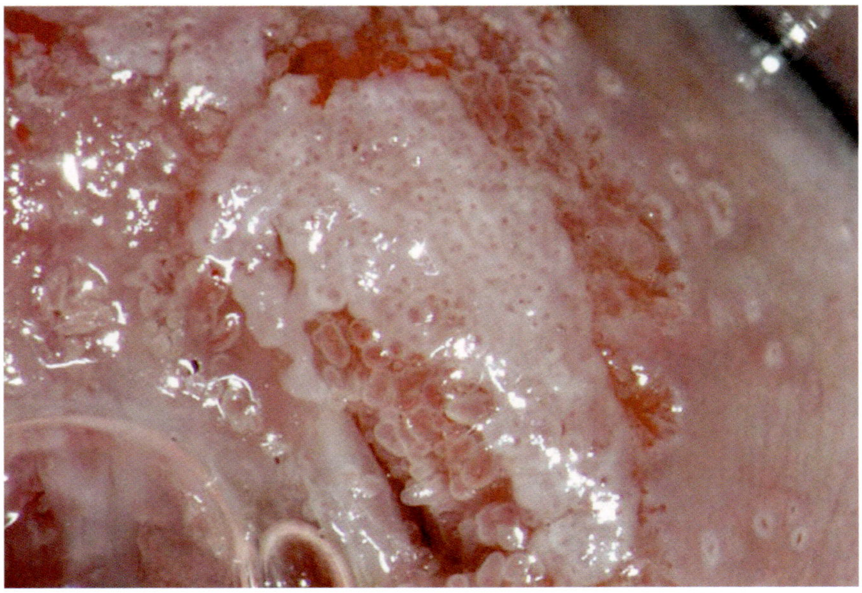

Figure 145 - Coarse red punctation on a dense acetowhite lesion.

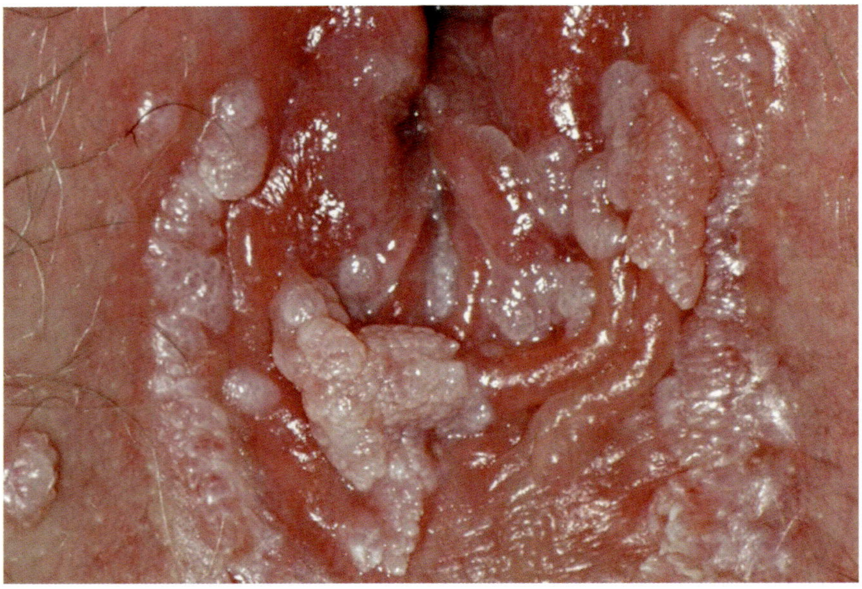

Figure 146 - Vestibular exophytic condyloma.

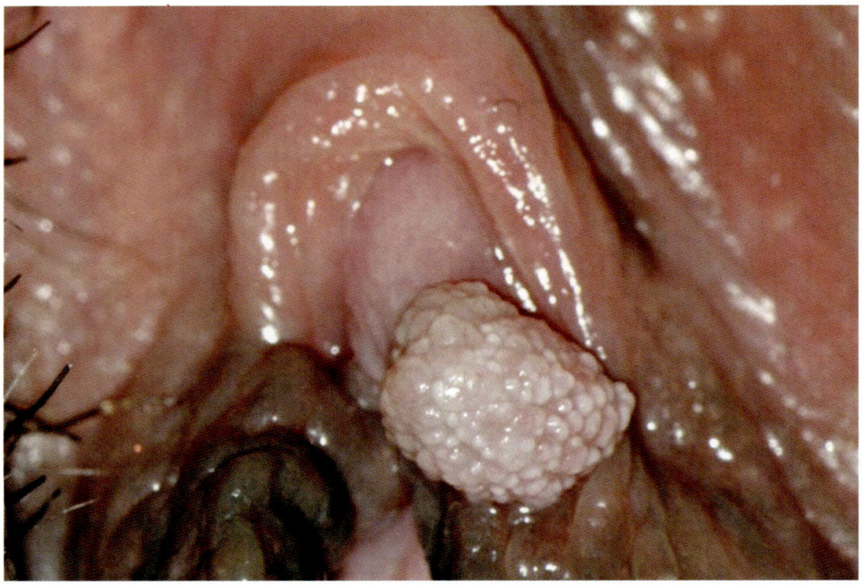

Figure 147 - Clitoral exophytic condyloma.

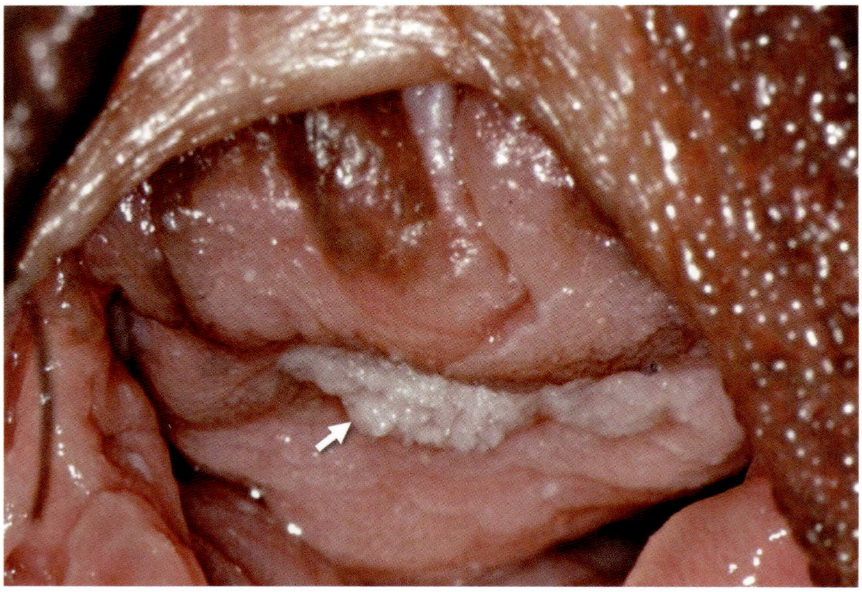

Figure 148 - Vaginal keratinized exophytic condyloma (→), next to urethra.

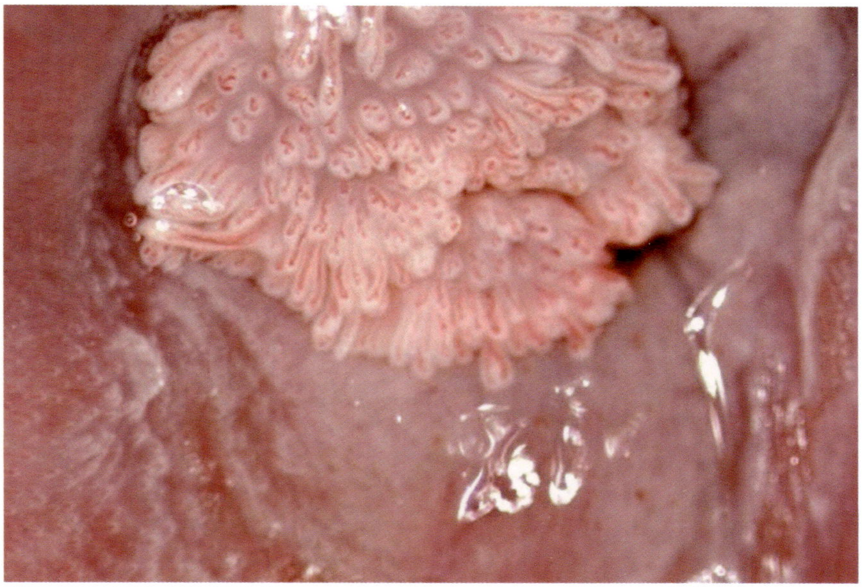

Figure 149 - Cervical exophytic condyloma.

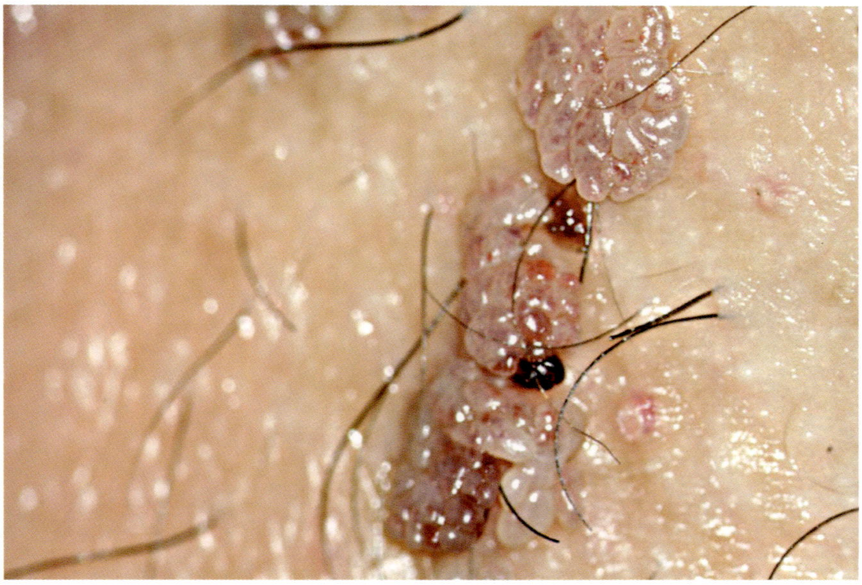

Figure 150 - Warts.

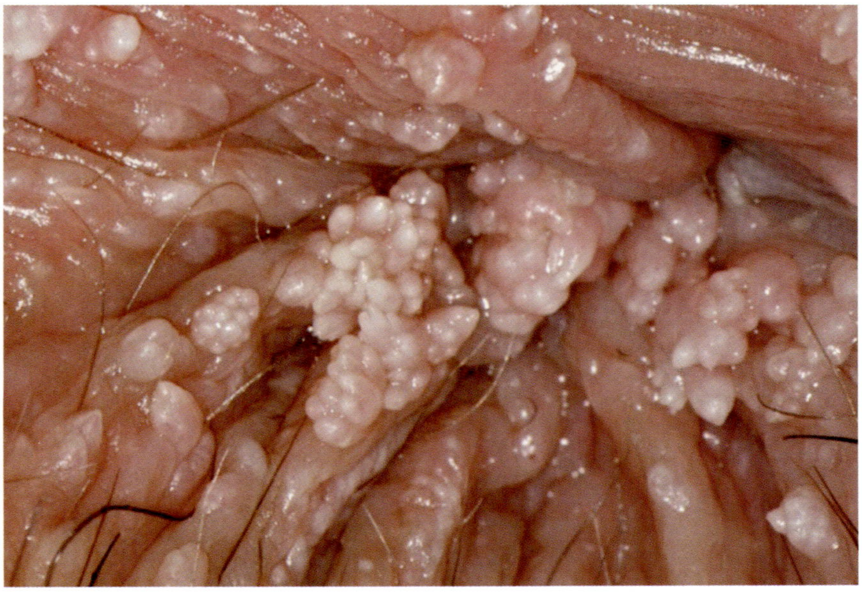

Figure 151 - Perianal exophytic condyloma.

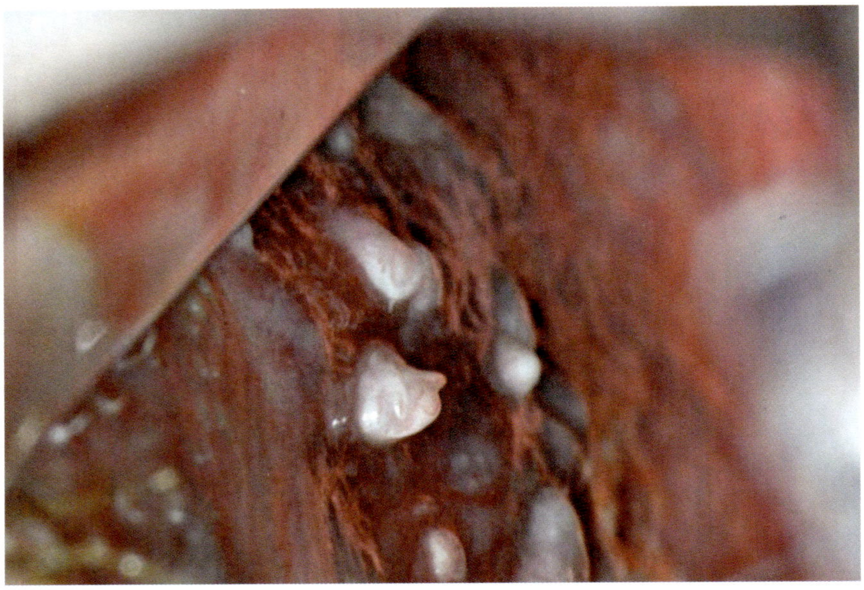

Figure 152 - Rectal condyloma.

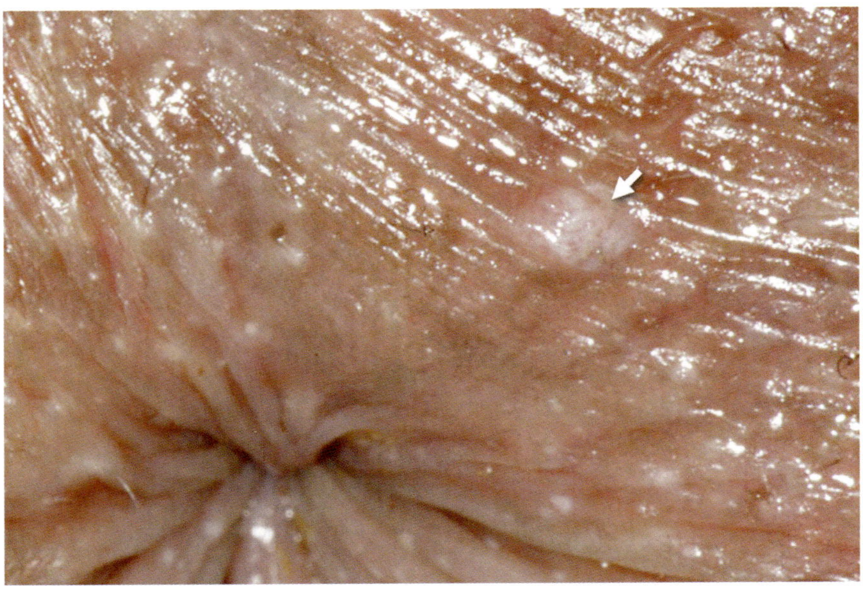

Figure 153 - Perianal micropapillary lesion (→).

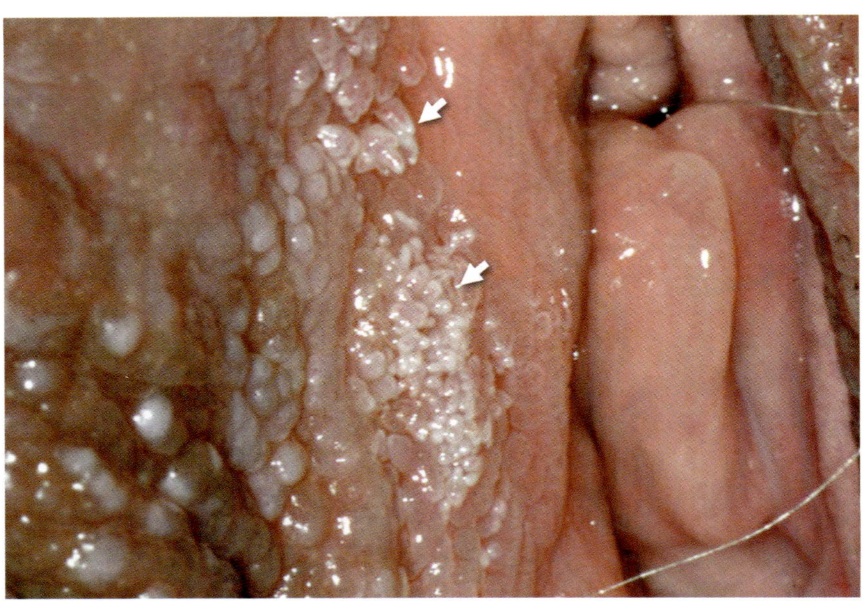

Figure 154 - Vestibular micropapillary lesions (→).

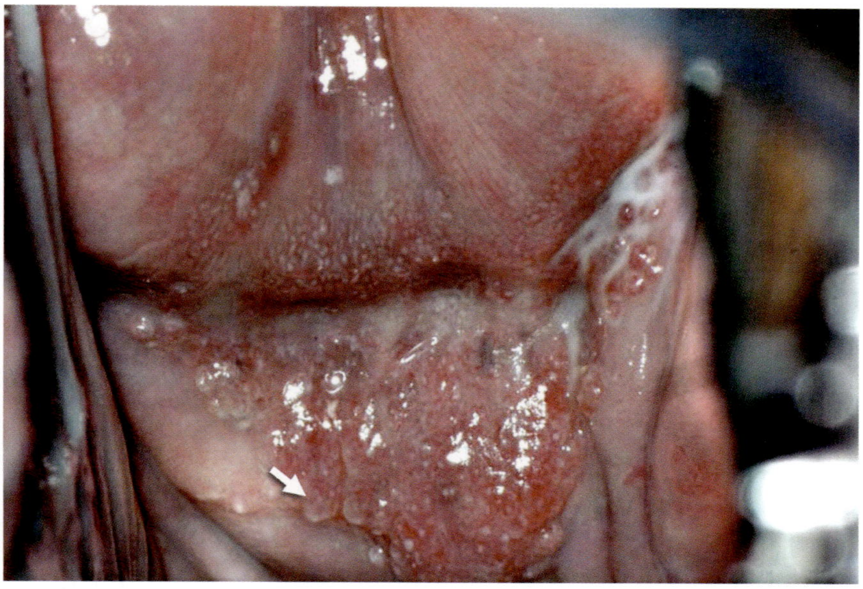

Figure 155 - Vaginal micropapillary lesion in the posterior fornix (→) (VaIN 3).

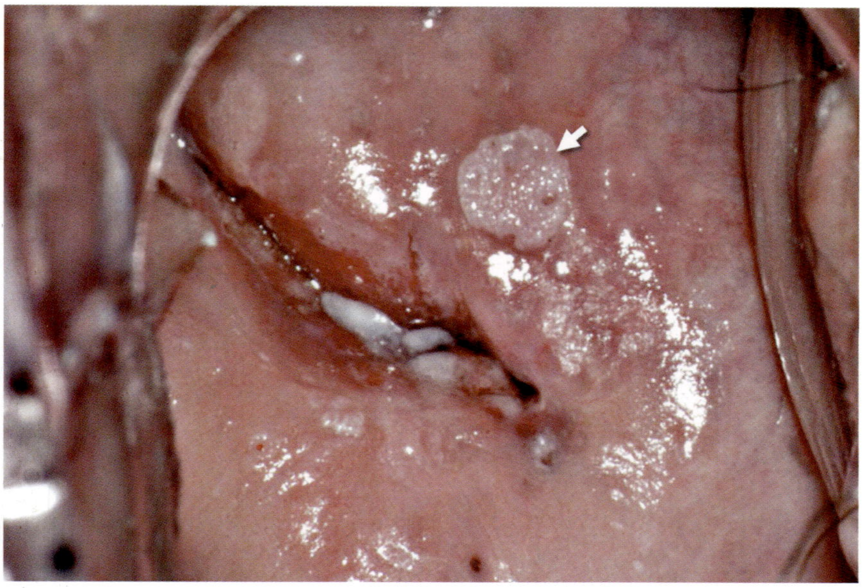

Figure 156 - Cervical micropapillary lesion (→).

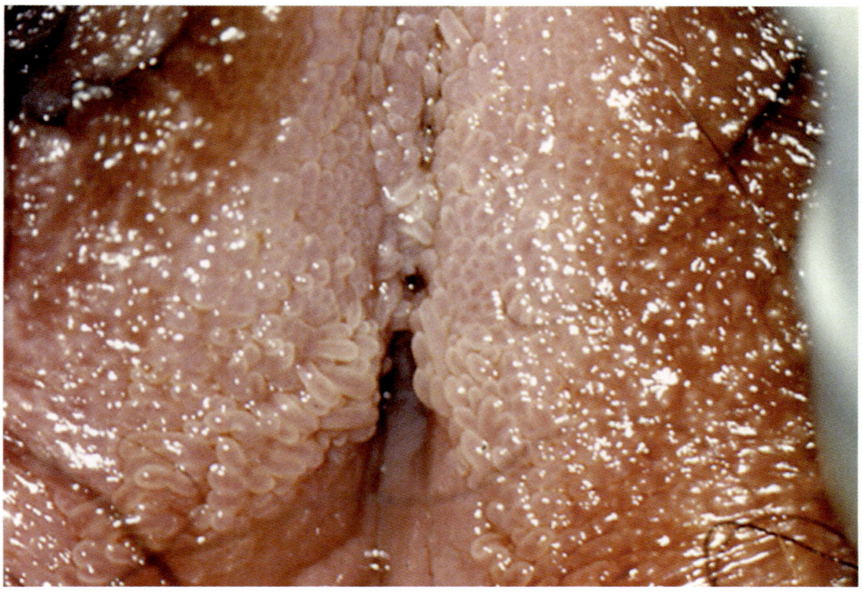

Figure 157 - Normal vestibular papillae.

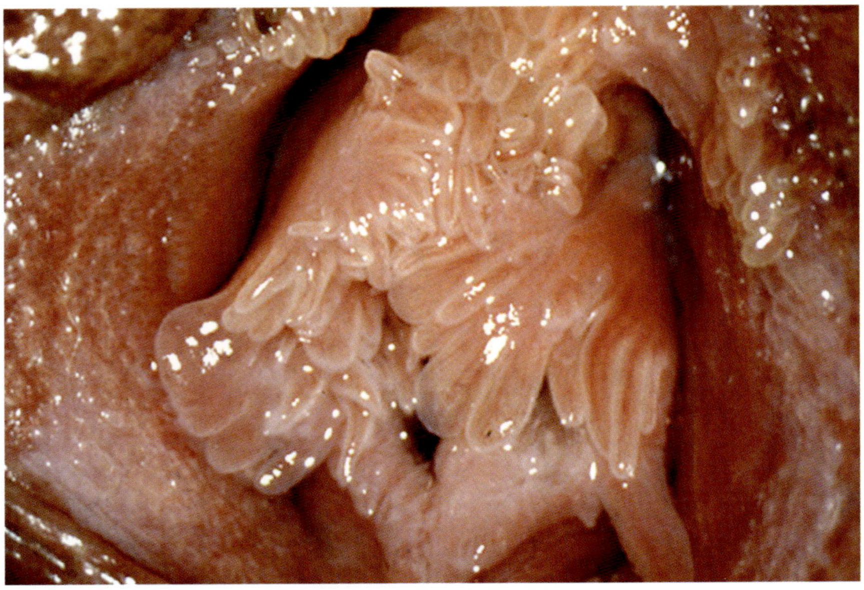

Figure 158 - Hymenal hypertrophic papillae.

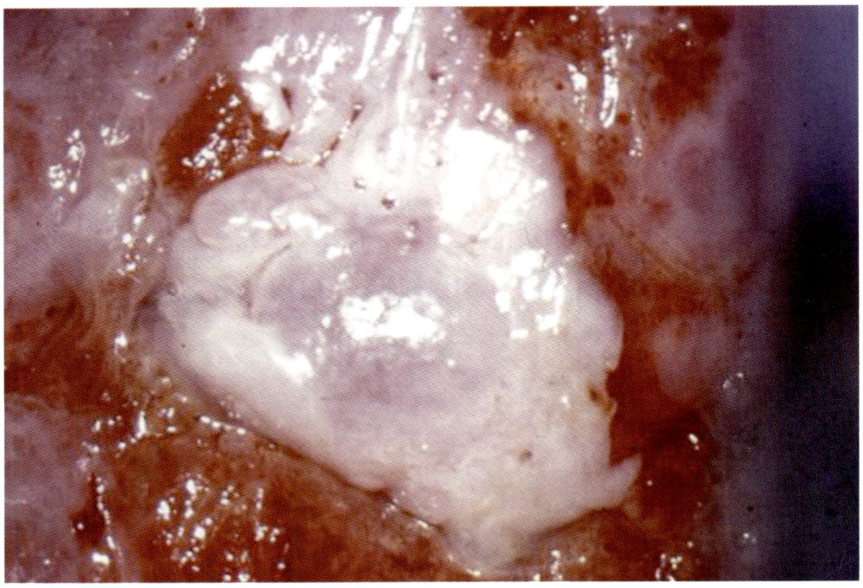

Figure 159 - Dense, chalky acetowhite lesion (CIN 3).

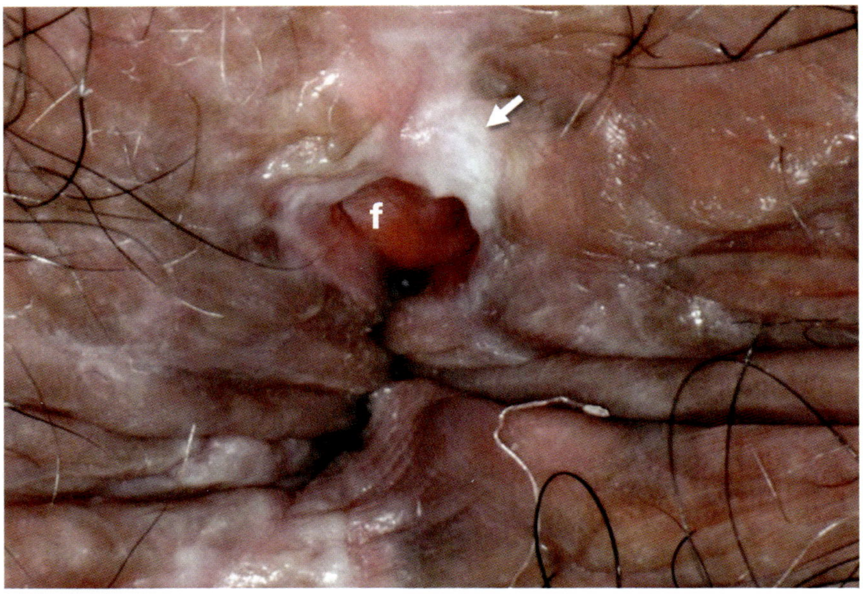

Figure 160 - Perianal intraepithelial lesion (→) and anal fissure (f).

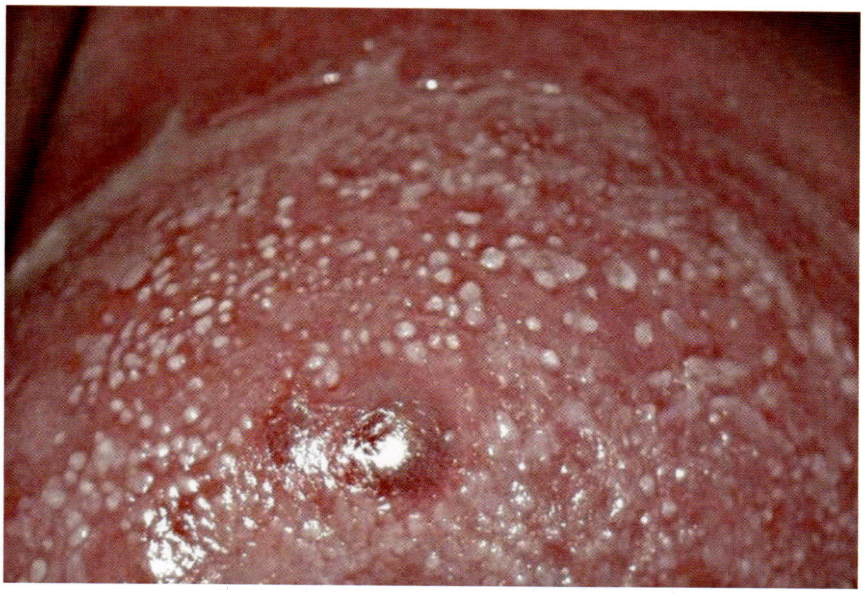

Figure 161 - Coarse and irregular viral white punctation.

vestibular (Figure 157) or hymenal (Figure 158) papillae which represent a variant in normal epithelium and may be caused by constant rubbing, even when they whiten after application of acetic acid.
Flat lesions are diagnosed colposcopically or by visual inspection with acetic acid (VIA), hence termed as subclinical papillomavirus infection (SPI). Flat lesions may be seen as flat, acetowhite lesions (Figure 159) or white punctation. Care must be taken with perianal acetowhite lesions because they may harbour intraepithelial lesions (Figure 160).
Viral white punctation (Figure 161) differs from fungal and metaplastic white punctation as it appears coarse and irregular.

Herpes Simplex Virus

Herpes Simplex Virus 1 and 2 (HSV-1 and HSV-2) belong to the large family of DNA viruses known as Herpesviruses and cause herpes simplex virus infection or simply herpes.
Cell changes induced by HSV are:

- polykaryocyte
- "ground glass" nuclei
- multiple intranuclear inclusions.

The *polykaryocyte* is a syncytium deriving from the merging of several cells (Figures 162a, 163), as a consequence to the introduction of virus-specific proteins in the cytoplasmic membranes of the infected cells. Once the syncytium is formed, nuclei are free in the cytoplasm but tend to gather (Figures 162b, 164). Finally, nuclei appear moulded, resembling a blackberry, and form the polykaryocyte (Figures 162c, 165).
After staining, *ground glass nuclei* appear hypochromatic due to the granular dispersion of the chromatin which is coarsely amassed on the nuclear membrane, whereas the nucleolus disappears. This finding depends on the increased production of deoxyribonucleic protein. The "ground glass" nucleus must be contrasted from the pale karyolitic nucleus due to degenerative changes, where one or two small nucleoli are always present.
Intranuclear inclusions (Figures 162c, 164) indicate a late stage of cell changes induced by HSV, after viral particles have left the cell; inclusions consist of residual nuclear material.
How can we differentiate multinucleation induced by HSV from multiple nuclei that may be encountered in Human Papillomavirus infection? Nuclei affected by HSV (Figure 166) often contain coarse intranuclear inclusions and always appear pale, with a "ground glass" aspect. On the contrary, HPV infection does not show hypochromatic nuclei, as they appear dark for condensed chromatin.
Herpes can involve the skin or mucous membranes of the mouth, lips, nose or genitals. HSV-1, also known as orolabial herpes, can cause fever blisters and cold sores around the mouth and on the face. HSV-2 is generally responsible for *genital*

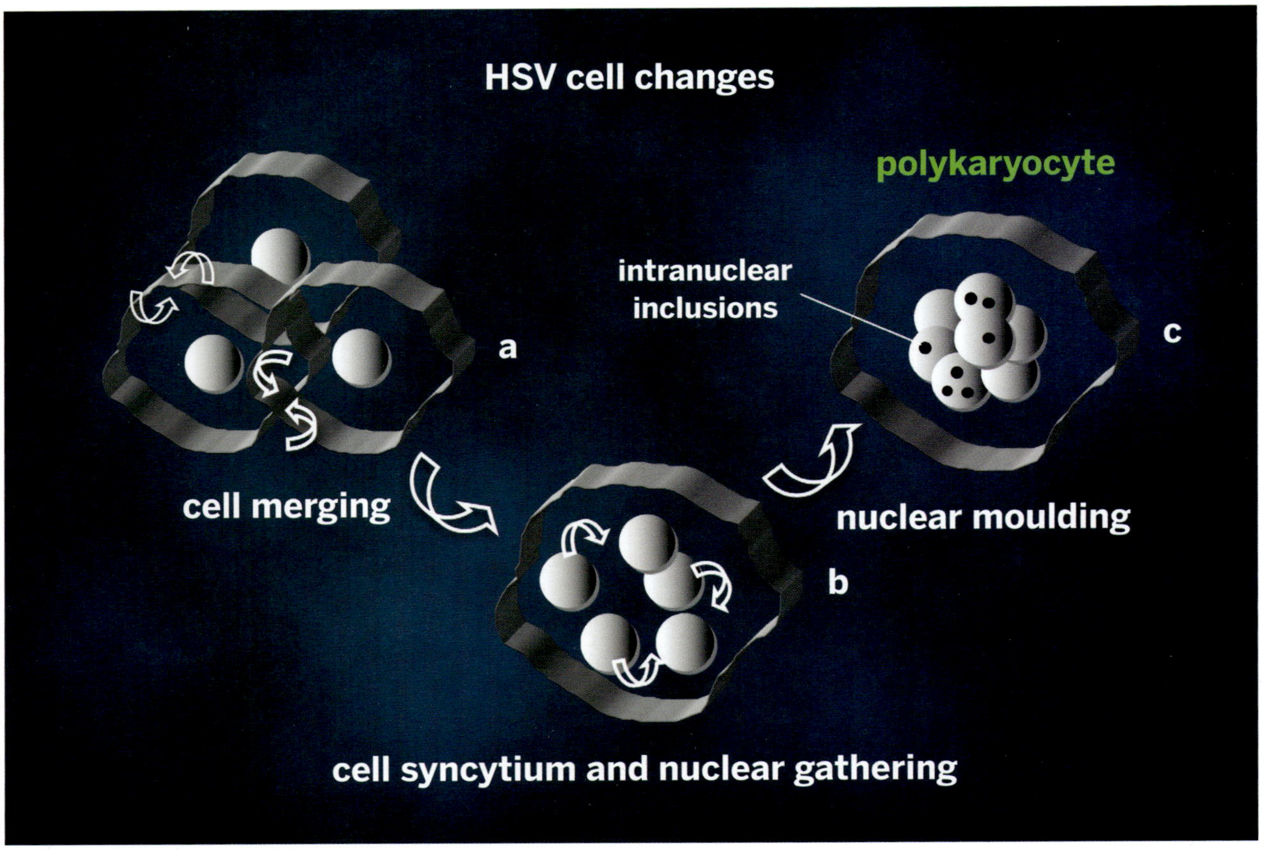

Figure 162 - Diagrammatic representation of cell changes induced by HSV.

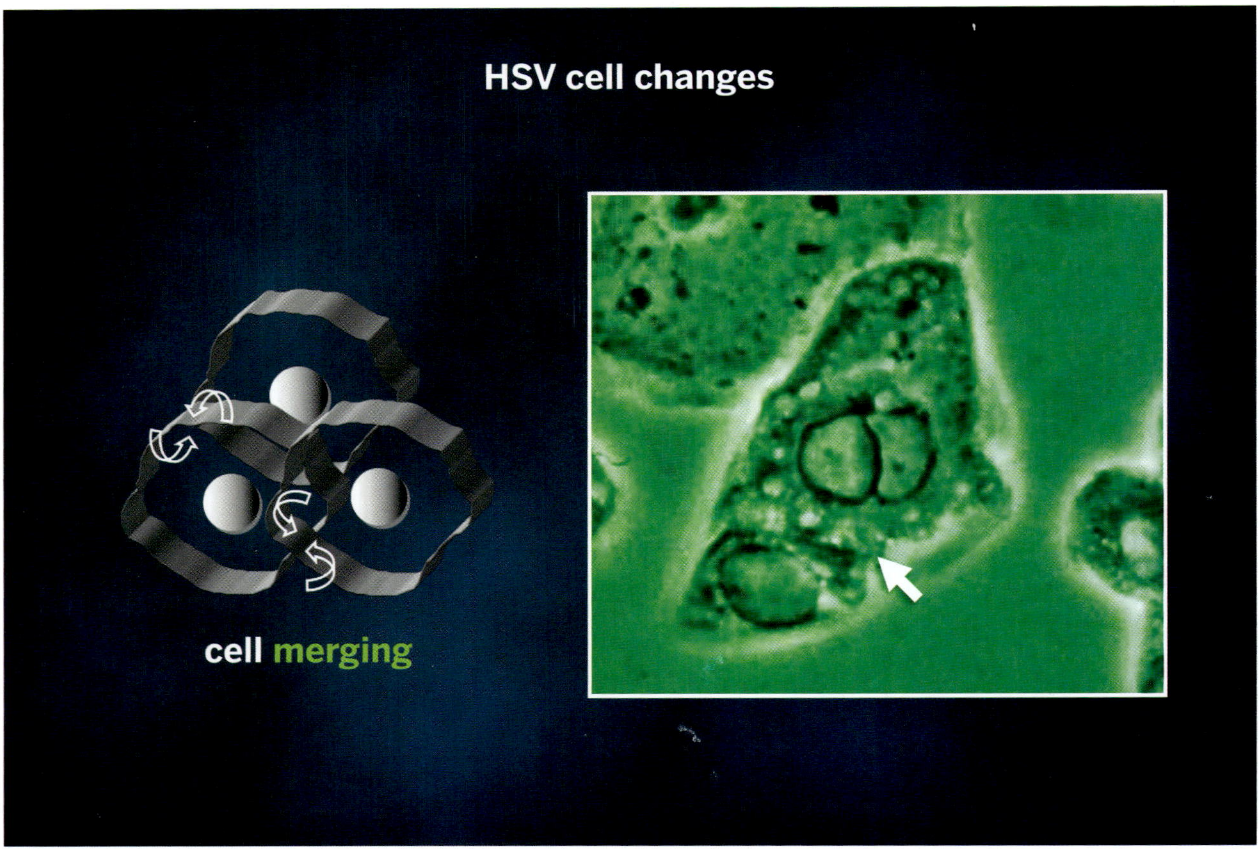

Figure 163 - Cell merging and formation of a cell syncytium.

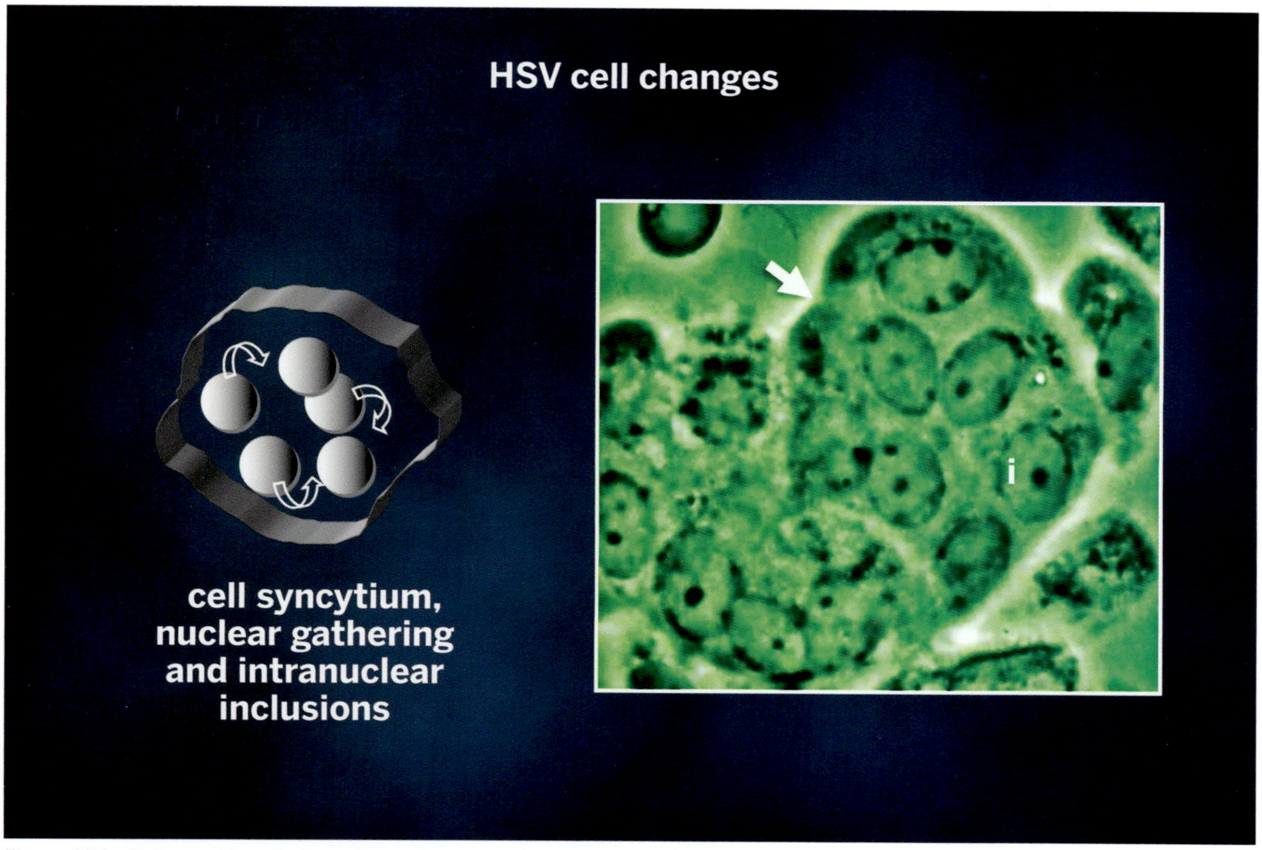

Figure 164 - Cell syncytium (→), nuclear gathering and intranuclear inclusions (i).

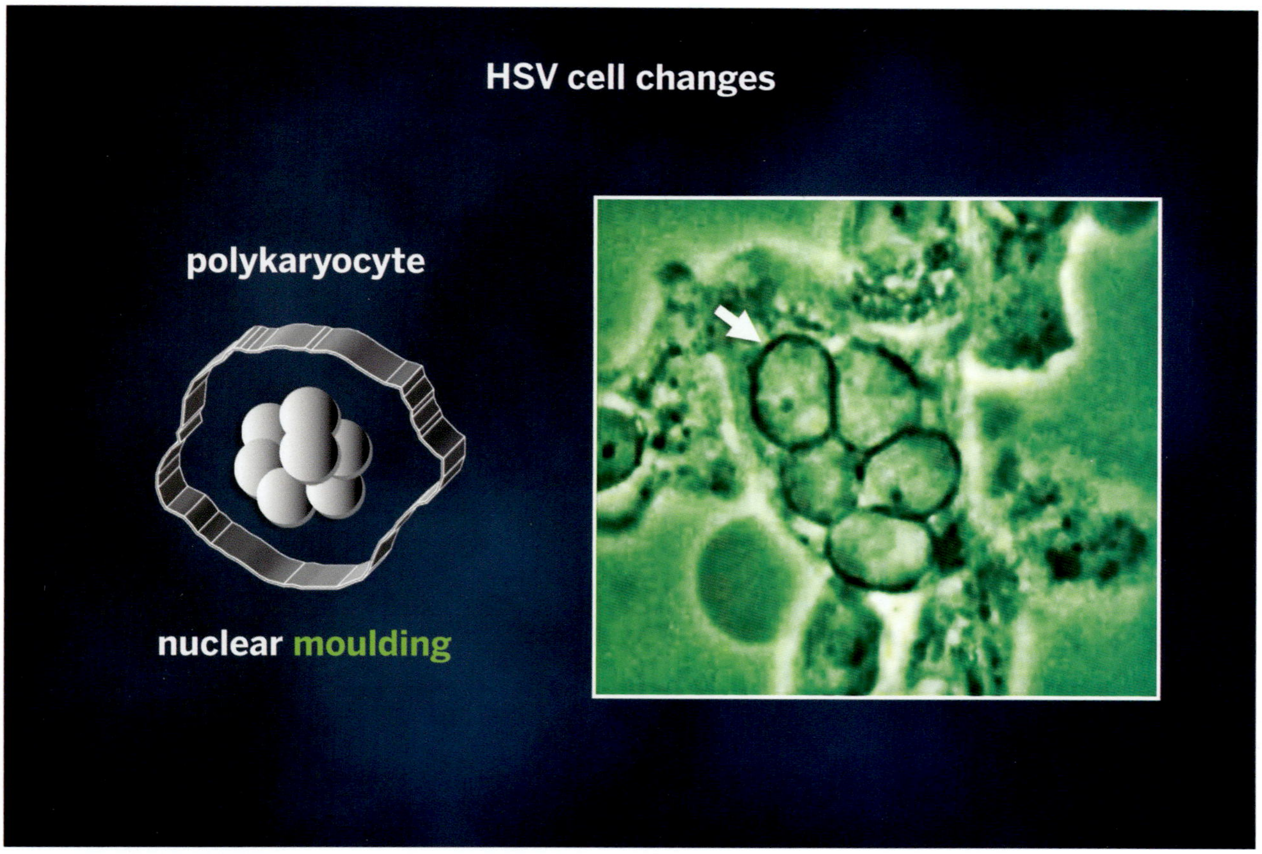

Figure 165 - Polykaryocyte.

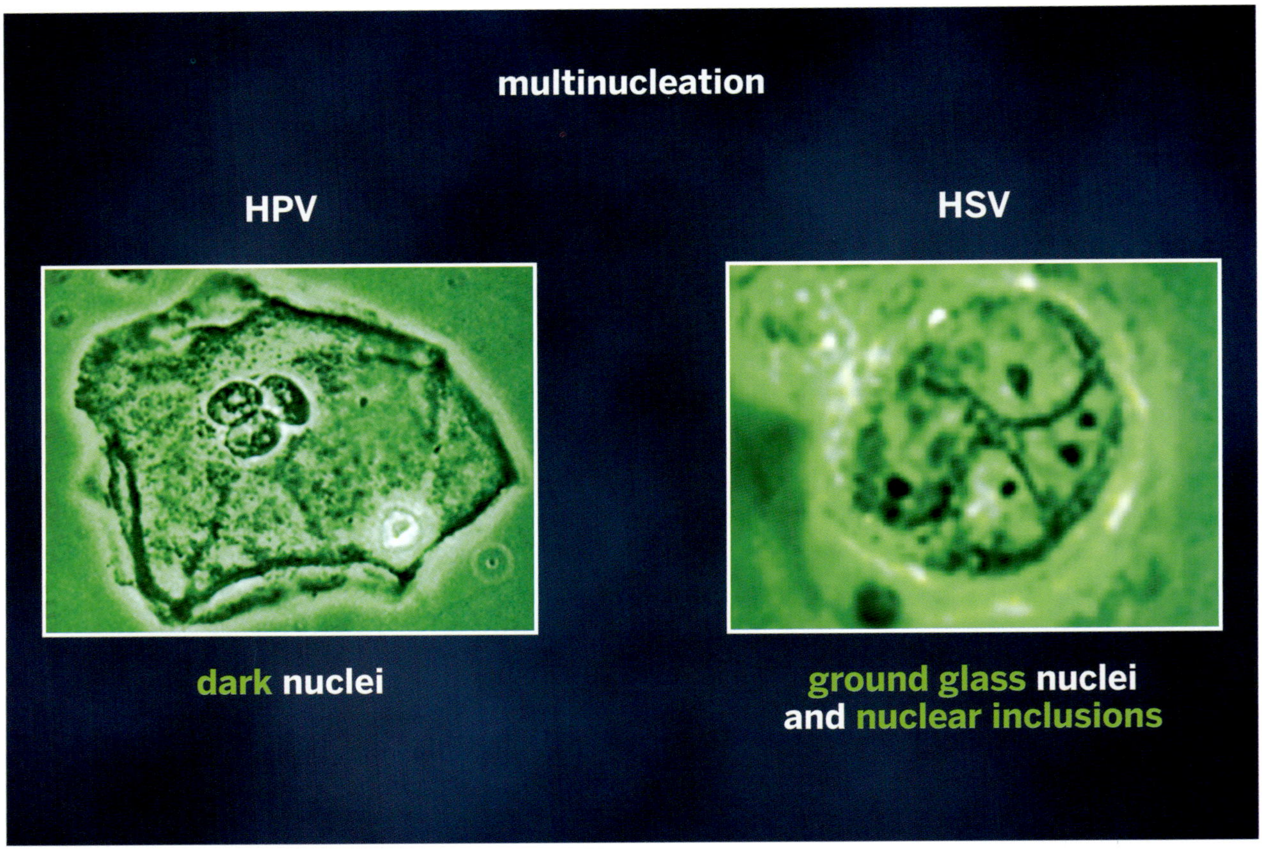

Figure 166 - Differential diagnosis of multinucleation.

herpes outbreaks. However, each serotype can cause the disease to manifest in either location. Genital herpes infections are extremely common worldwide and more than 90% of adults have been infected by at least one of these viruses. After the initial or *primary* infection, some infected people experience sporadic episodes of viral reactivation. Most people with HSV-2 do not realize that they are infected because they experience no symptoms at all, or barely noticeable symptoms that go unrecognized or are mistaken for different conditions, like insect bite or rash.

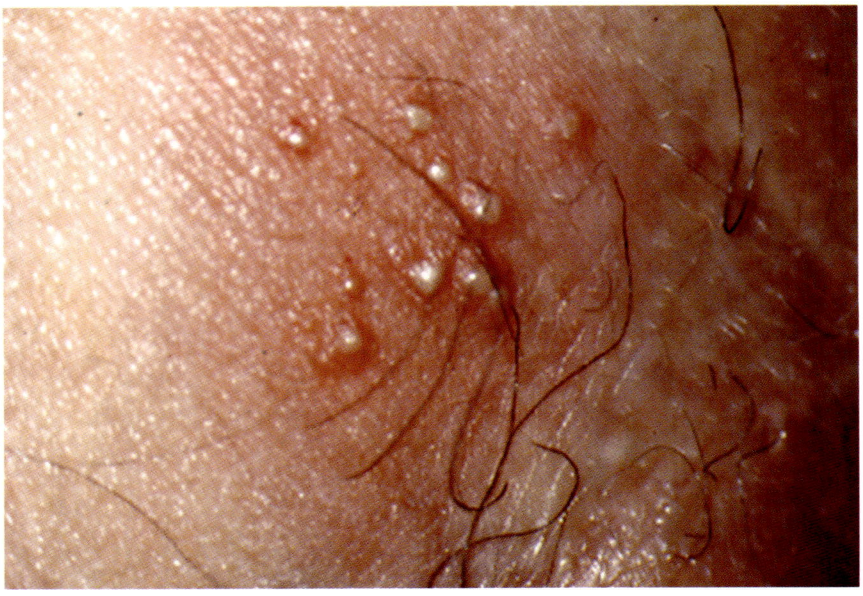

Figure 167 - Vulvar blisters by HSV.

During the first outbreak, some people experience flu-like symptoms including fever, swollen lymph nodes (near the groin), headache, muscle aches, tiredness, nausea and lack of appetite. Urogenital symptoms may be present in form of painful urination, abnormal vaginal discharge and tingling, burning or itching sensation in the area where blisters will appear. Genital herpes symptoms usually develop about 1-2 weeks after exposure to an infected person. Sometimes a shooting pain may precede the appearance of blisters. In women, these blisters can appear on the labia, inside the vagina and on the cervix, groin (Figure 167) and thighs, on the buttocks and around the anus. During genital herpes infection, vagina and cervix may appear inflamed or may exhibit blisters surrounded by a hyperemic area (Figures 168, 169).

Later blisters open into sore ulcers, involving genital skin (Figures 170, 171) and labia. As the outbreak progresses, the ulcers turn into scabs and heal without causing any scarring. These lesions may take from two to four weeks to fully heal.

It is possible to develop lesions in areas where there was no direct contact. For example, it is possible for lesions to appear around the anus (Figure 172) without having had anal sex.

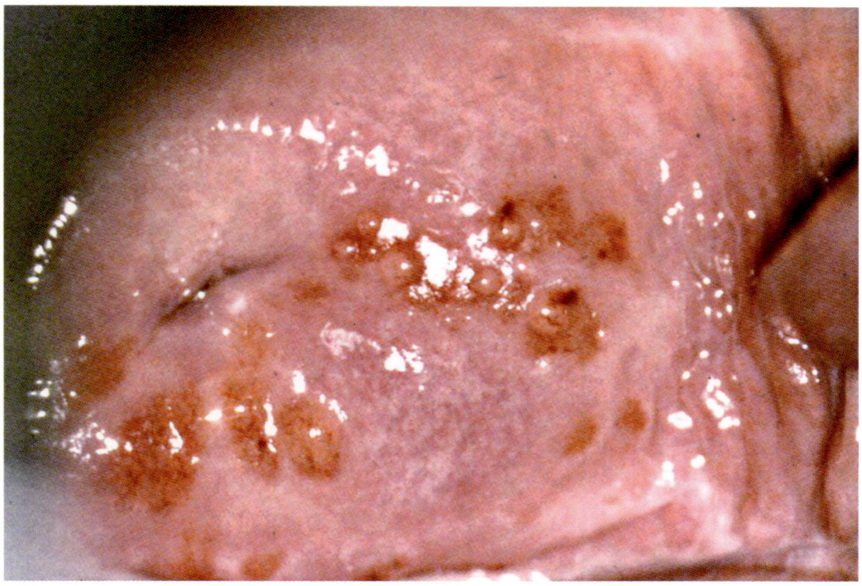

Figure 168 - Cervical blisters with hyperemic base by HSV.

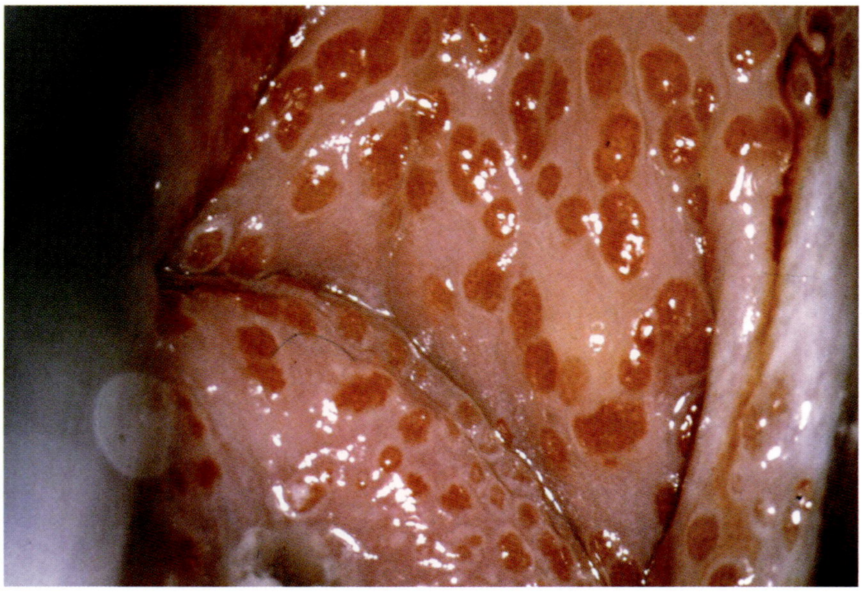

Figure 169 - Blisters with hyperemic base by HSV involving cervix and vagina.

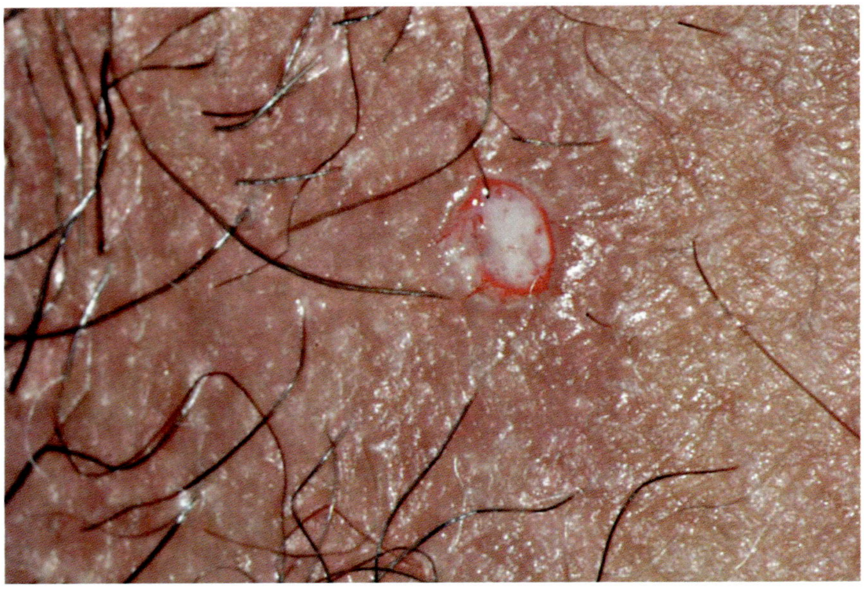

Figure 170 - HSV sore on genital skin.

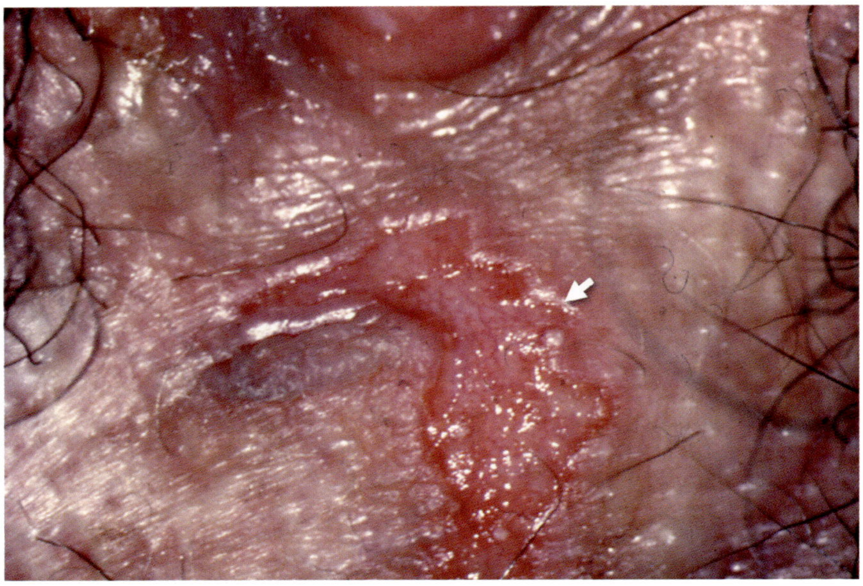

Figure 171 - HSV sore (→) involving perineal area.

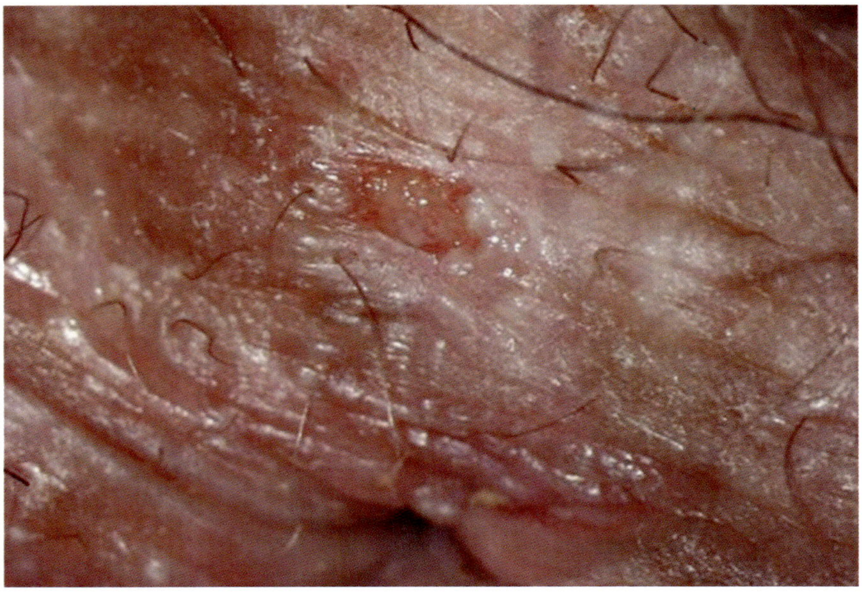

Figure 172 - HSV perianal sore.

Cytomegalovirus

Cytomegalovirus (CMV) infection is a common herpesvirus infection. Over half of adults by age 40 have been infected with CMV. This virus is easily spread through sexual and nonsexual contact with body secretions. Once the virus enters a person's body, it stays there for life and may reactivate. All herpesviruses share a characteristic ability to remain latent within the body over long periods.

Cytomegalovirus is responsible for a single and large intranuclear inclusion body which gives the nucleus a characteristic aspect of "owl's eye" (Figure 173). There is usually some clearing around the inclusion and the chromatin tends to condense around the peripheral area of the nucleus. Owl's eye appearance of intranuclear inclusion body is highly specific for CMV infection.

Although the virus may be found throughout the body, CMV infection is frequently associated with the salivary glands. People infected with CMV show a wide range of symptoms: from no symptoms to fever and fatigue (resembling infectious mononucleosis) to severe symptoms involving the eyes, the brain, or other internal organs.

This infection can cause serious health problems for patients with weakened cell-mediated immunity, as well as babies infected with CMV before they are born (congenital CMV). In fact, cytomegalovirus remains the most common congenital infection worldwide, with approximately 1% of all newborns infected in utero. Of those infected in utero, approximately 10% will show signs and symptoms of cytomegalovirus infection at birth and develop sequelae, especially mental retardation, hearing deficit, or both. CMV infection has been associated with an increased risk of in situ/invasive carcinoma development, as a cofactor to high-risk types of Human Papillomavirus.

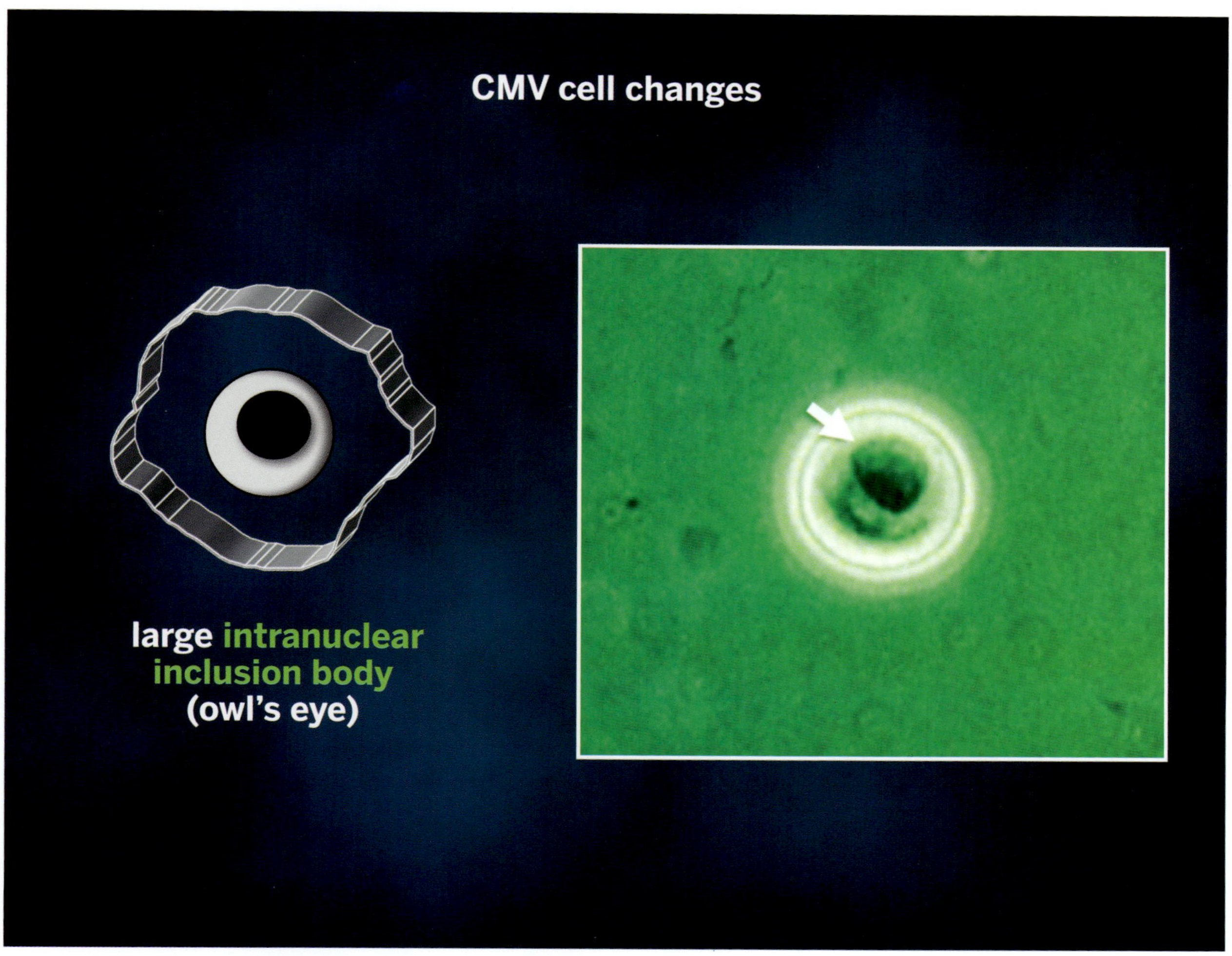

Figure 173 - Large intranuclear inclusion (→) by CMV (owl's eye).

Squamous metaplasia

Metaplasia is usually an adaptive change that occurs in reaction to chronic irritation, or in response to estrogen stimuli.

The cervix is composed by two regions (Figure 174): the ectocervix and the endocervix. The ectocervix is lined by a nonkeratinized stratified squamous epithelium, whereas the endocervix is lined by a monolayered columnar epithelium. There is a sharp border between these two regions, called squamocolumnar junction (SCJ) because it clearly separates squamous epithelium from columnar epithelium.

The squamocolumnar junction is not static because high levels of estrogens are responsible for the eversion of the cervical os, which in turn causes the fragile glandular epithelium to be exposed to a more acidic environment in the vagina. This eversion, or ectropion, is sometimes incorrectly referred to as a "cervical erosion" because of its appearance as a red rim surrounding the cervical os.

Estrogen stimulation may be observed during intrauterine life, menarche, oral contraceptives intake, first pregnancy and luteal insufficiency.

The eversion of the cervical os causes columnar epithelium to be exposed (Figure 175). The stromal papillae of the ectopic columnar epithelium have a grape-like aspect. Within the endocervix itself, the papillae are broader and less grape-like in appearance. After the application of acetic acid, columnar grape-like villi of the ectopic columnar epithelium whiten and are more easily recognized.

Phase contrast microscopy enables an immediate evaluation of different cell stages through which metaplasia takes place.

The low ph of vagina causes the shedding of fragile columnar cells on exposed villi (Figure 176) and in a variable time the columnar epithelium is replaced by a newly developed tissue, called *immature metaplastic epithelium*.

This immature metaplastic epithelium (Figure 177) may turn into a typical mature metaplastic epithelium and the area where this transformation occurs is

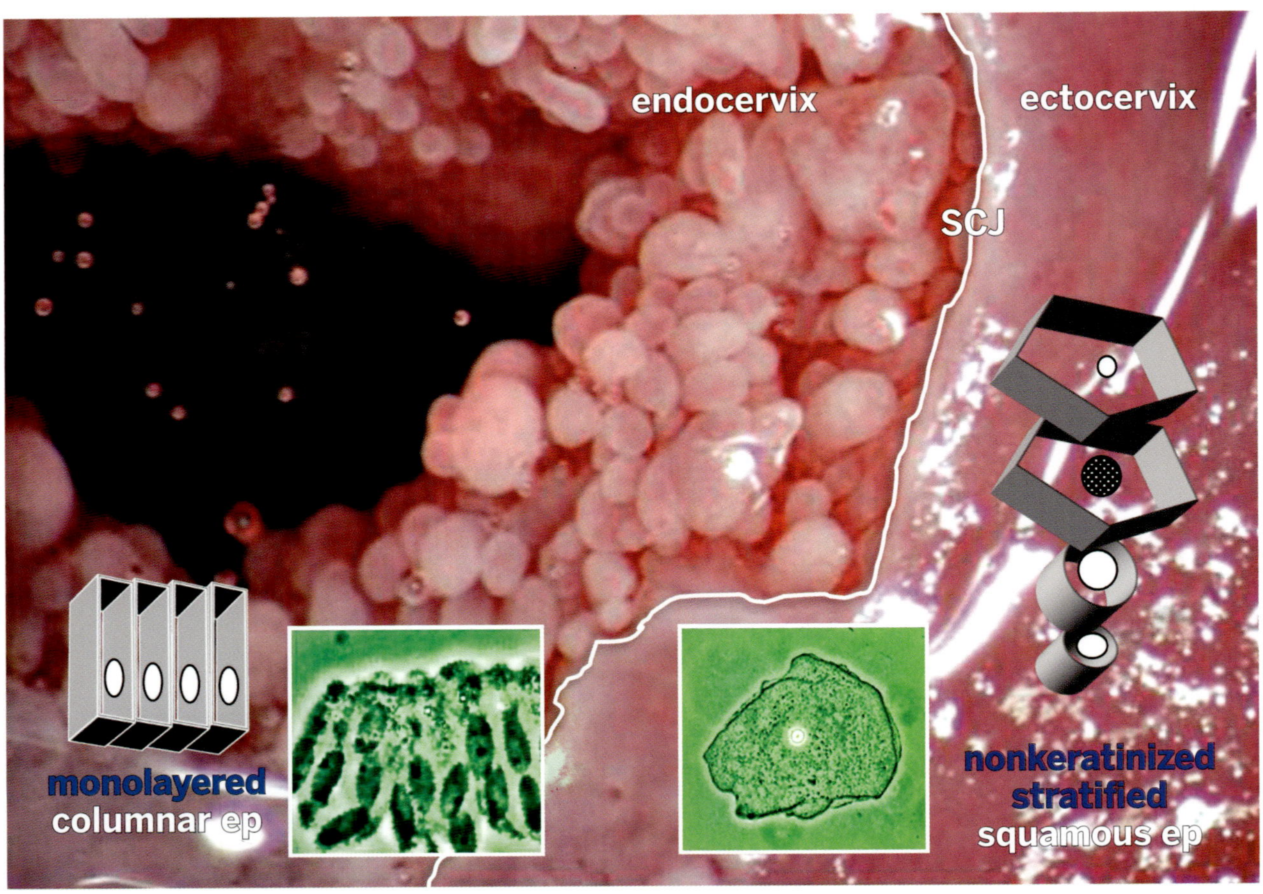

Figure 174 - Regions of the cervix and lining epithelia.

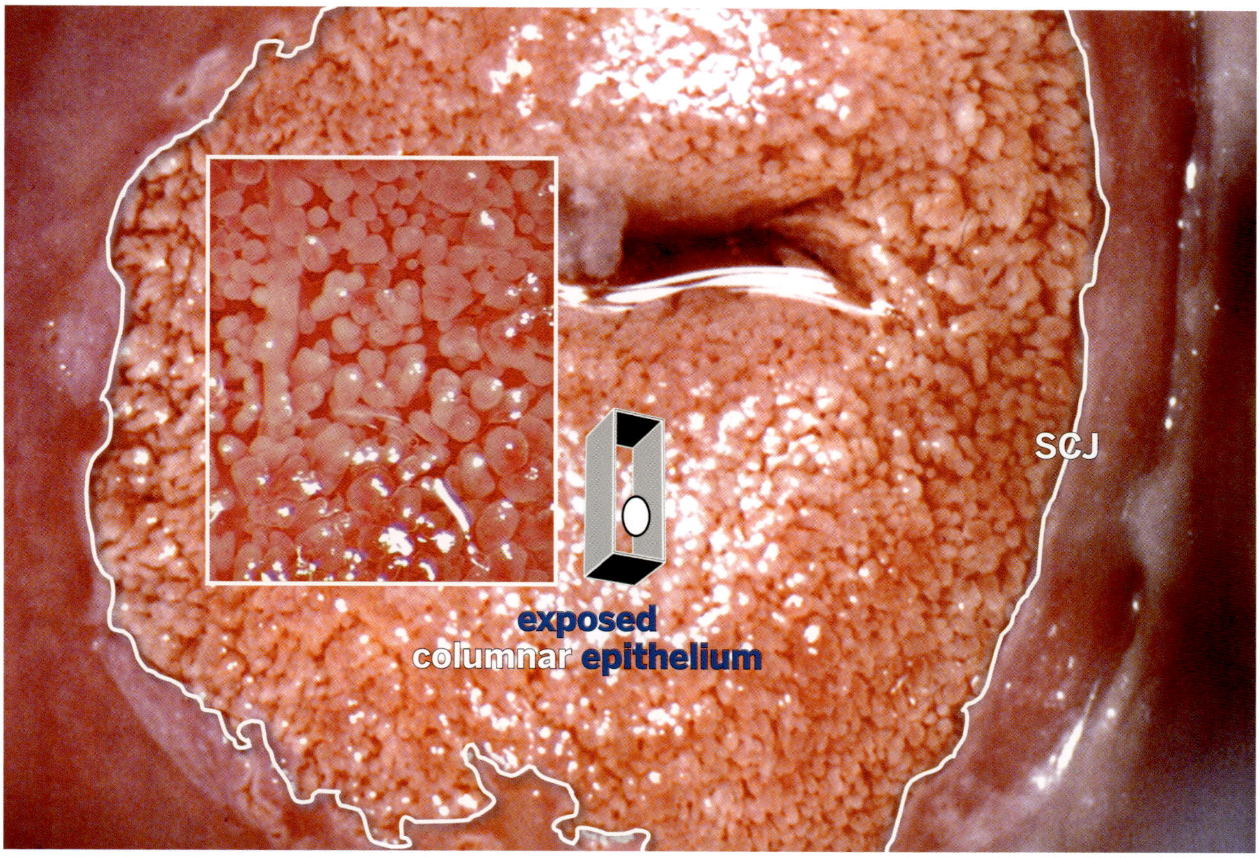

Figure 175 - Grape-like aspect of exposed columnar epithelium after application of acetic acid.

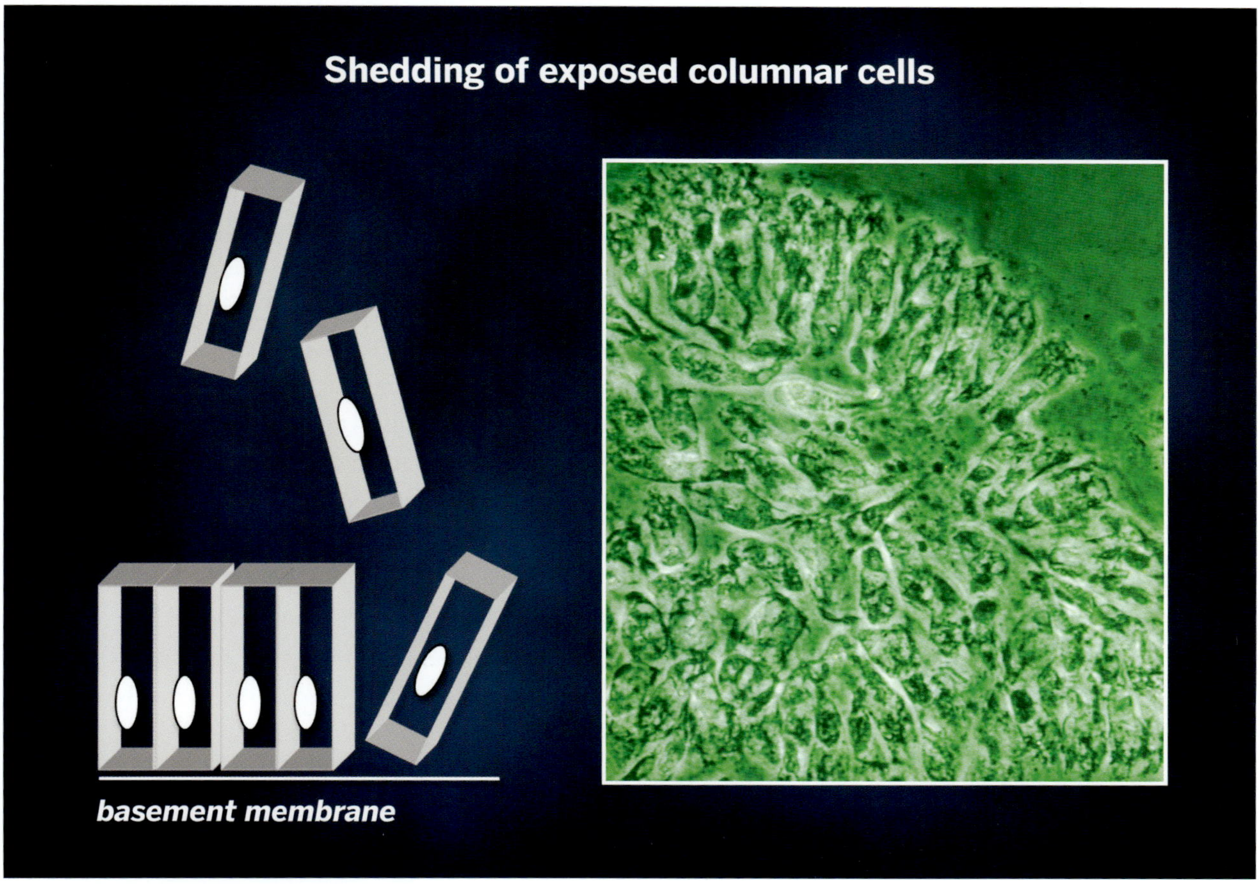

Figure 176 - Shedding of exposed columnar cells.

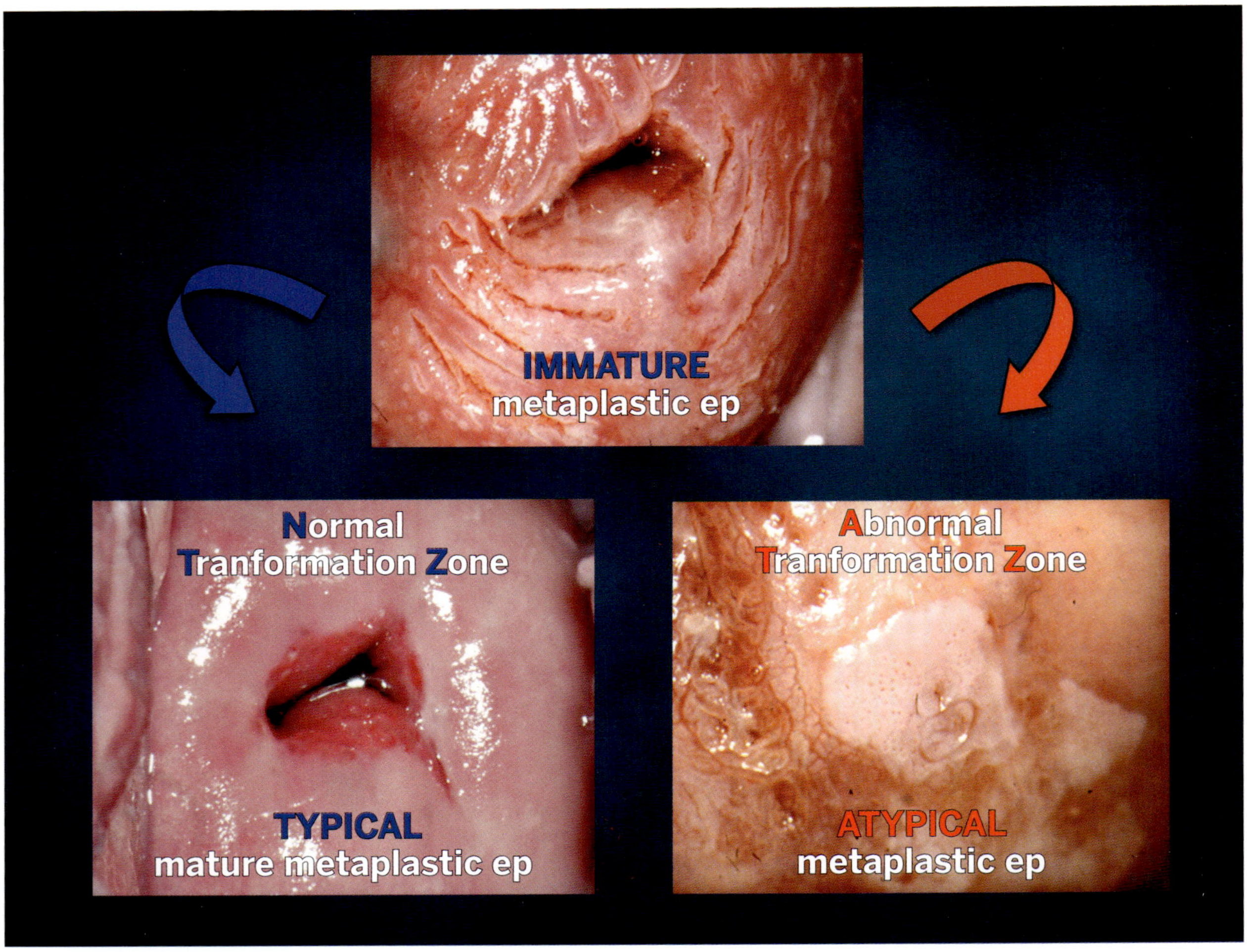

Figure 177 - Evolution of immature metaplastic epithelium.

termed as the normal transformation zone (NTZ). Otherwise, the metaplastic epithelium may become atypical within an abnormal transformation zone (ATZ).

The behaviour of squamous metaplasia holds the key to the understanding of cervical oncogenesis.

At the beginning of the metaplastic process this multilayered but still undifferentiated epithelium caps the villus and causes some opaqueness at the tip of the villus after application of acetic acid (Figure 178). Later, this epithelium extends into the clefts of two adjacent villi, until a smooth surface is produced within the original columnar epithelium (Figure 179). It must be pointed out that wedge-shaped offshoots originating from the original squamocolumnar junction that finally eventually join to intra-junctional metaplastic patches, are called epithelialization (Figure 180).

An excessive surface maturation occurring during metaplastic process may block a cript opening, and thus an epithelial pearl is formed (Figure 181). These benign epithelial pearls must be distinguished from malignant epithelial pearls, characterized by concentric cells different in shape and containing abnormal nuclei (Figure 182).

The acetowhite metaplastic epithelium over the villi may exceed in height the smooth surface, developing white punctation (Figure 183), colposcopically distinguishable from the other white punctations (fungal and viral) because it appears fine and contiguous to the squamocolumnar junction.

How may a monolayered columnar epithelium turn into a thick stratified squamous tissue?

If we consider columnar villi, each villus contains one or more capillary loops with an overlying single layer of columnar cells. The low vaginal pH causes the shedding of columnar cells.

Squamous metaplasia is preceded by the appearance of cuboidal cells between columnar cells and basement membrane, termed as subcolumnar reserve

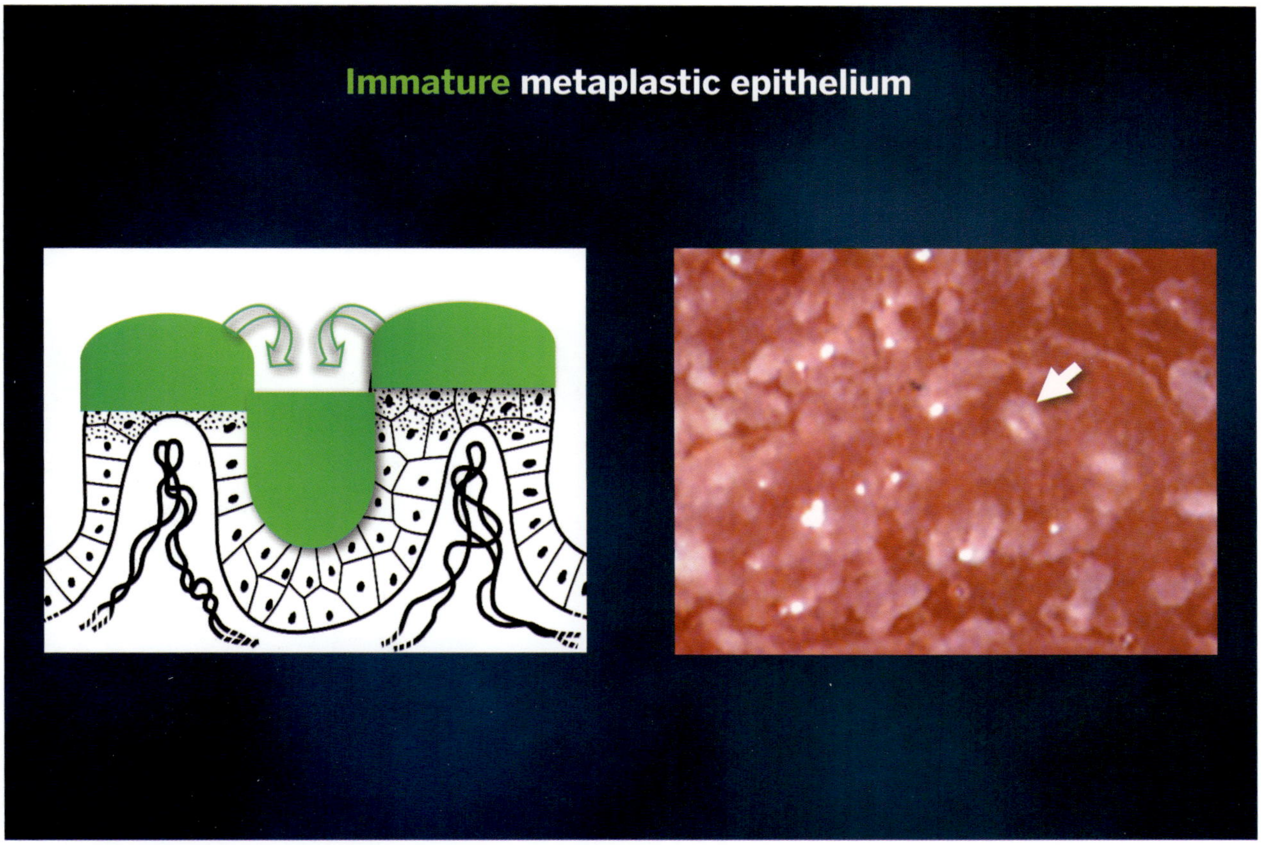

Figure 178 - Acetowhite immature metaplastic epithelium caps the villi (→).

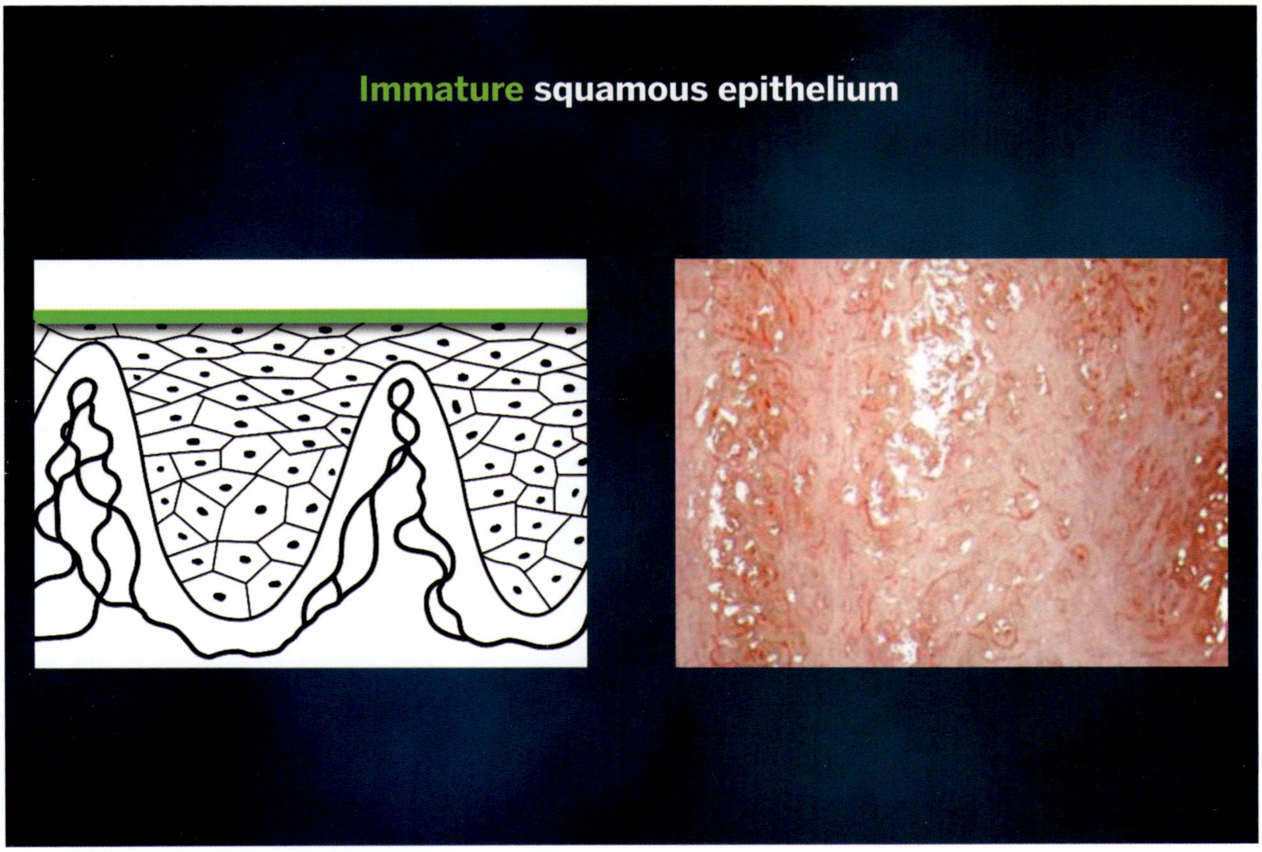

Figure 179 - Smooth immature metaplastic epithelium.

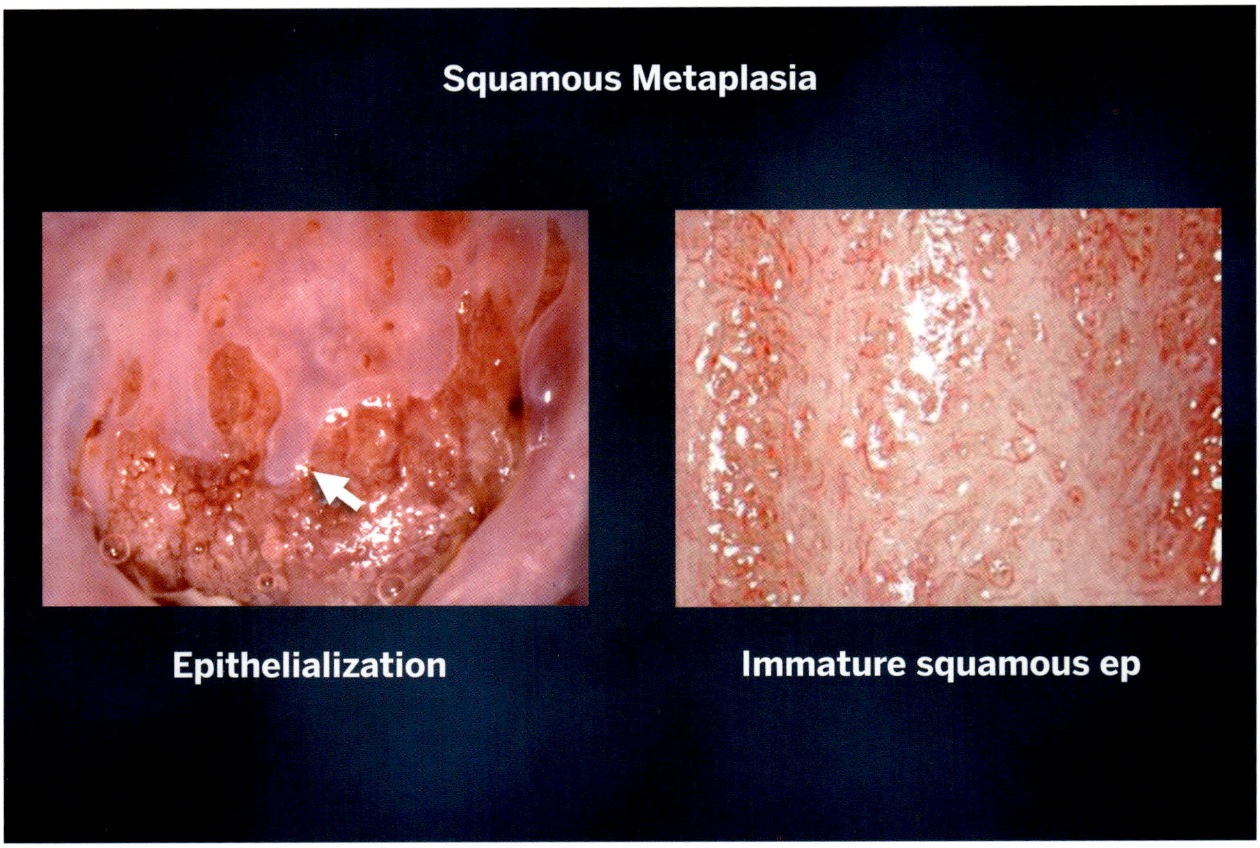

Figure 180 - Difference between epithelialization and immature metaplastic epithelium.

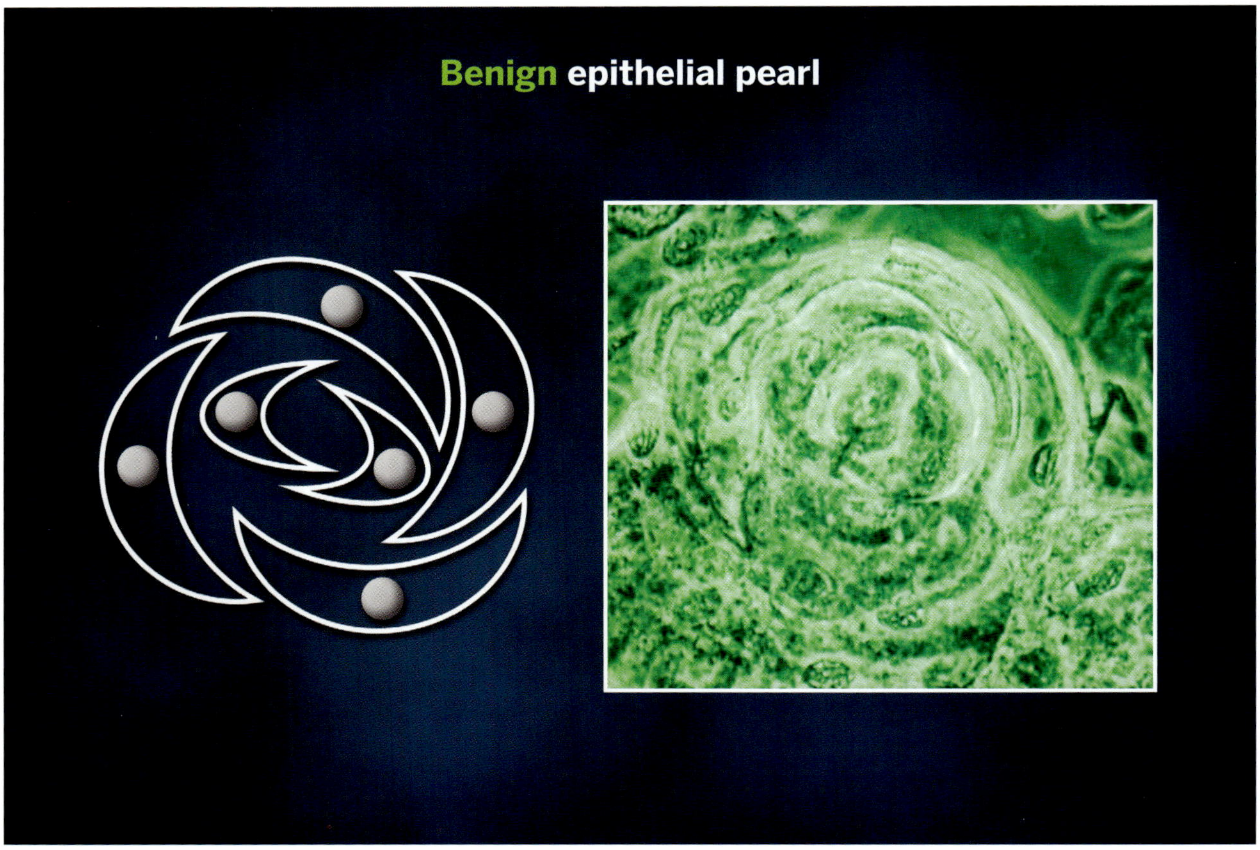

Figure 181 - Benign epithelial pearl.

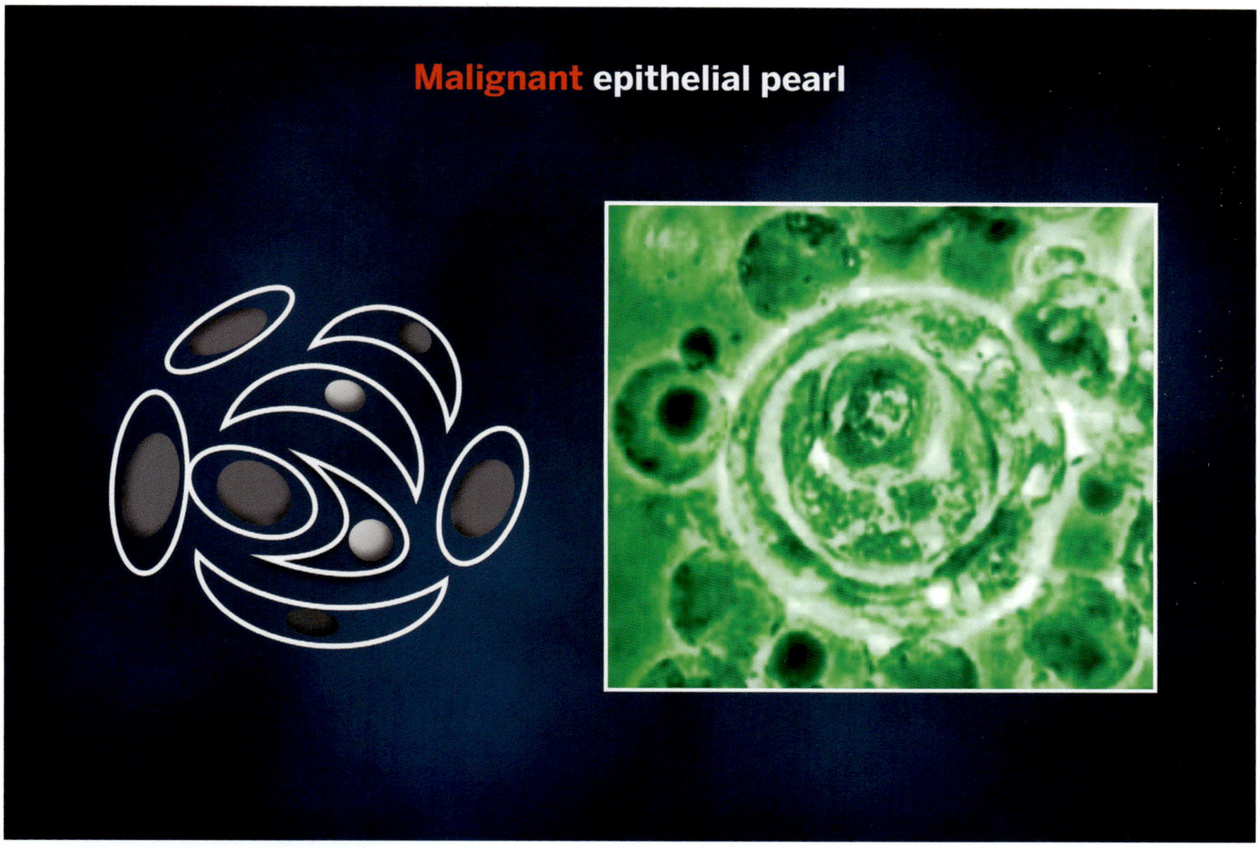

Figure 182 - Malignant epithelial pearl.

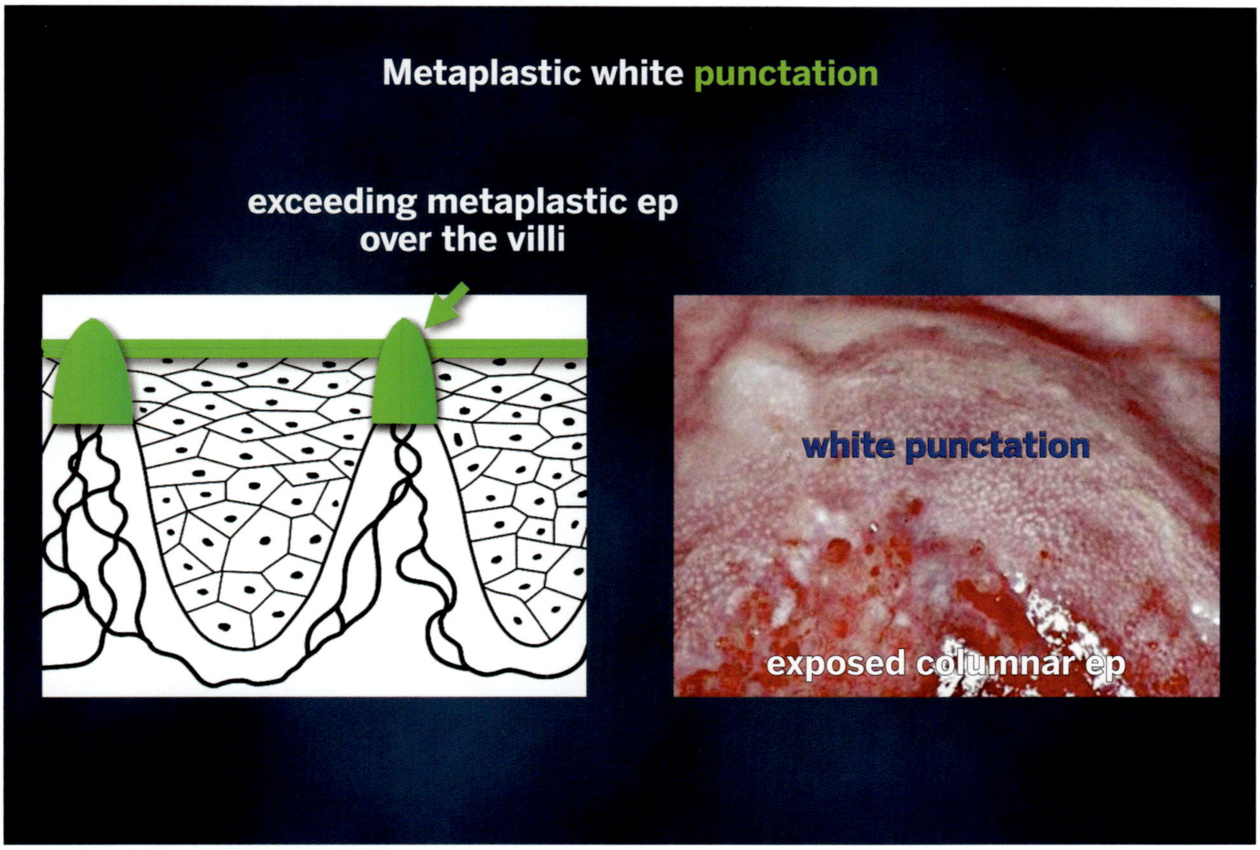

Figure 183 - Formation of metaplastic white punctation.

cells (Figure 184). At the beginning of squamous metaplasia, reserve cells appear interspersed with the predominant columnar cells when seen end on. Later, reserve cells multiply and gradually substitute columnar cells (Figure 185) almost completely. The original columnar epithelium sometimes remains atop these new elements and is later shed.

The following step is represented by the maturation of reserve cells in metaplastic cells which leads to the formation of a multilayered but still undifferentiated epithelium, named as *immature metaplastic epithelium* (Figure 186).

Finally, in normal conditions, this immature epithelium will turn into to a *mature squamous epithelium*, practically indistinguishable from the original squamous epithelium.

What is the composition of immature metaplastic epithelium?

In 1998, the Author proposed his classification of metaplastic maturation. Proceeding from the basement membrane towards the surface, metaplastic maturation is represented by different cell types (Figure 187):

- *Reserve* cell
- *Immature* metaplastic cells
  - Parabasal-like cell
  - Spider cell
  - Tadpole cell
- *Maturing* metaplastic cell
- *Premature* metaplastic cells.

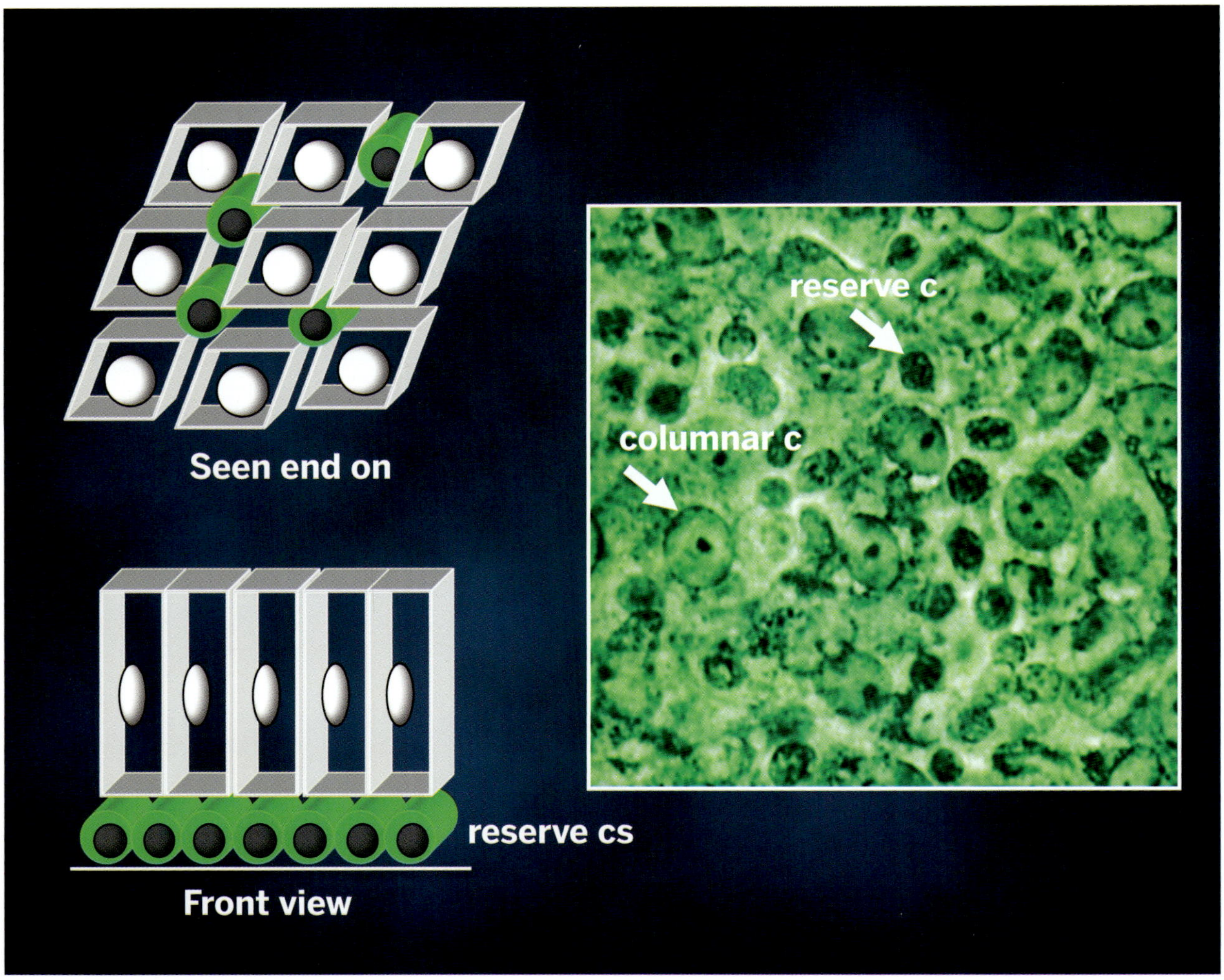

Figure 184 - Few reserve cells are interspersed among predominant columnar cells.

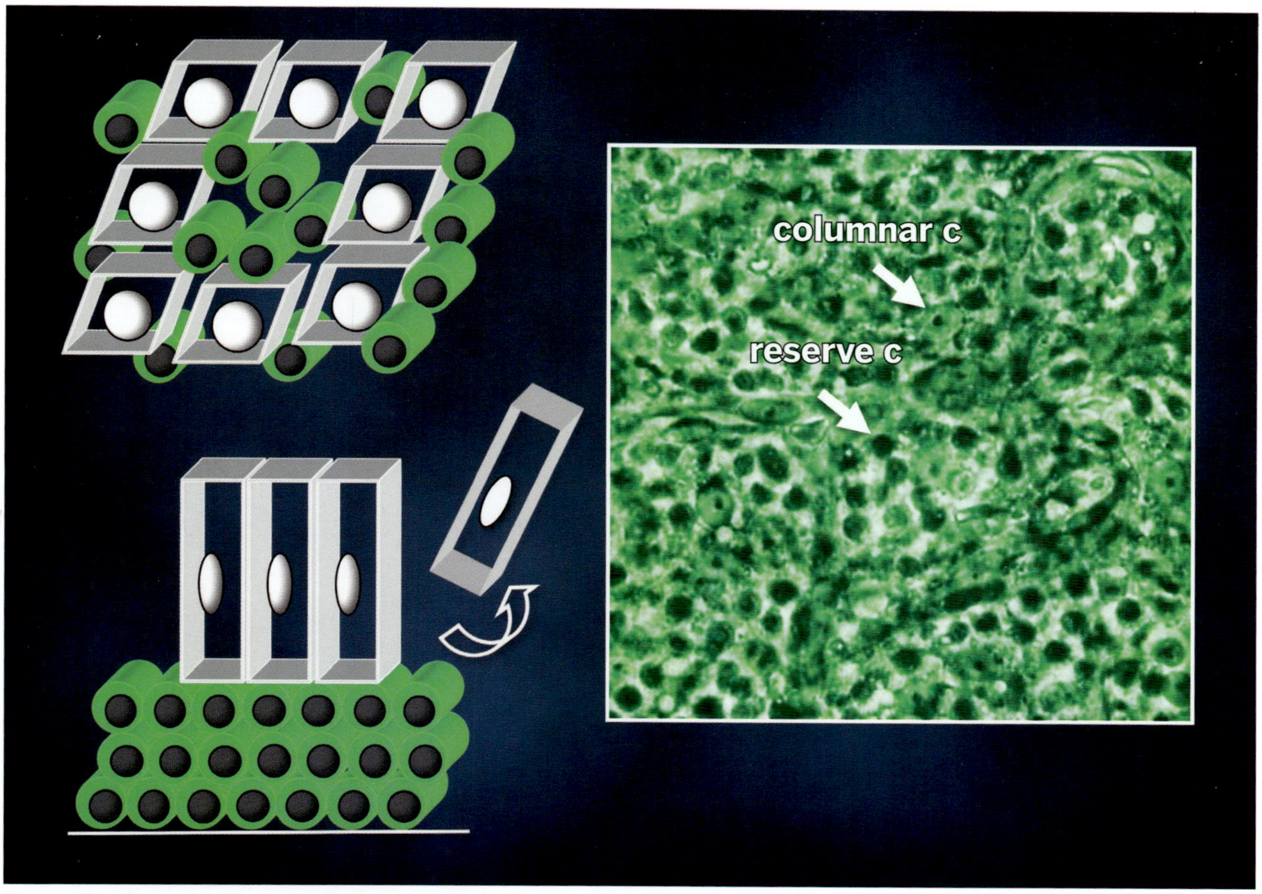

Figure 185 - Reserve cells predominate on residual columnar cells.

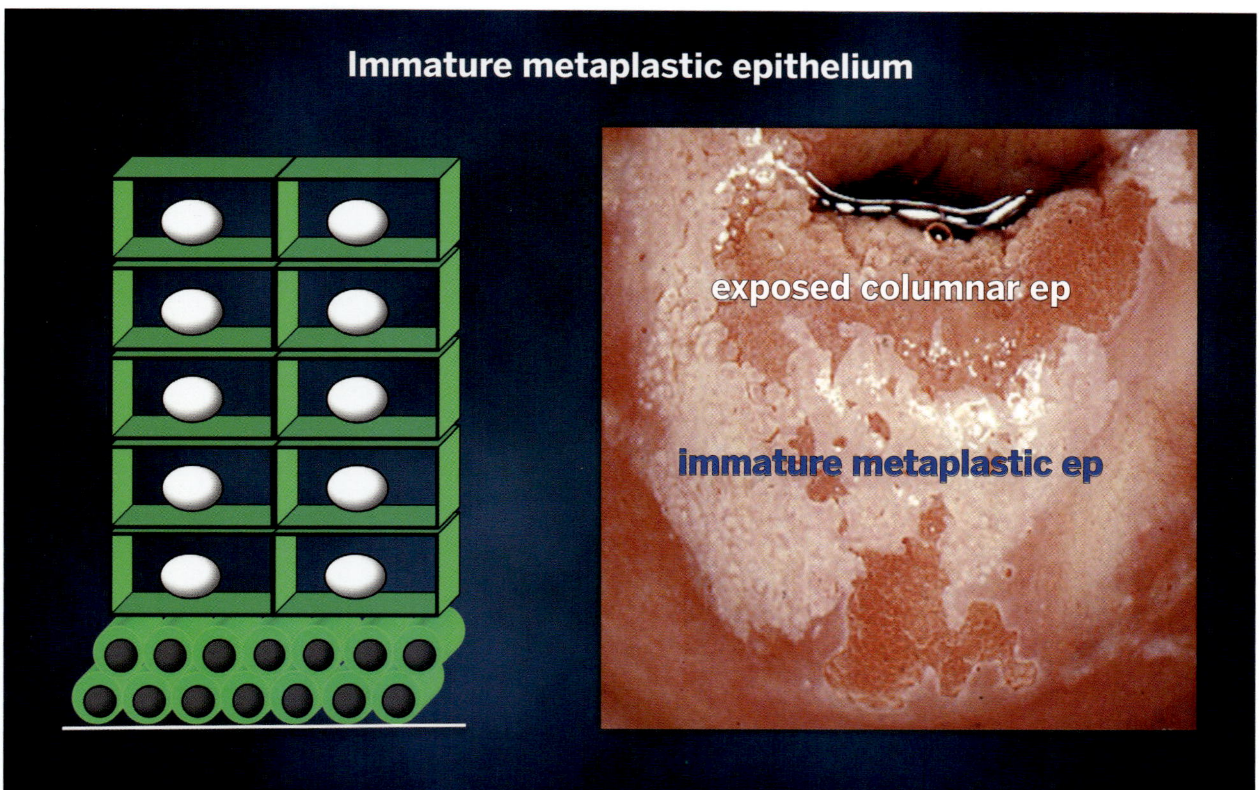

Figure 186 - Stratified but not differentiated immature metaplastic epithelium.

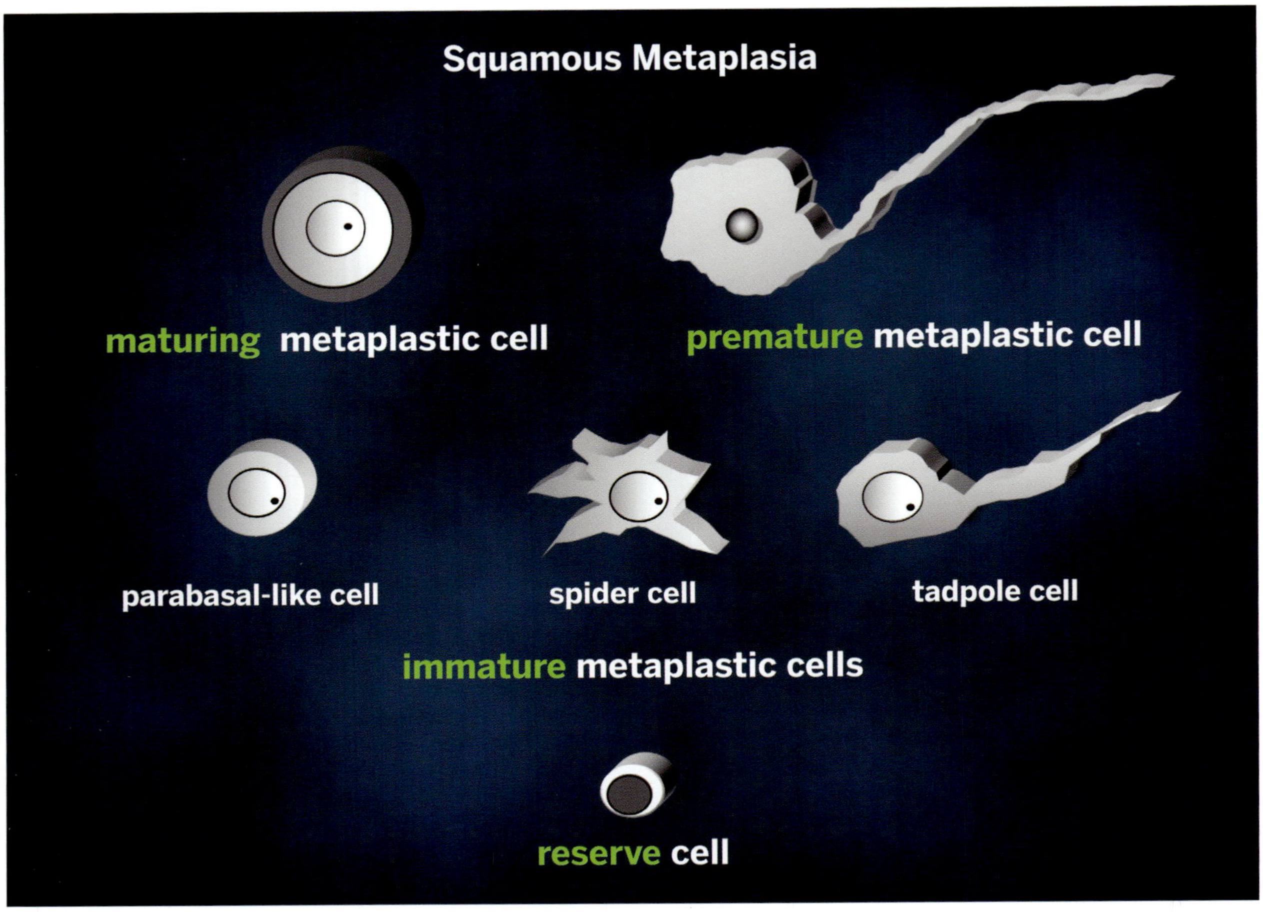

Figure 187 - Diagrammatic representation of squamous metaplasia.

Reserve cells (Figure 188) appear small, roundish and contain a dark and homogeneous nucleus surrounded by a thin cytoplasmic ring. The maturation of reserve cells towards the immature metaplastic cells is revealed by the progressive enlargement of the cell body (Figure 189) and later by the clearing of the nuclear chromatin texture due to granular dispersion (Figure 190).

Immature metaplastic cells show a pale nucleus because of granular dispersion and margination of the chromatin, and an evident nucleolus (immature nucleus). Immature metaplastic cells include three cell types (Figure 187):

- parabasal-like cell
- spider cell
- tadpole cell.

Parabasal-like cells (Figure 191) are quite similar to parabasal cells belonging to squamous epithelium, but they can be easily differentiated because the latter are deeply nestled in the thick squamous epithelium, overlayed by intermediate and superficial cells, and cannot be shed.

Spider cells show multiple spider-like cytoplasmic projections (Figure 192). Spider cells may appear connected through their cytoplasmic processes (Figure 193).

Tadpole cells exhibit a long, single cytoplasmic projection (Figure 194). These cytoplasmic processes may be so long, that they cross the entire epithelial thickness (Figure 195).

Maturing metaplastic cells (Figure 196) show the same nuclear patterns of immature metaplastic cells, but are easily detectable in wet mount preparations for a characteristic sharp border between the dark viscous esoplasmic ring and the pale endoplasmic area. Before turning into a premature cell, the viscous esoplasmic ring gets progressively clearer (Figure 197).

The immature metaplastic cells and maturing metaplastic cells, although keeping part of their characteristic morphology, become larger and turn into

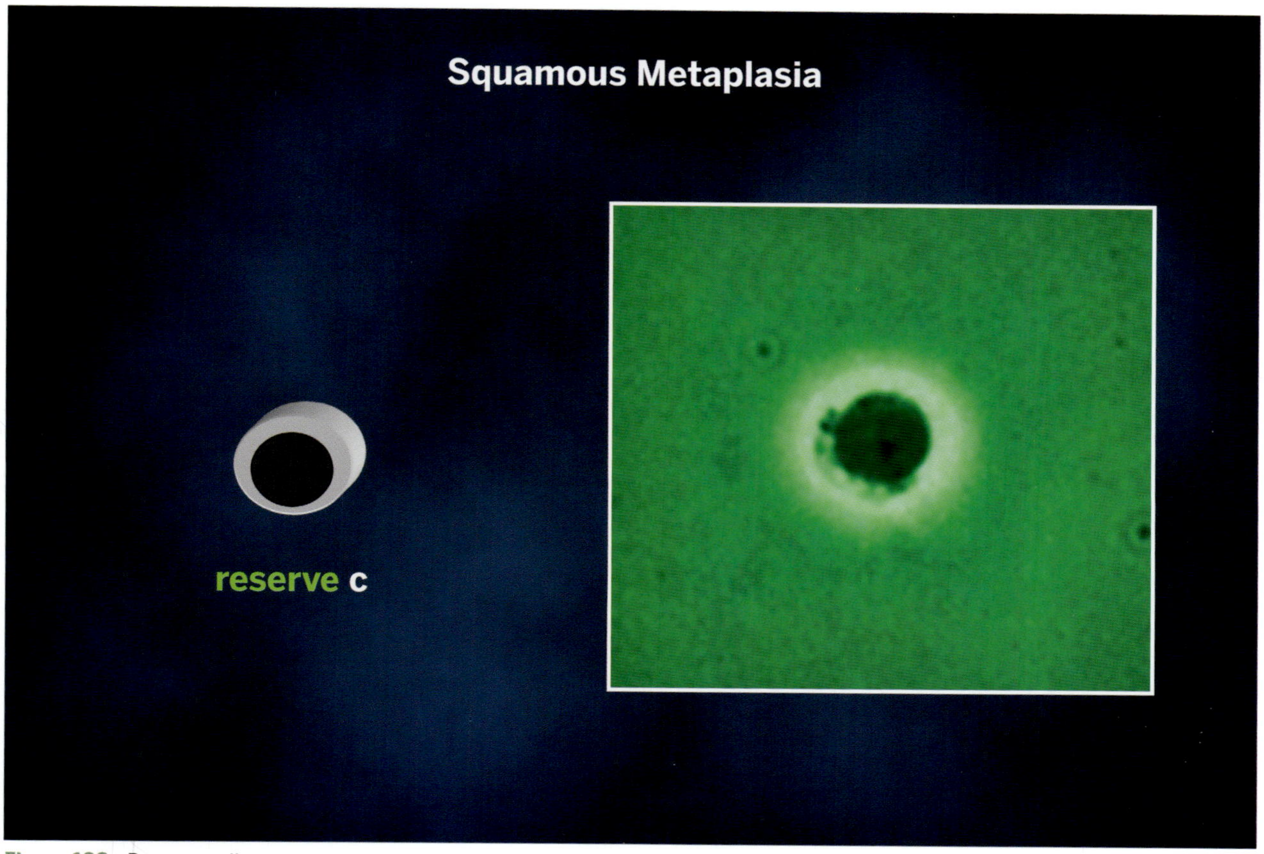

Figure 188 - Reserve cell.

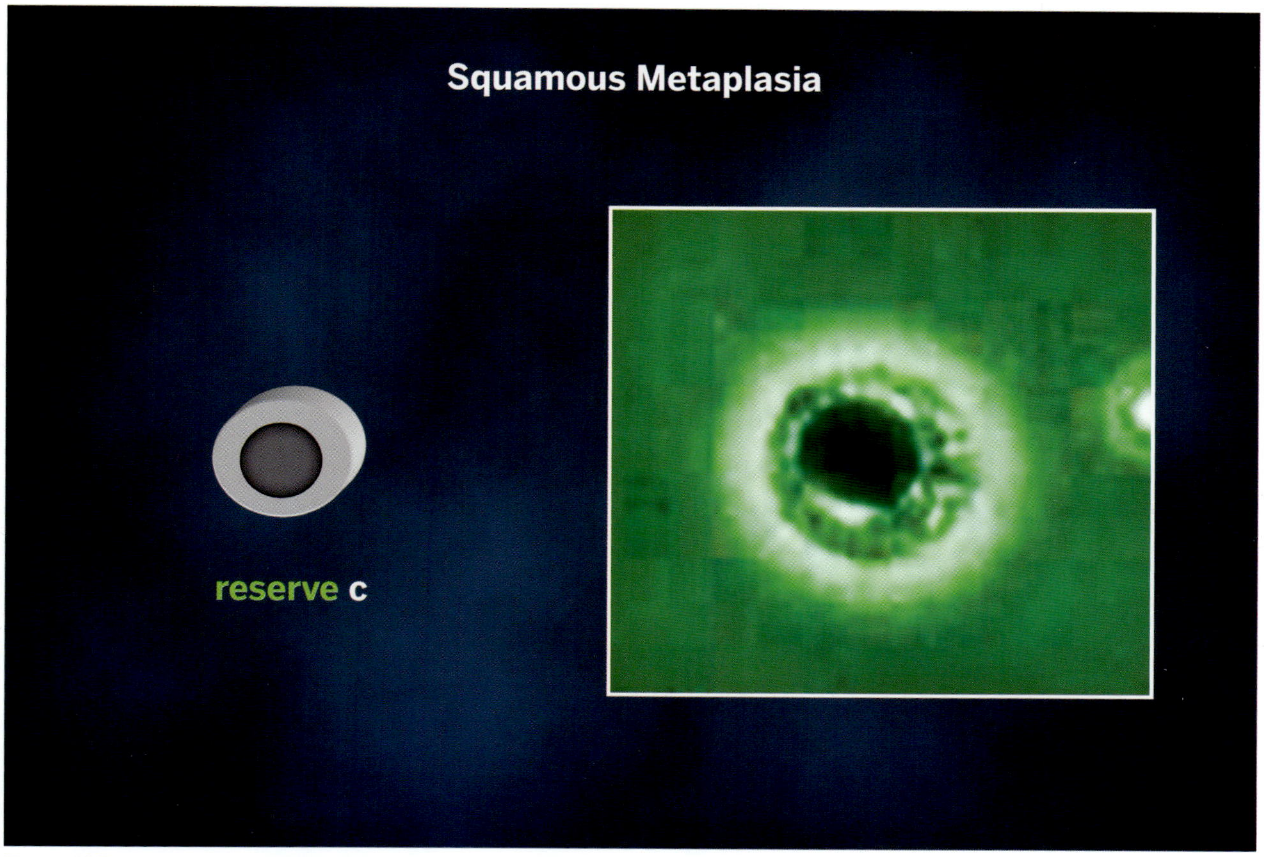

Figure 189 - Initial maturation of reserve cell is revealed by the enlargement of cytoplasm.

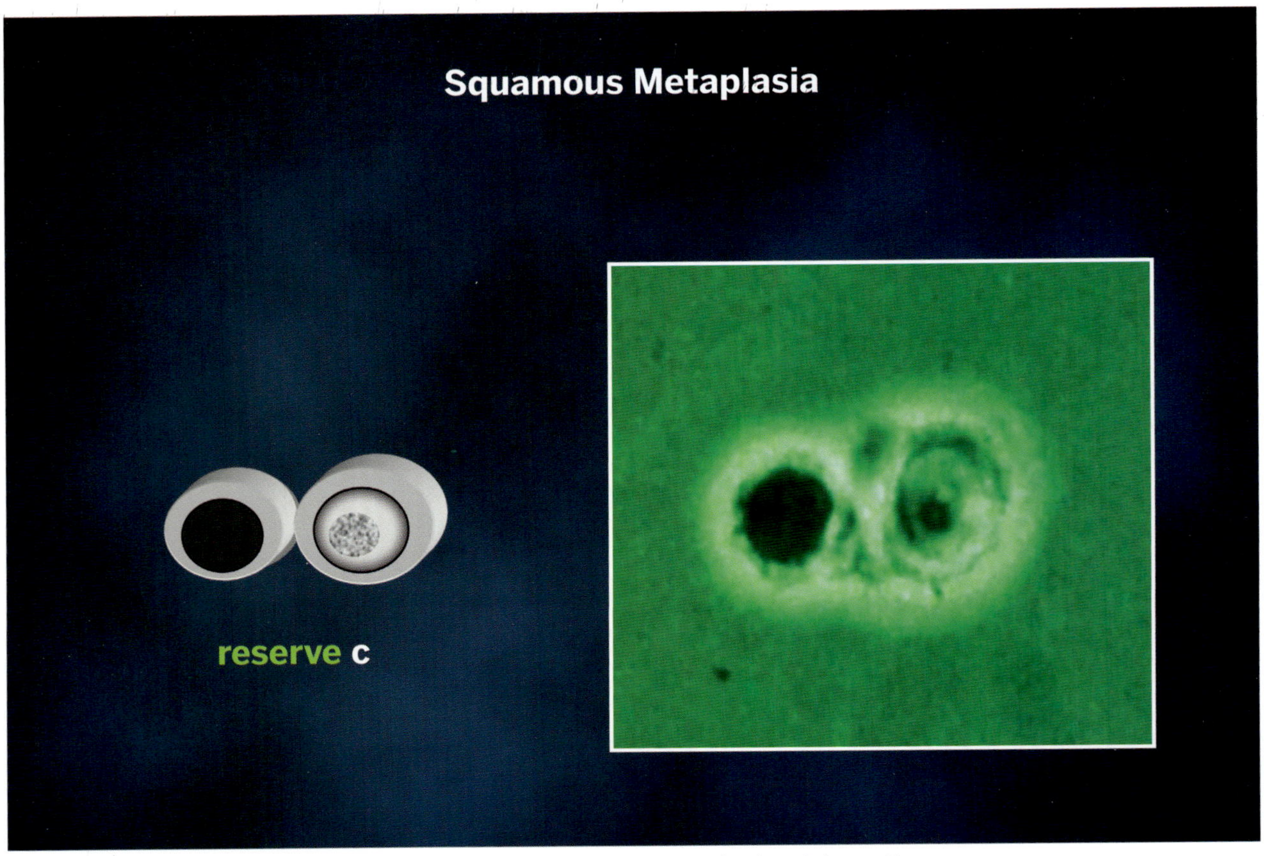

Figure 190 - Maturation of reserve cell is characterized by the progressive clearing of chromatin.

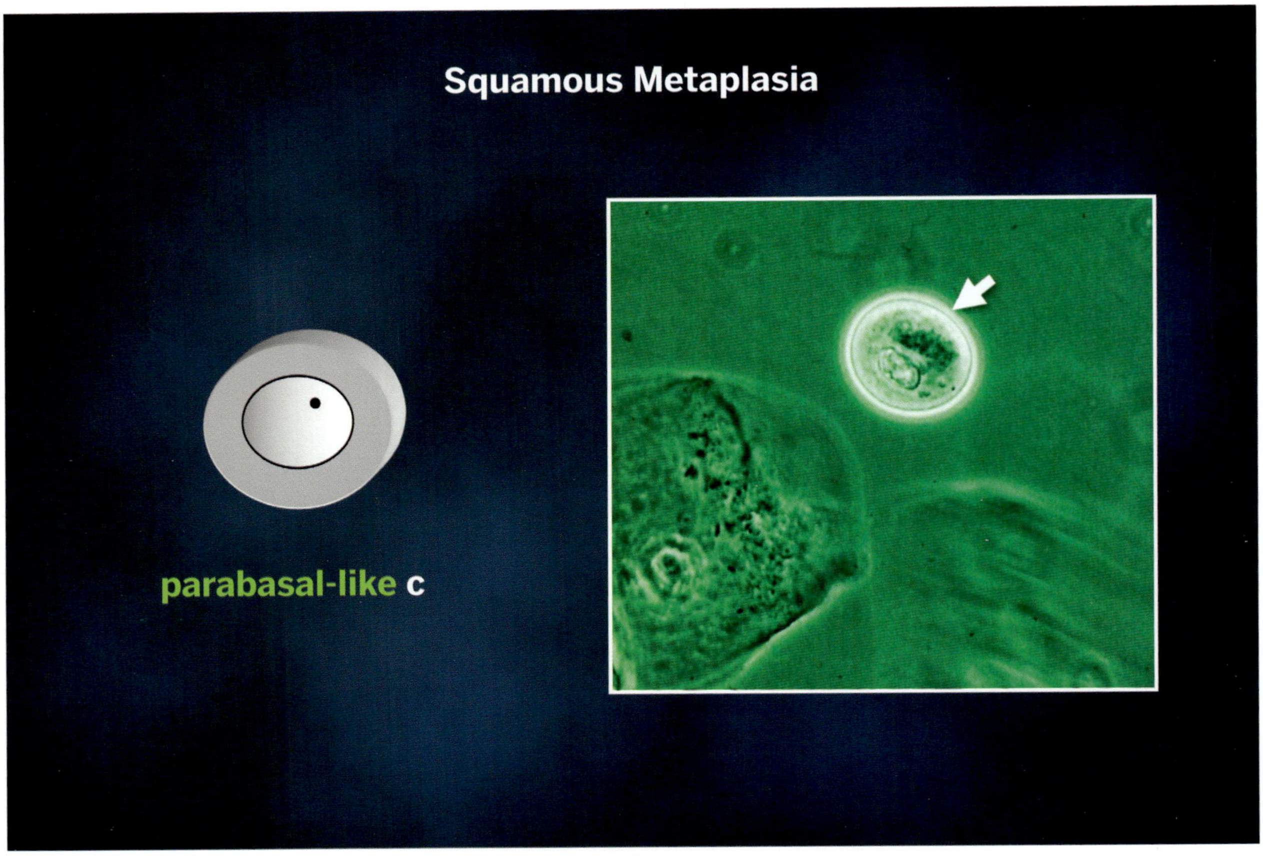

Figure 191 - Parabasal-like immature metaplastic cell.

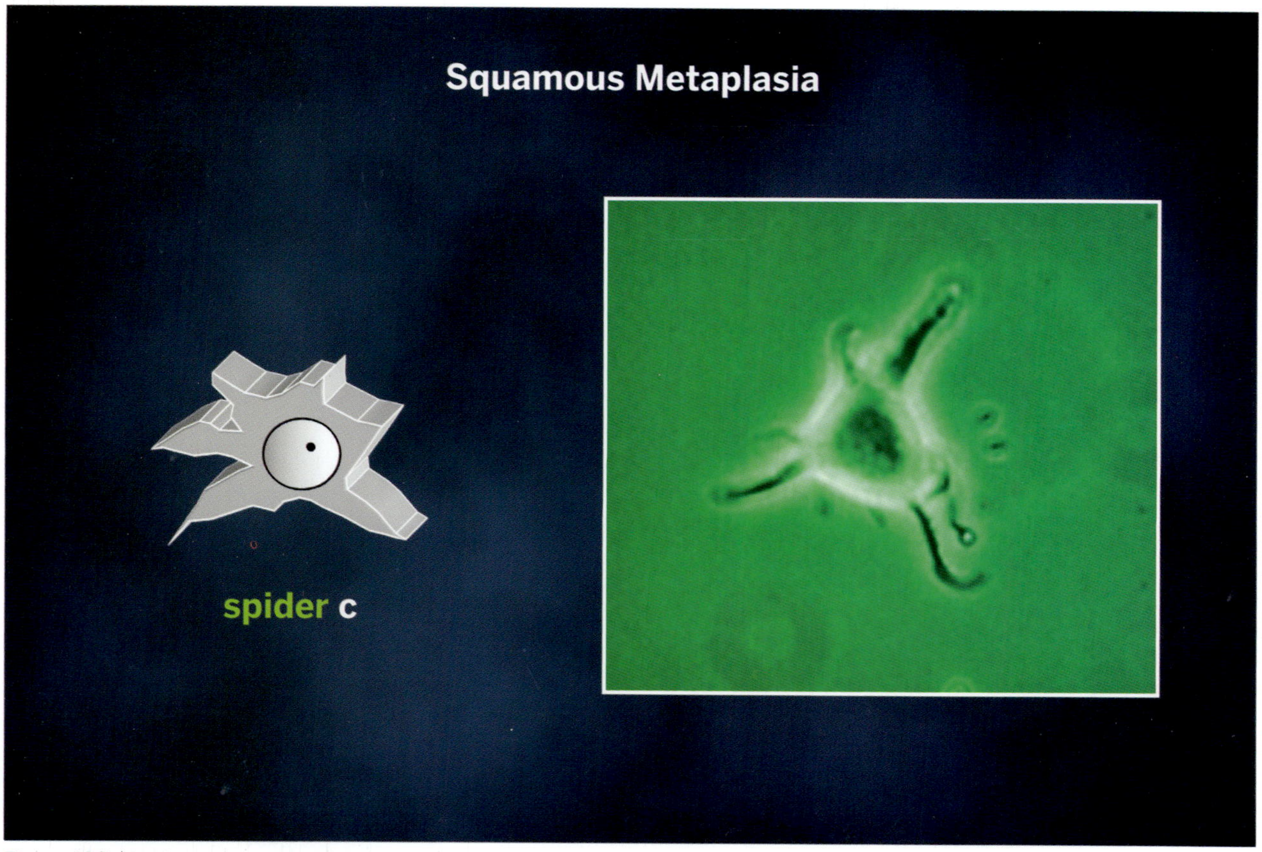

Figure 192 - Spider immature metaplastic cell.

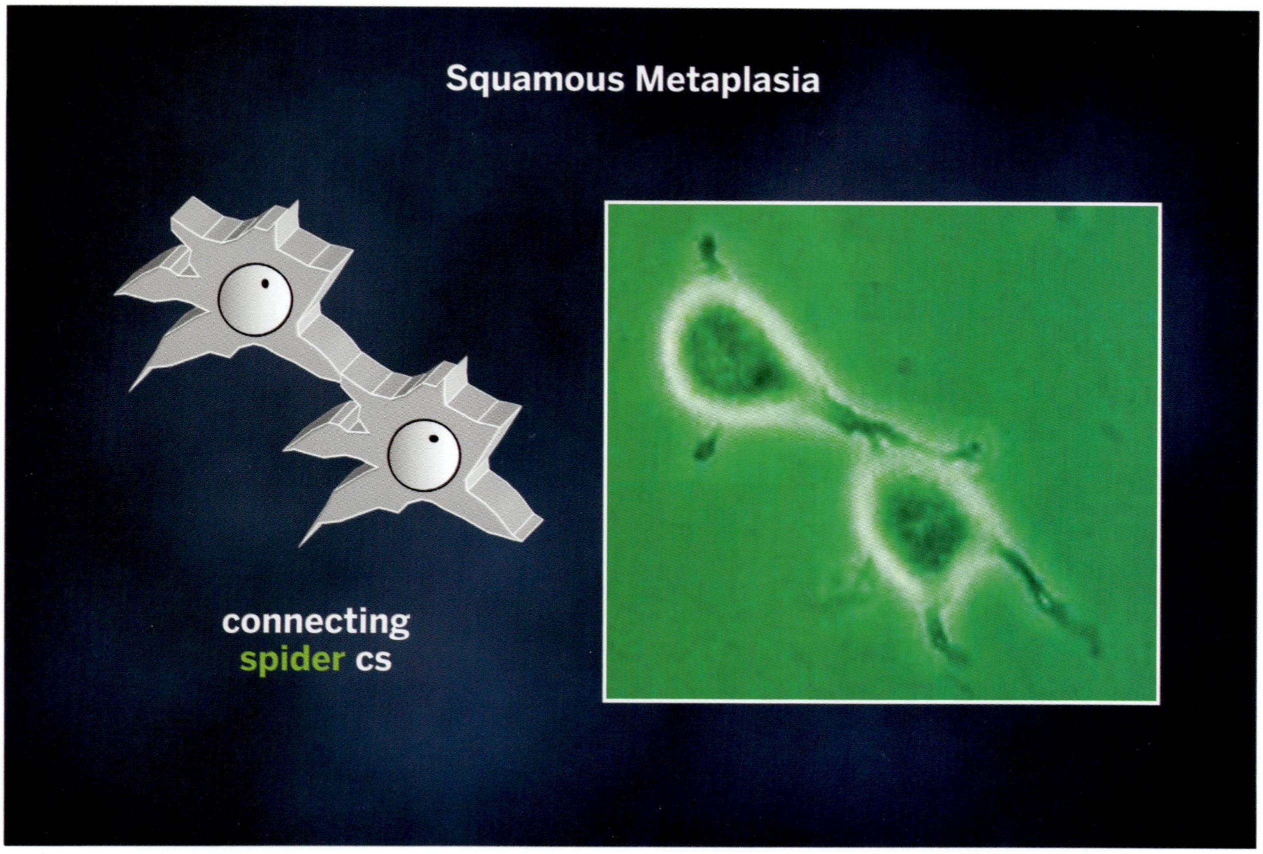

Figure 193 - Connecting spider immature metaplastic cells.

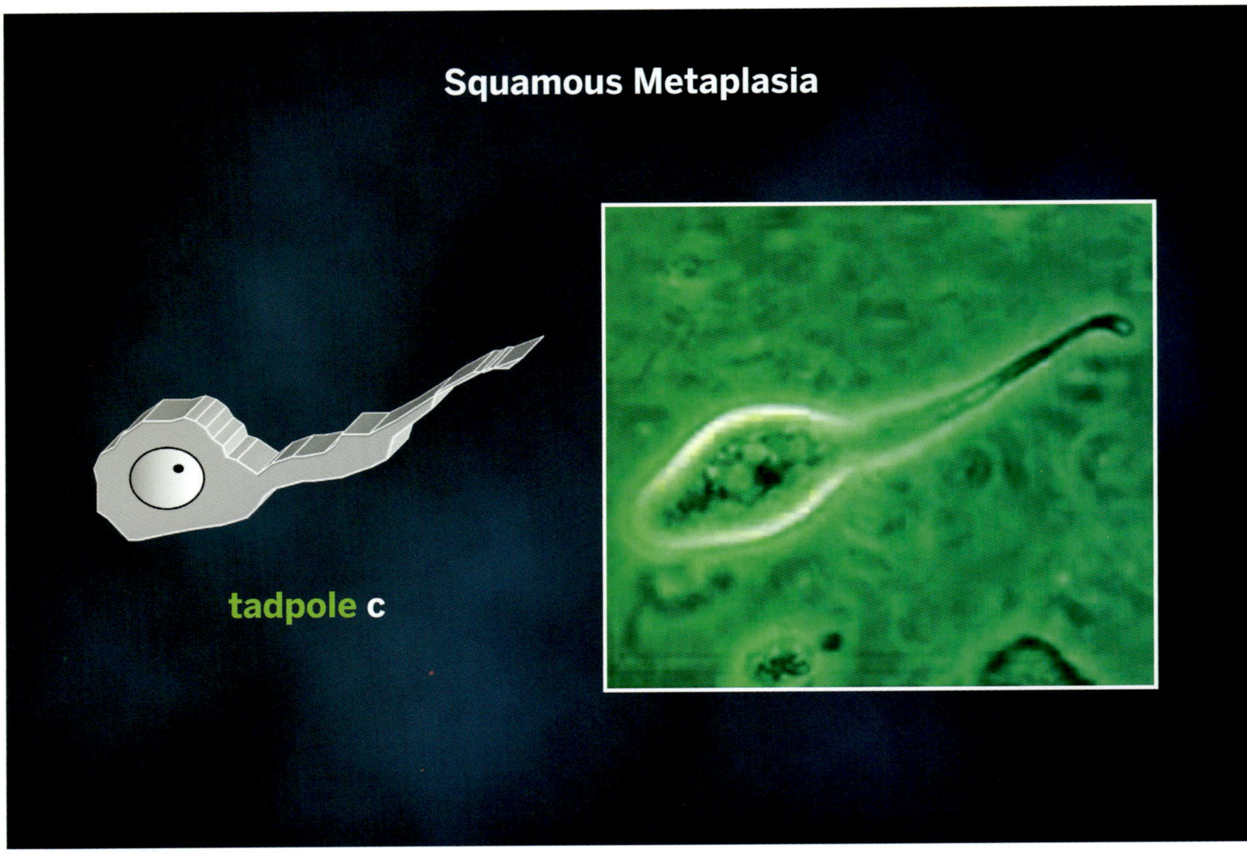

Figure 194 - Tadpole immature metaplastic cell.

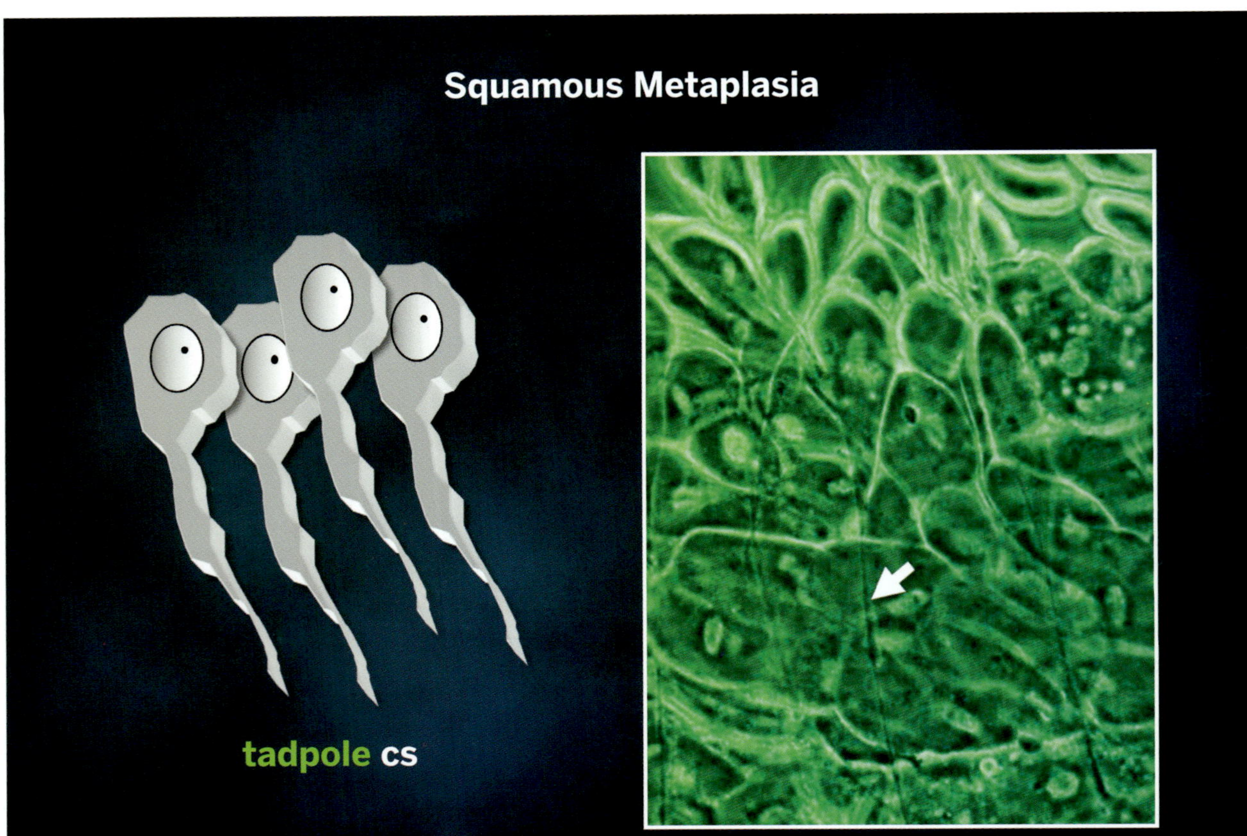

Figure 195 - The cytoplasmic processes (→) of the tadpole immature metaplastic cells cross the entire epithelial thickness.

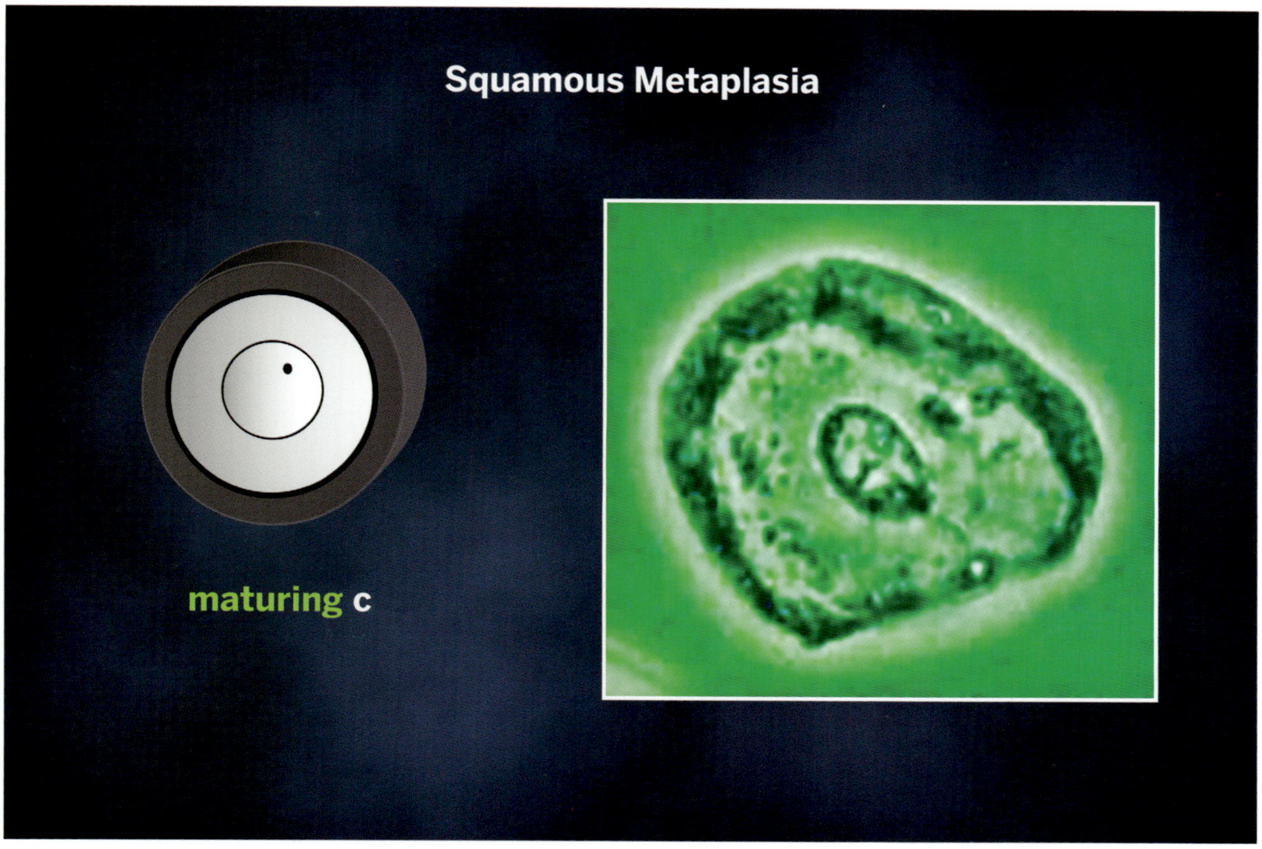

Figure 196 - Maturing metaplastic cell.

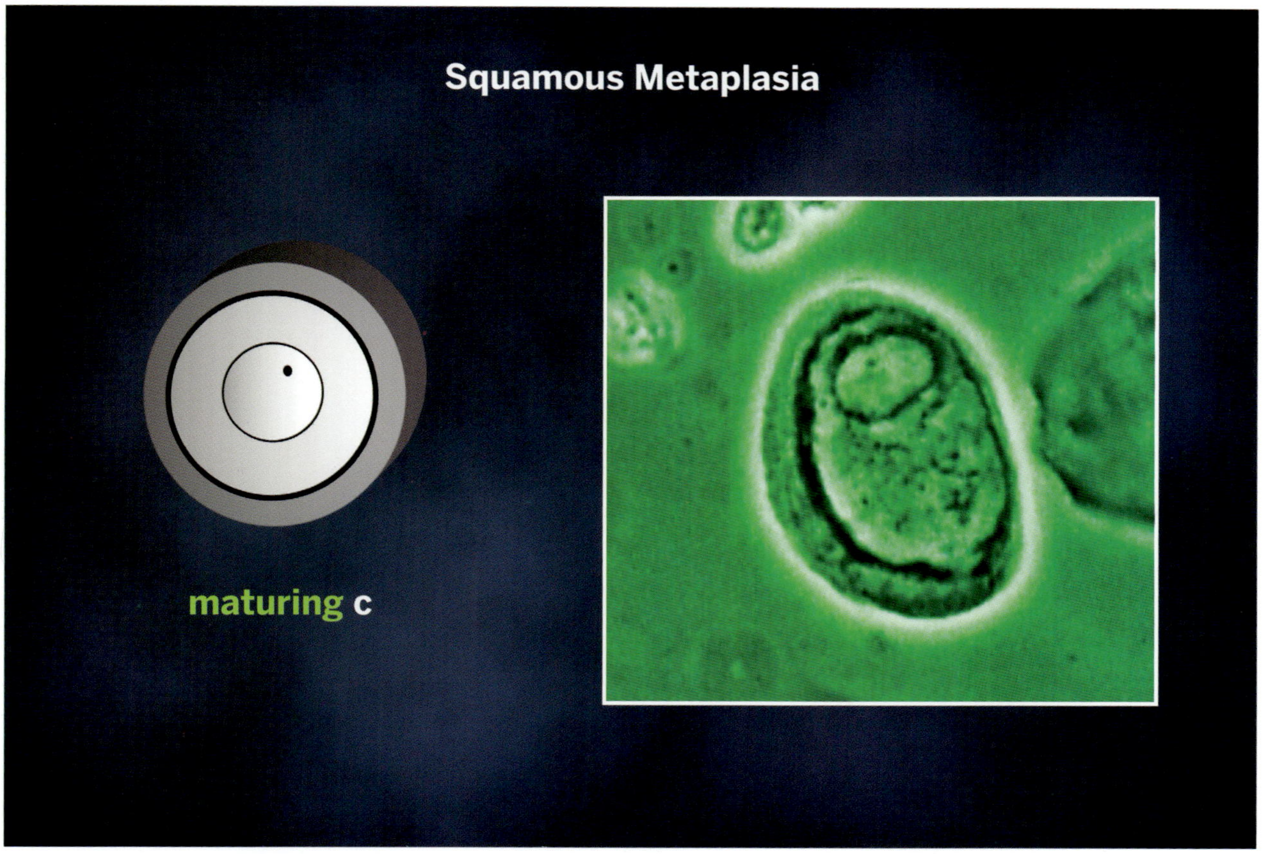

Figure 197 - Maturation of the maturing metaplastic cell is revealed by the peripheral clearing of its viscous esoplasmic ring.

premature metaplastic cells, characterized by the contemporary presence of both an immature and a mature element either in the nucleus or in the cytoplasm (Figure 198).
Premature metaplastic cells are respectively distinguished in four types (Figure 199):

- the first morphotype (Figures 199a, 200) may present the same cytoplasmic body as a native squamous cells, although it has a roundish shape, but contains an immature nucleus
- the second morphotype (Figures 199b, 201) resembles a spider cell but is larger and contains a mature nucleus
- the third morphotype (Figures 199c, 202) of premature metaplastic cells derives from an immature tadpole cell; its cytoplasmic body and nucleus are virtually identical to those of a native squamous cell and the long cytoplasmic projection is the only feature that enables its recognition as a metaplastic cell
- the fourth morphotype (Figures 199d, 203) of premature metaplastic cells exibits the same cytoplasmic body and nucleus of native squamous cells, although it keeps the residual border between the ectoplasmic ring and the endoplasmic area of the maturing cell from which it derives.

The metaplastic process is completed by the formation of a mature metaplastic epithelium which is nearly indistinguishable from the original squamous epithelium. Only the eventual presence of gland openings or nabothian cysts – when the new tissue blocks the openings of the cervix's glands, trapping their mucous secretion in tiny pockets under the epithelium – can reveal its origin from a columnar epithelium (Figure 204).
Abnormal gland openings can be noticed predominantly in carcinomas in situ (Figure 205).
Mature metaplasia is a permanent condition but immature metaplastic changes make epithelium

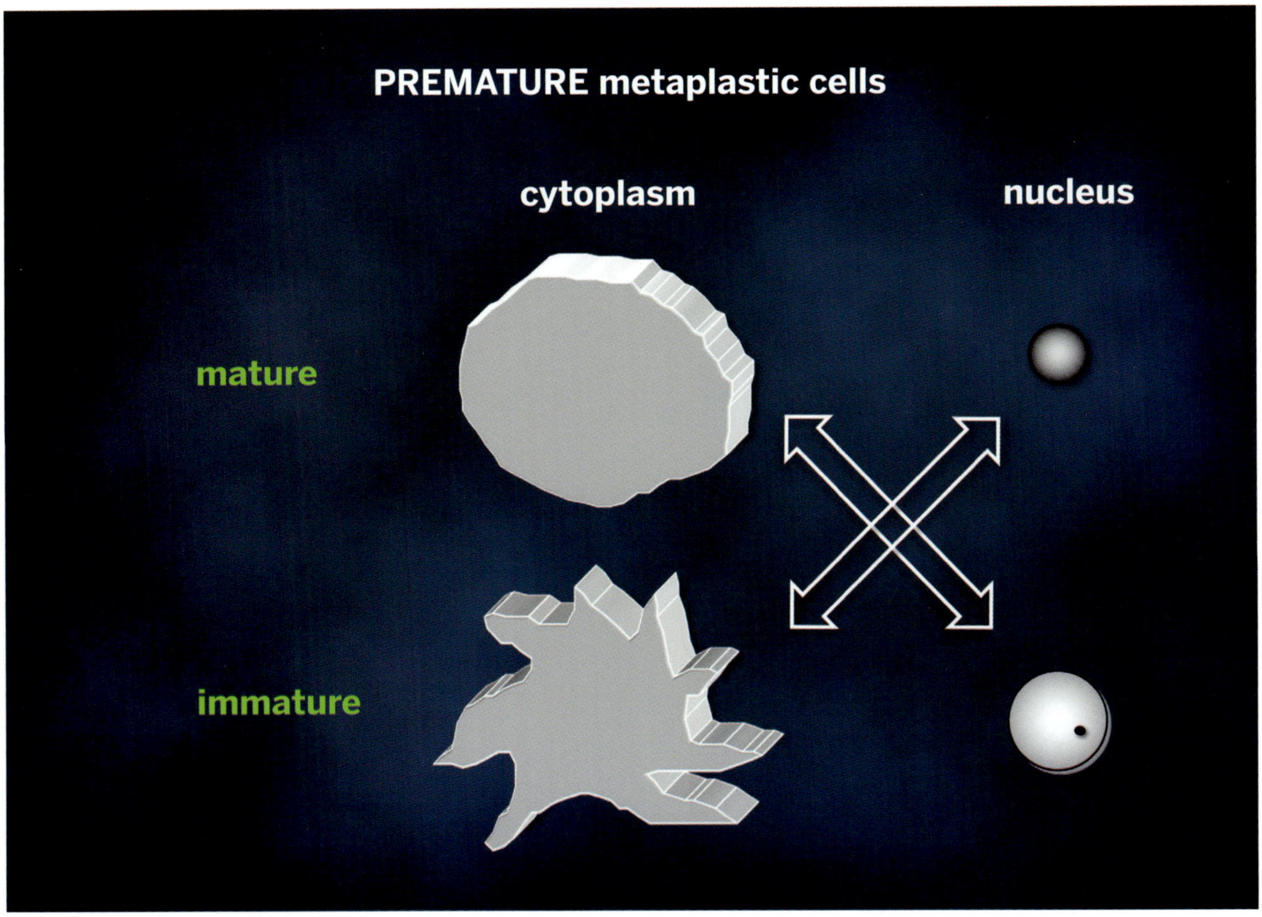

Figure 198 - Premature metaplastic cells are characterized by the contemporary presence of both an immature and a mature element either in the nucleus or in the cytoplasm.

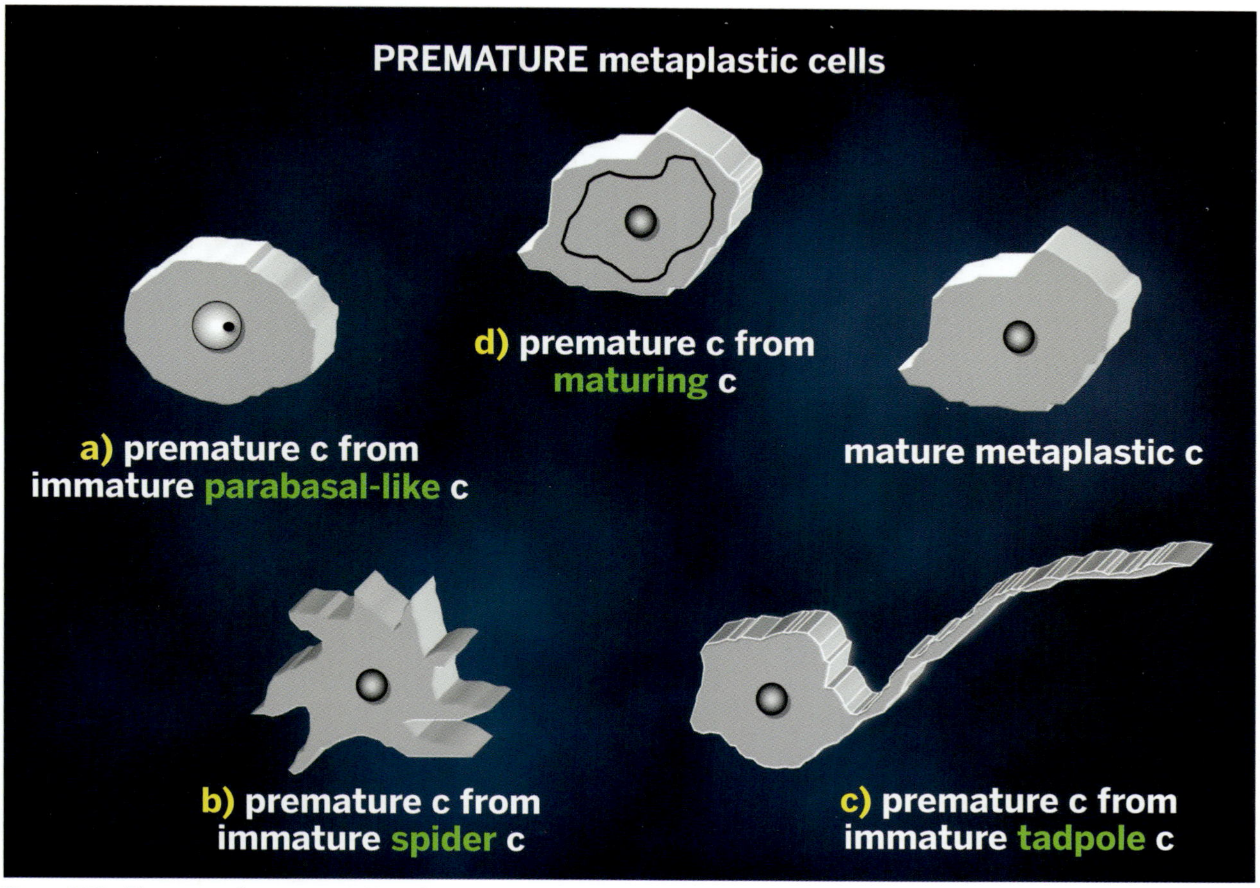

Figure 199 - Diagrammatic representation of premature metaplastic cells.

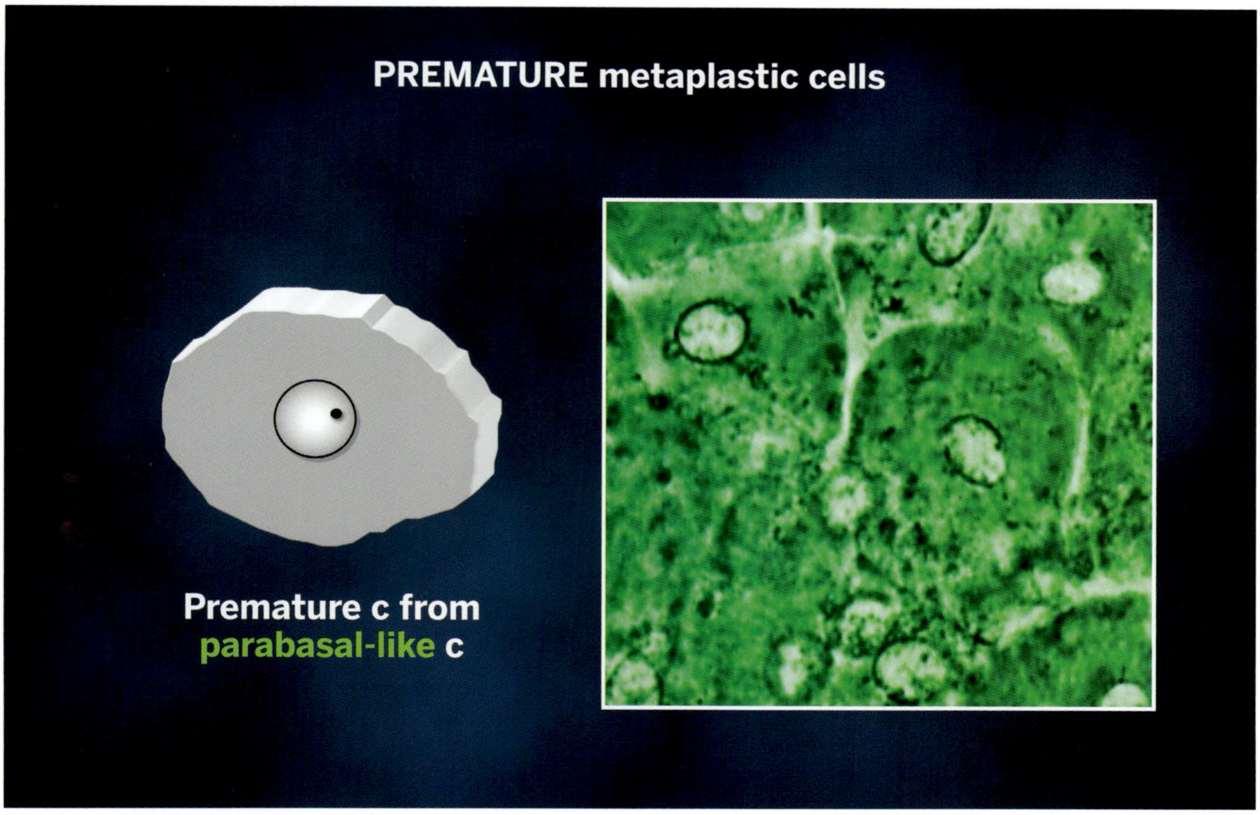

Figure 200 - Premature metaplastic cell deriving from a parabasal-like immature metaplastic cell.

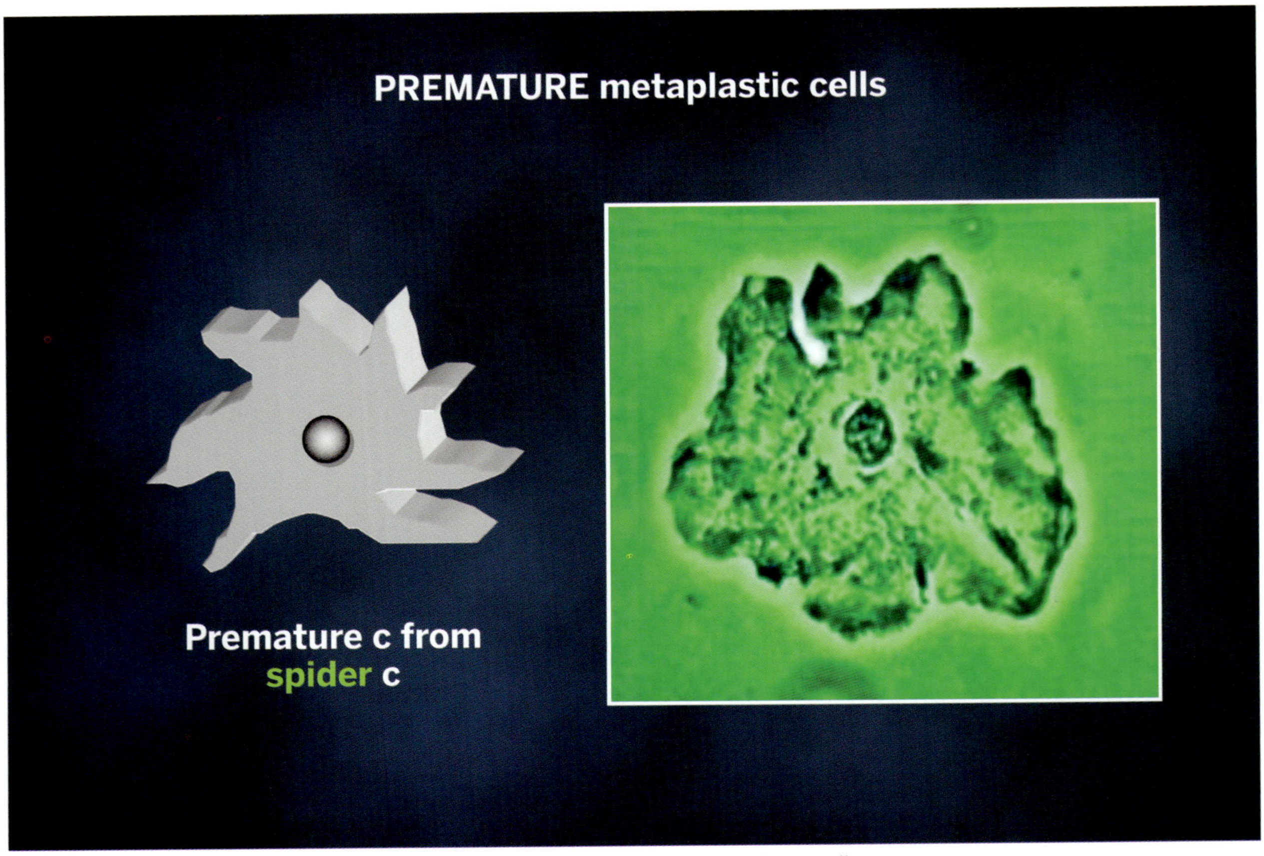

Figure 201 - Premature metaplastic cell deriving from a spider immature metaplastic cell.

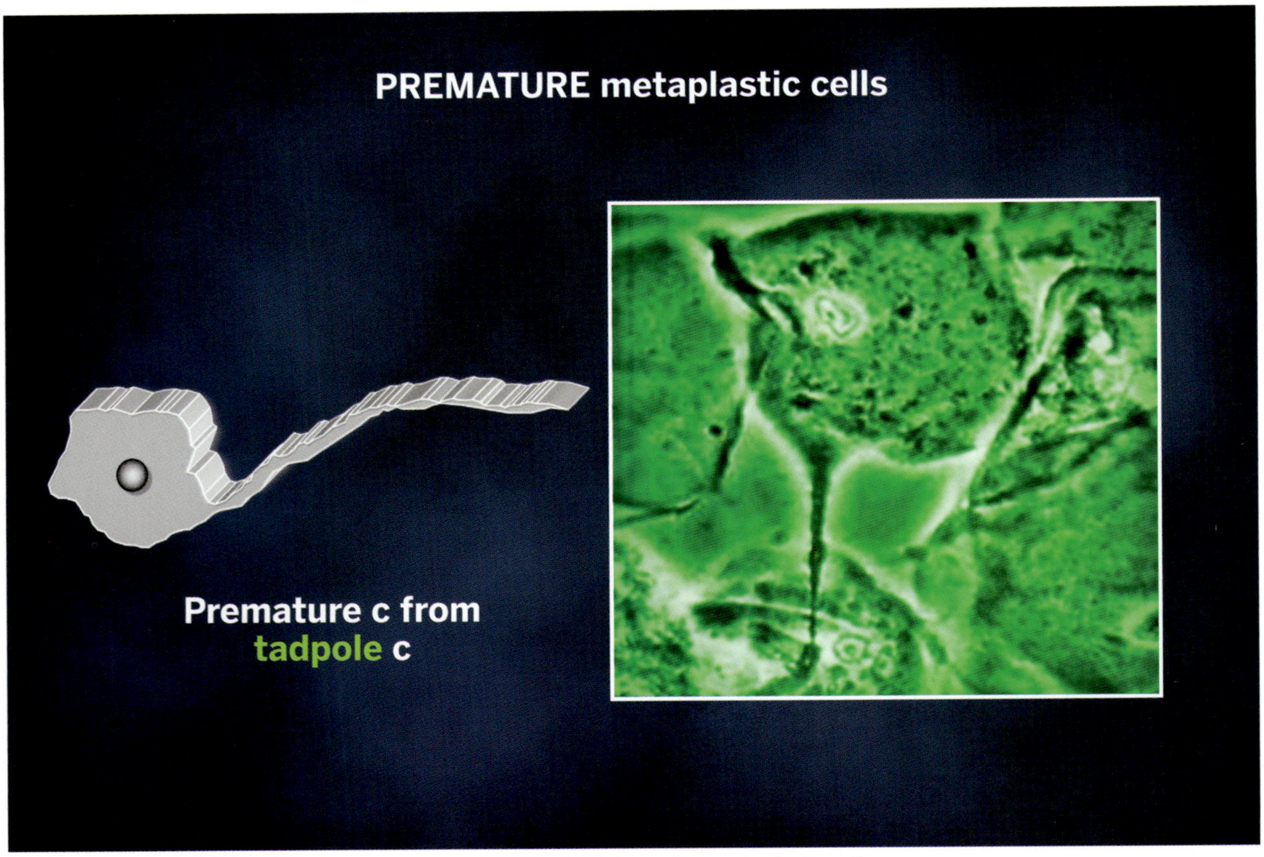

Figure 202 - Premature metaplastic cell deriving from a tadpole immature metaplastic cell.

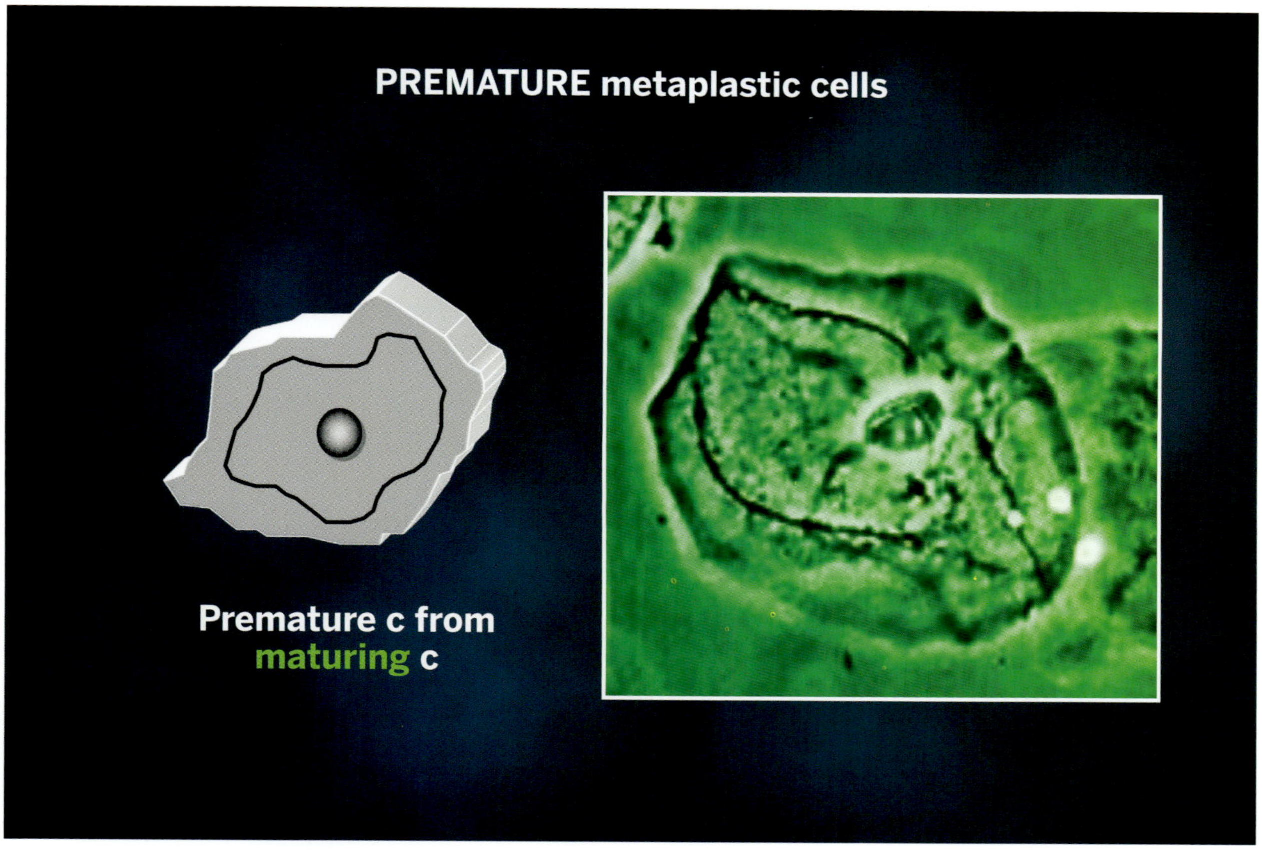

Figure 203 - A residual sharp line between the ectoplasmic ring and the endoplasmic reveals that this premature metaplastic cell derives from a maturing metaplastic cell.

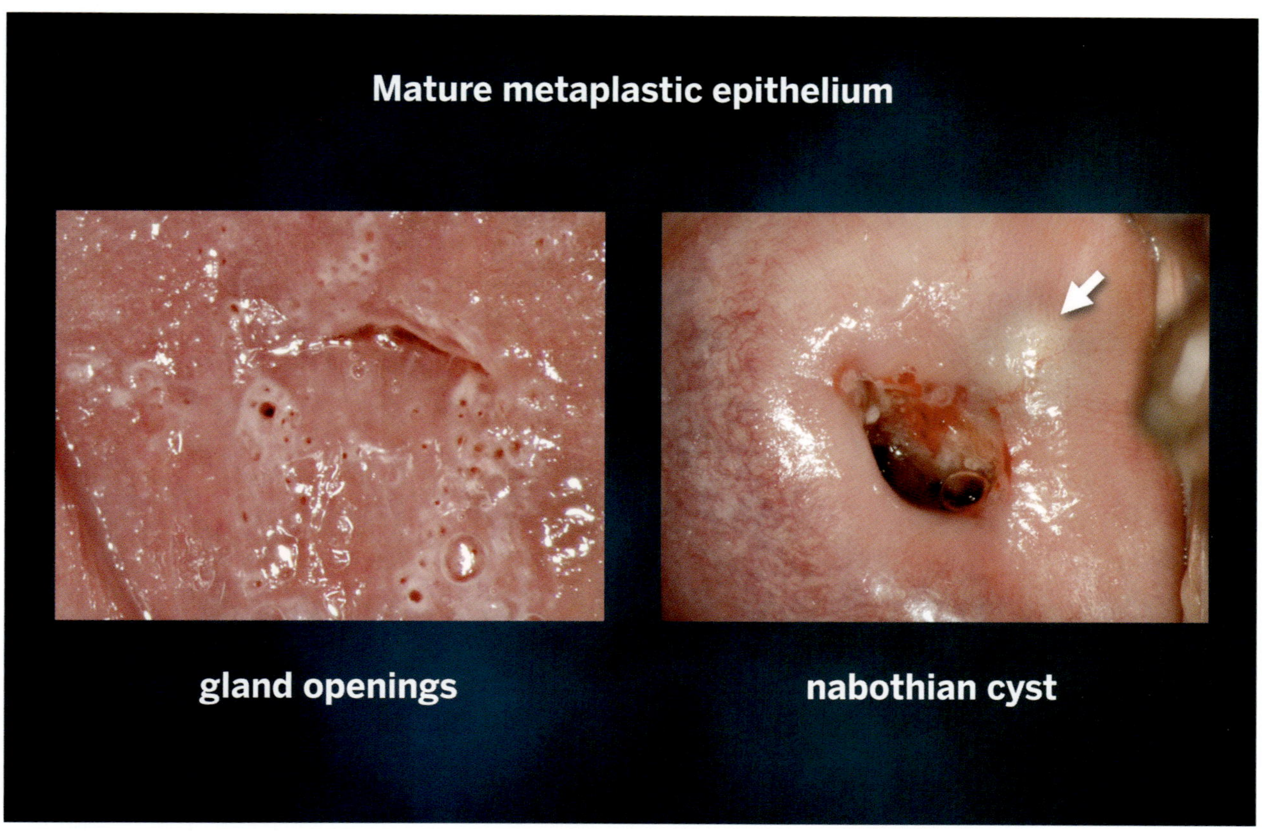

Figure 204 - Only the presence of gland openings and nabothian cysts differentiates mature squamous epithelium from original squamous epithelium.

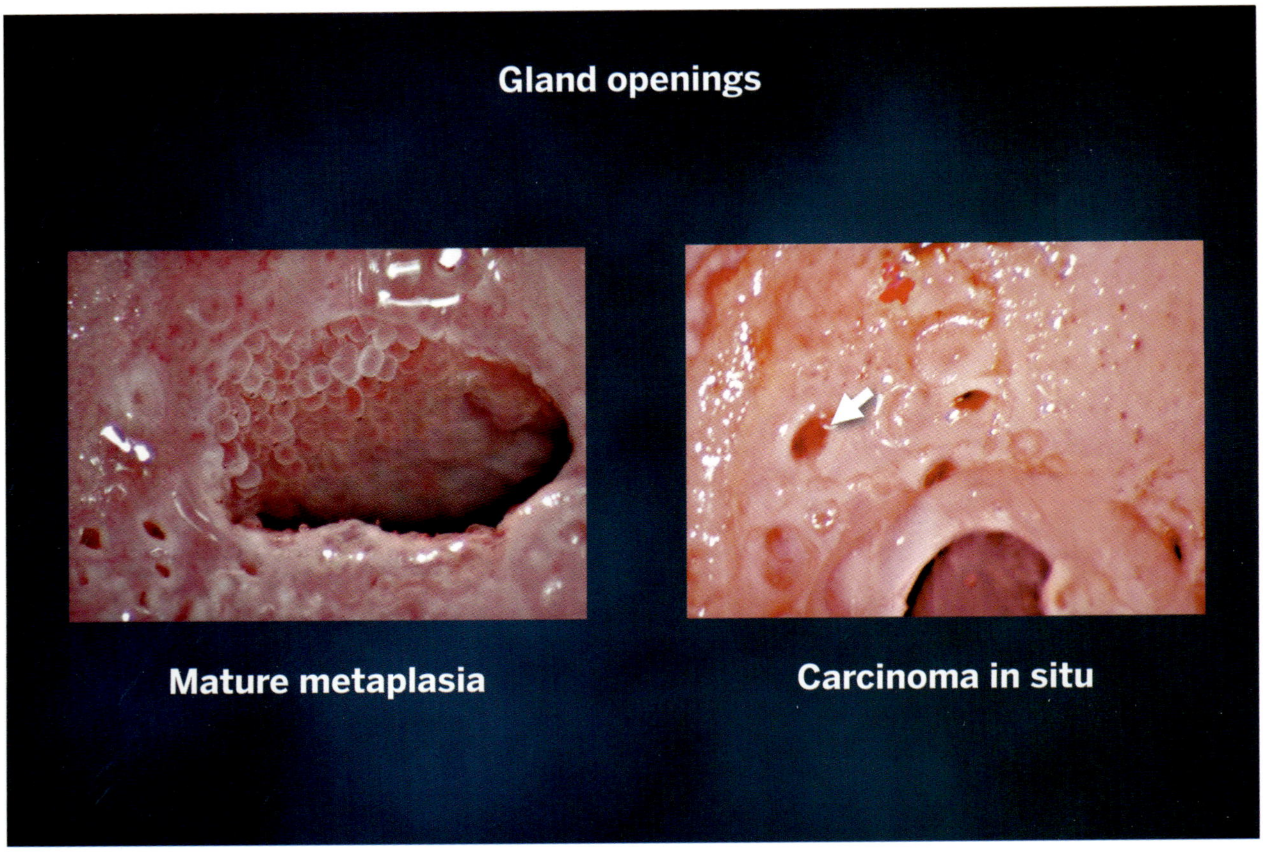

Figure 205 - Abnormal gland openings (→) in carcinoma in situ.

liable to potential neoplastic noxae. In fact, the transformation zone, the area in the columnar epithelium where a new squamous metaplastic epithelium forms, is the site where cervical intraepithelial neoplasia (CIN) originates.

Cell-mediated immunity

Leukocytes or white blood cells are actively engaged in the destruction or neutralization of invading microorganisms and are quickly transported by the blood stream to the proximity of the infection or the inflammation.
White blood cells may be classified in two main groups:

- *Granular leukocytes*
  - Neutrophils
  - Eosinophils
  - Basophils
- *Nongranular leukocytes*
  - Lymphocytes
  - Monocytes.

In contrast to erythrocytes, leukocytes recur to amoeboid movement to move from the blood vessel wall to the site of injury. The granulocytes and monocytes are termed as phagocytes because they swallow the foreign particles (cell debris, microbes, dead or dying cells) they come in contact with. Macrophages are produced by the differentiation of monocytes in tissues.
Wet mount microscopy enables the direct observation of all viable cells contributing to cell mediated immunity. It is possible to recognize lymphocytes, granulocytes and macrophages (Figure 206).
Lymphocytes are smaller than the other leukocytes, and contain a predominant roundish nucleus and a small rim of cytoplasm.
Granulocytes are characterized by the presence of granules in their cytoplasm. They are also called polymorphonuclear leukocytes because of the varying shapes of the nucleus, which is usually lobed into three segments. In common parlance, the term polymorphonuclear leukocytes often refers specifically to neutrophil granulocytes, the most

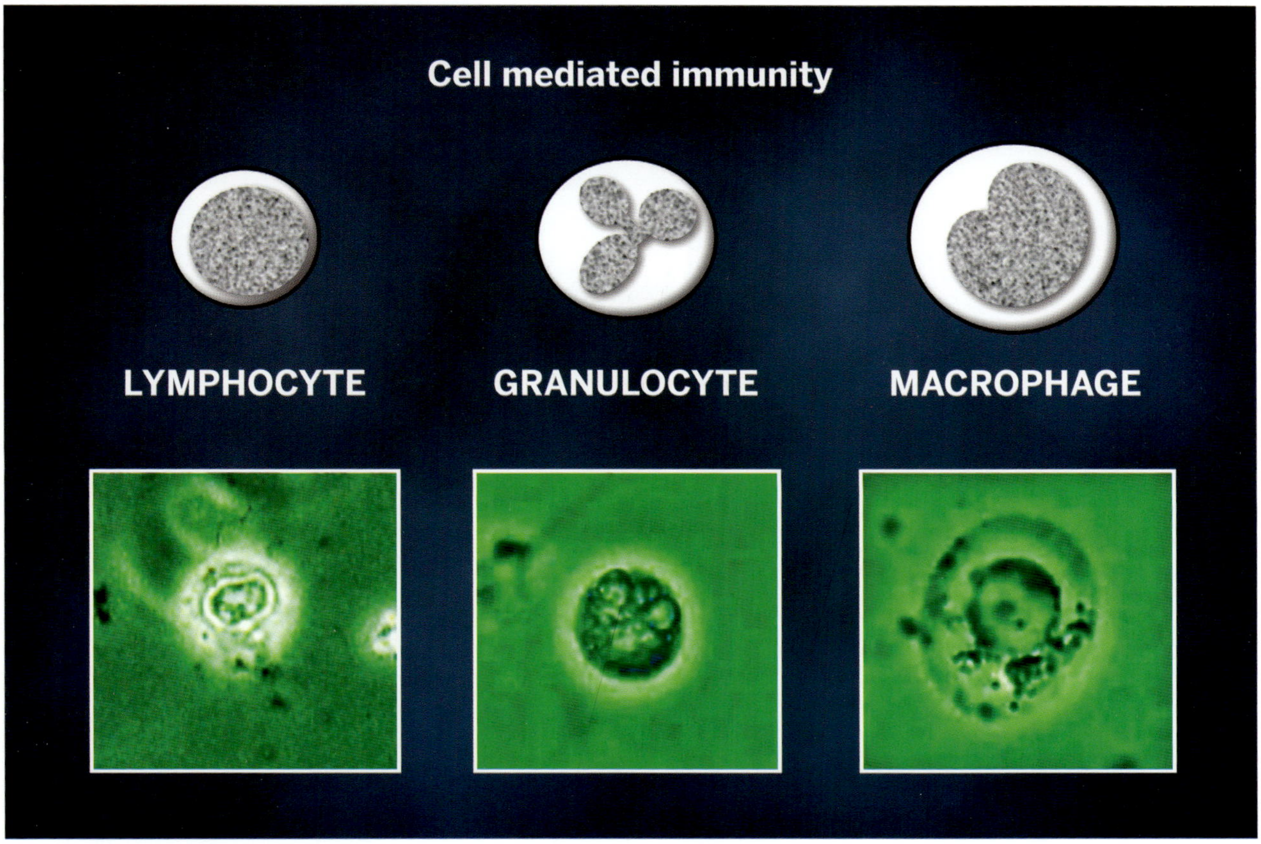

Figure 206 - Leukocytes.

abundant of the granulocytes. The other types (eosinophils and basophils) have lower numbers. In presence of acute inflammation, granulocytes are so tightly clustered that they assume an "epithelial" aspect (Figure 207) or appear adhered to epithelial cells (Figure 208). This finding is easily distinguishable from multinucleation for the characteristic nuclear shape of neutrophils. Sometimes neutrophils align tightly in contact, in order to convey their immunologic information (Figure 209).

Macrophages (Figure 206) are the largest leukocytes seen in microscopic field and are observed in chronic inflammation. They have the size of basal cells, but are distinguished from the latter by the presence of cytoplasmic inclusions or vacuoles. Macrophages, called also histiocytes, show a large roundish or kidney-shaped nucleus with a finely granular chromatin.

Phagocytes are provided with temporary projections of the cytoplasm, known as pseudopods and filopods (Figures 210, 211).

Pseudopods appear as short and plump cytoplasmic projections and serve in locomotion and *phagocytosis.*

Filopods are slender and club-shaped cytoplasmic projections that act as phagocytic tentacles to grasp foreign particles and pull them towards the cell for phagocytosis Figure 212).

The process of phagocytosis takes place when the organism comes in contact with foreign material. The phagocytes in the immune system get activated by the presence of certain particles lying on the surface bacterial cells, inflammatory cells or other foreign bodies. As soon as phagocytes detect a foreign particle, they produce surface glycoprotein receptors, that increase their ability to adhere to the particle surface. The phagocyte slowly attaches to the surface of the foreign particle. The engulfment of foreign material is facilitated by actin-myosin contractile system. It allows the cell membrane to expand in order to engulf the particle and then to contract immediately, ingesting it.

The cell membrane of the phagocyte begins to expand and forms a cone around the foreign particle.

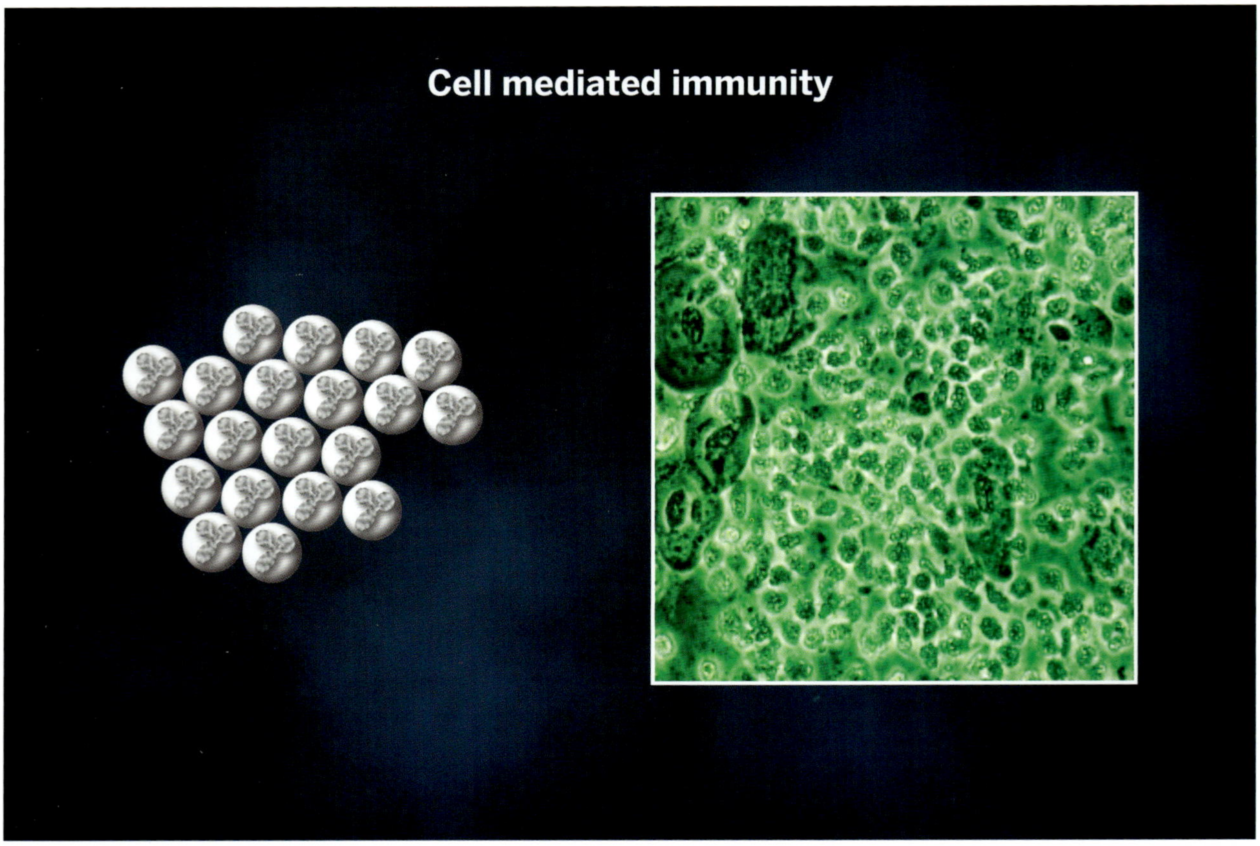

Figure 207 - Clustered neutrophils with epithelial aspect.

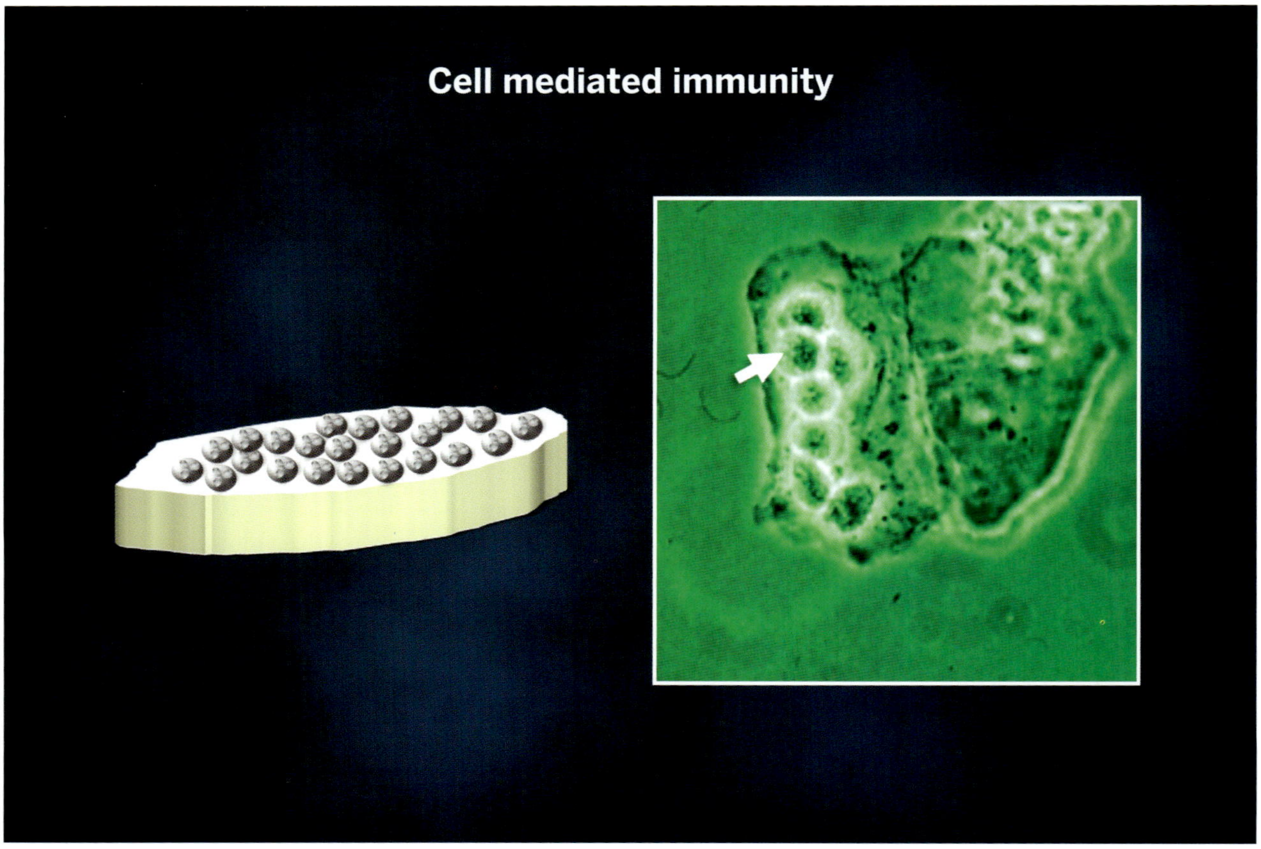

Figure 208 - Neutrophils adhered to an epithelial cell (→).

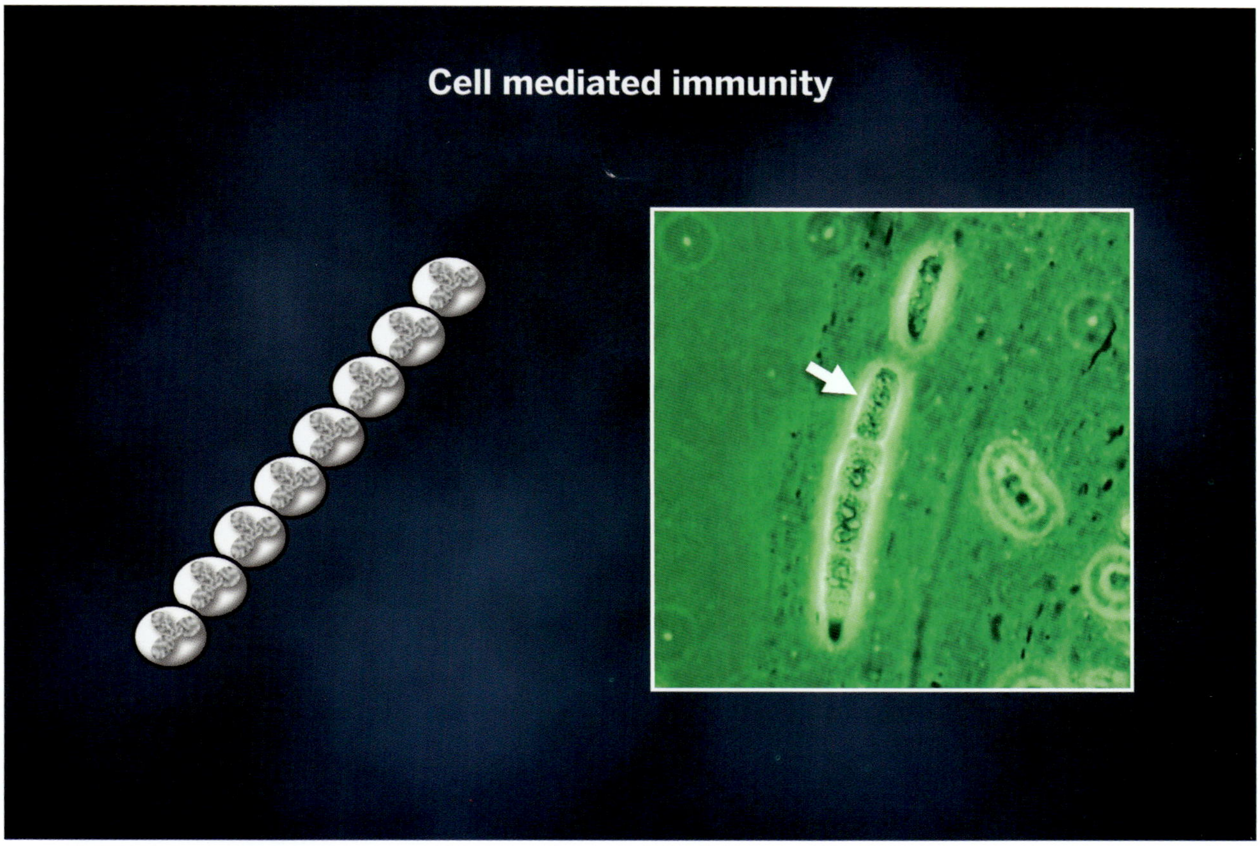

Figure 209 - Train of neutrophils (→).

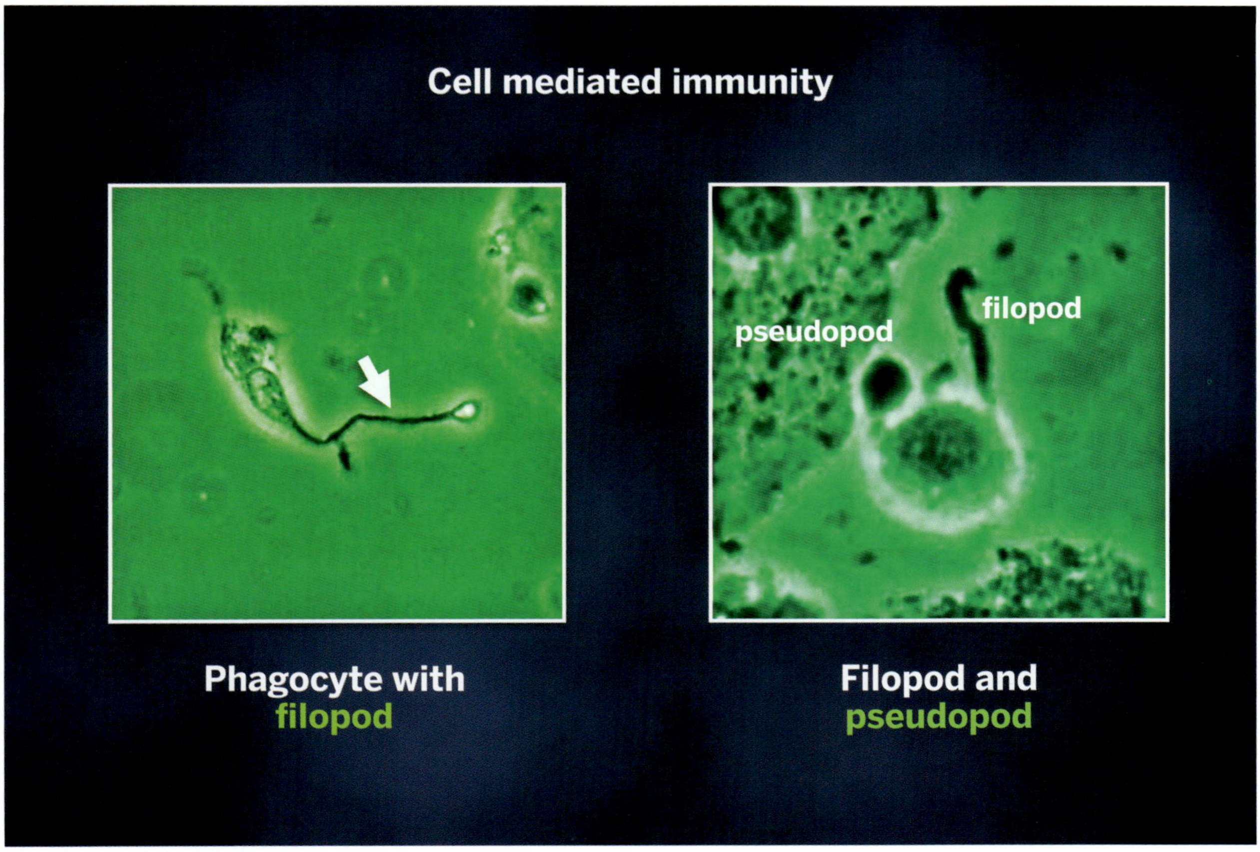

Figure 210 - Filopods and pseudopods.

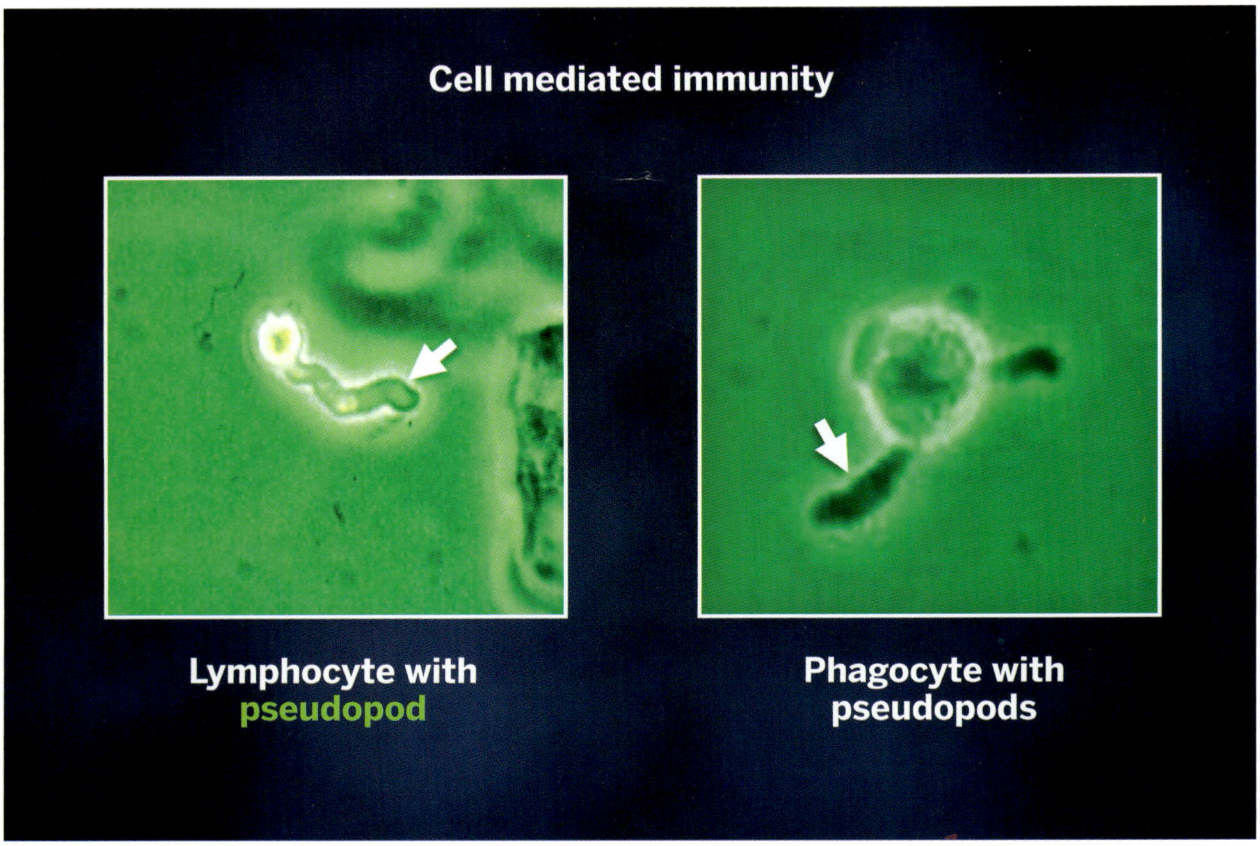

Figure 211 - Pseudopods.

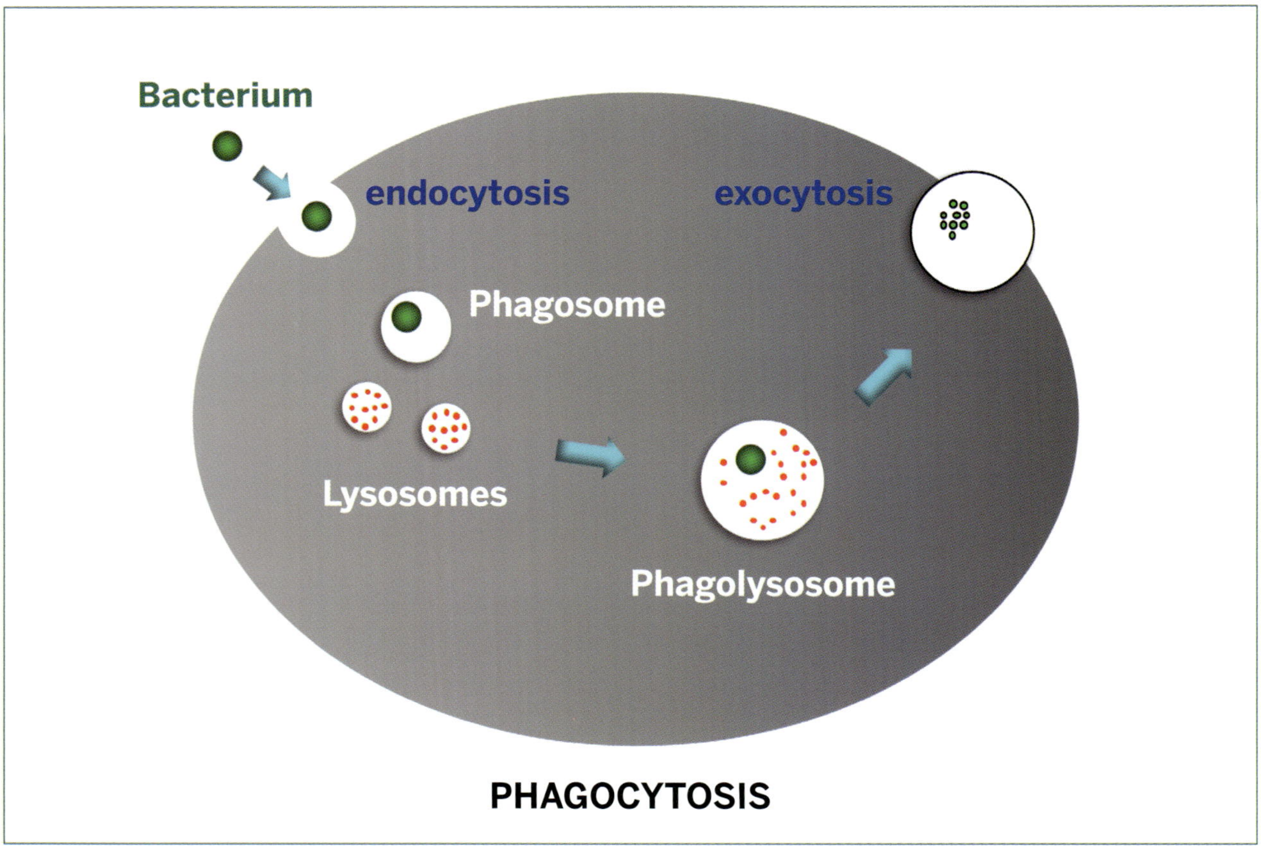

Figure 212 - Diagrammatic representation of phagocytosis.

The cell membrane surrounds the foreign particle from all sides to create a vacuole, known as phagosome or food vacuole. The phagosome is then passed into the cell for absorption. Now comes the role of the lysosomes, specific cell structures specialized in digesting the particles that enter the cell through the cell membrane. Phagosomes fuse with cellular lysosomes, forming phagolysosomes, where pathogenic microorganisms or other foreign particles can be killed and digested. The lysosomes break the food vacuole or phagosome into its component materials. The essential nutrients, if any, are absorbed in the cell, and the rest is expelled as waste matter by exocytosis (Figures 213, 214). In case of the immune system, the cell creates a peroxisome, a special structure that helps the body to get rid of the toxins.

During the process of phagocytosis, the phagocytes themselves are destroyed and release free phagolysosomes (Figure 215).

The detection of leukocytes in a vaginal wet mount, associated with different physiological and pathological conditions, may be a useful clue that helps the evaluator in making a correct diagnosis (Table 2).

The appearance of granulocytes is hormone-dependent and under normal conditions their number progressively increases from the early secretory phase.

In presence of an exposed epithelium, leukocytes may be numerous and activated, despite a concomitant vaginal bacterial flora represented by Lactobacilli (Figure 216).

Bacterial vaginosis is characterized by a background of different free-floating and cyto-adhered bacteria (clue cells) but its diagnosis relies also on the absolute absence of leukocytes, as opposed to aerobic vaginitis.

Vaginal colonization of enteric bacteria does not require pharmacological treatment and is revealed by the detection of rods or cocci concomitant with no significant leukocyte presence.

Last, candidiasis and trichomoniasis usually show Candida vegetative forms or cytopathy and mobile protozoas together with numerous activated leukocytes.

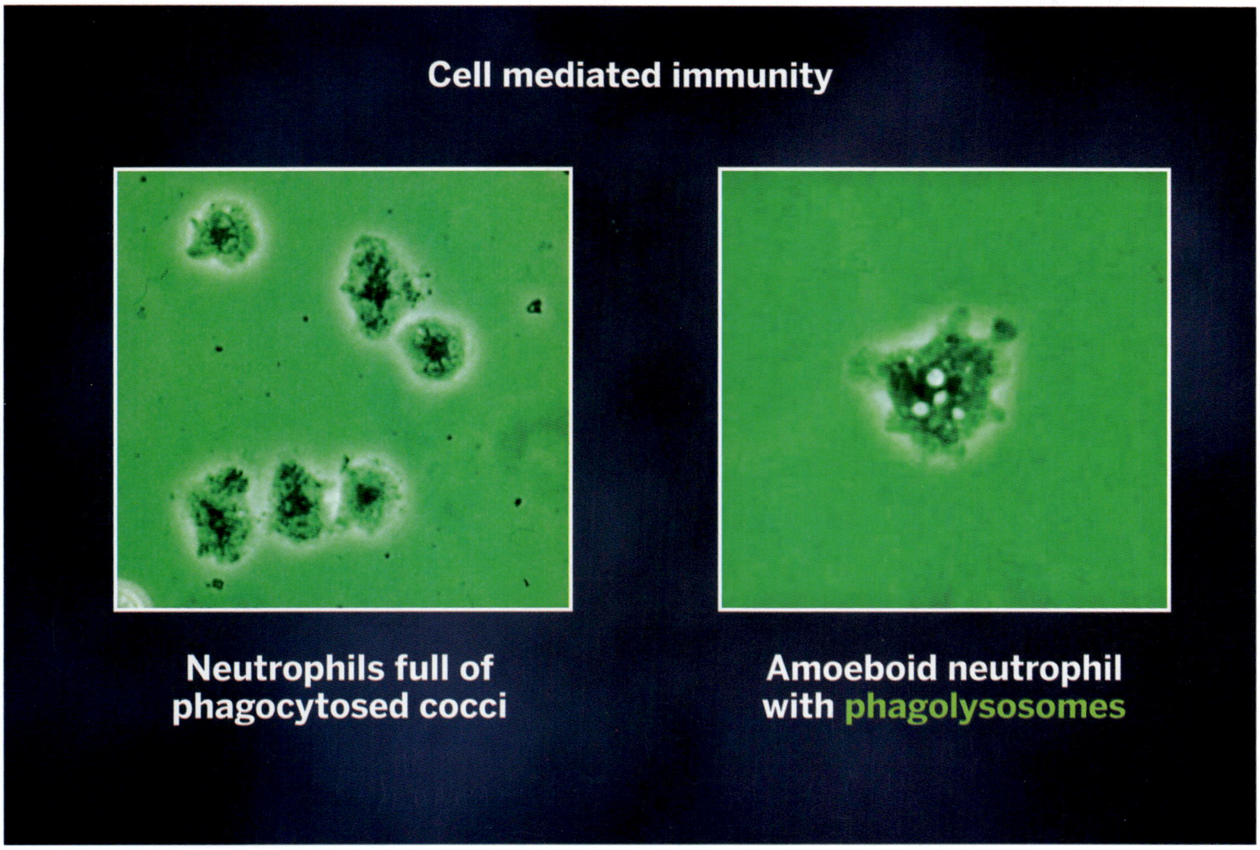

Figure 213 - Activated neutrophils.

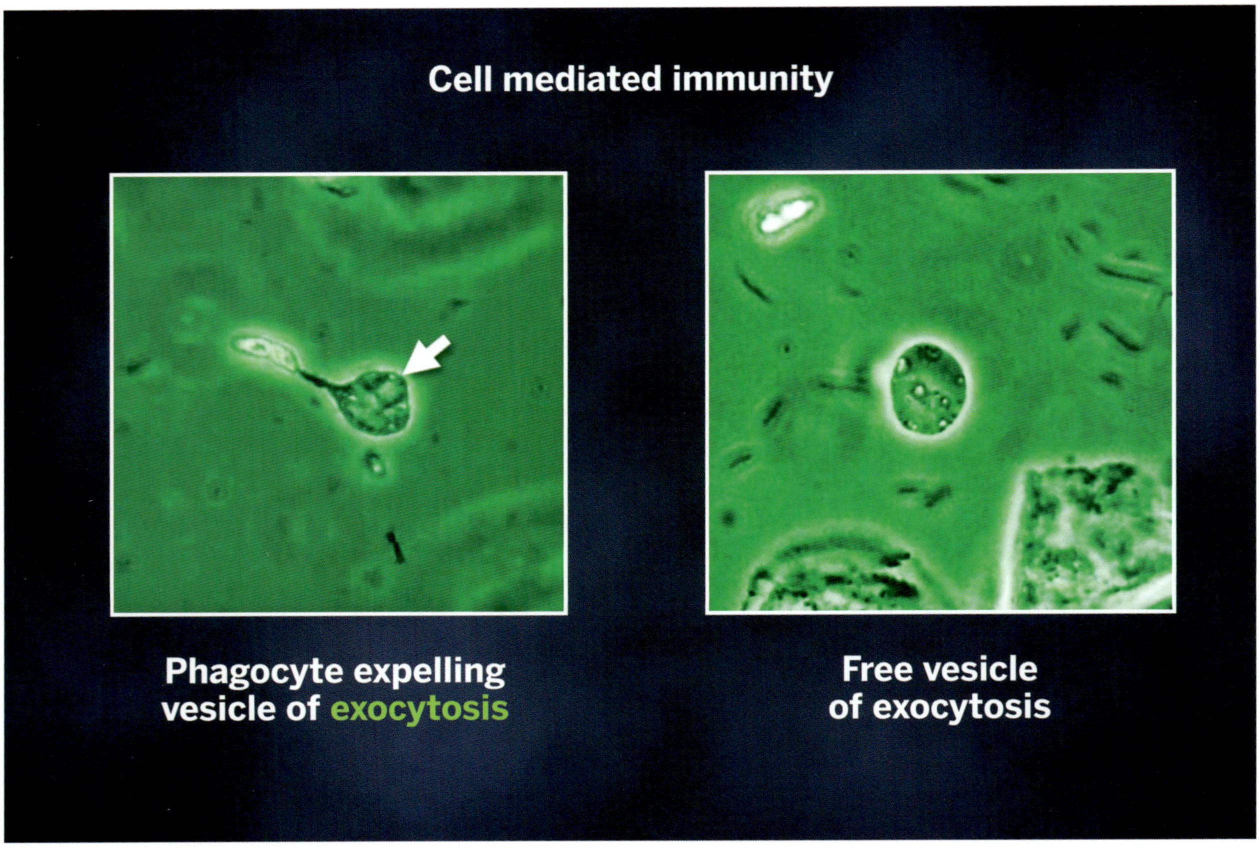

Figure 214 - Steps of exocytosis.

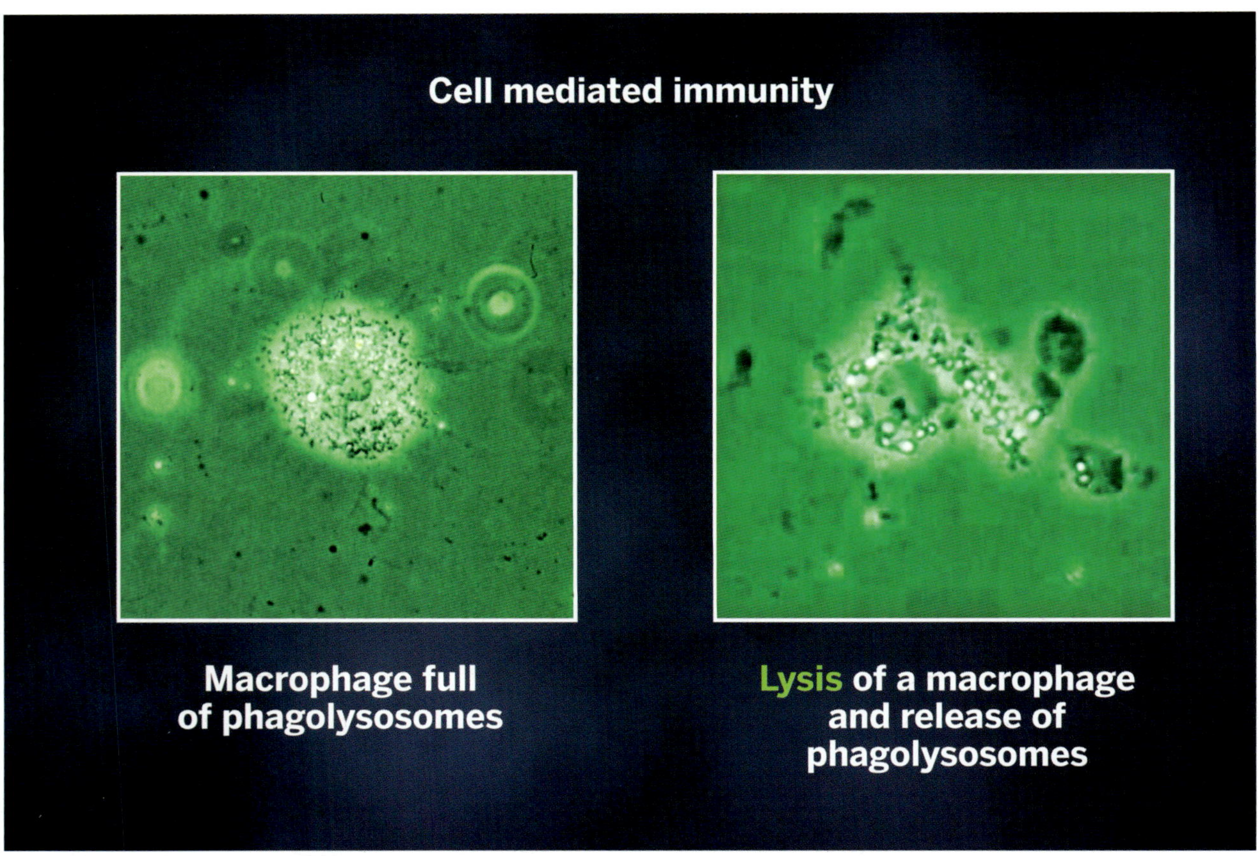

Figure 215 - Phagolysosomes in macrophage.

TABLE 2 - Presence of leukocytes in different conditions

	LEUKOCYTES	Lactobacilli	Pathogens
Secretory phase	+	+	-
Exposed epithelium	+	+	-
Bacterial vaginosis	-	-	+
Aerobic vaginitis	+	-	+
Enterics colonization	-	-/+	+
Candidiasis and trichomoniasis	+	-	+

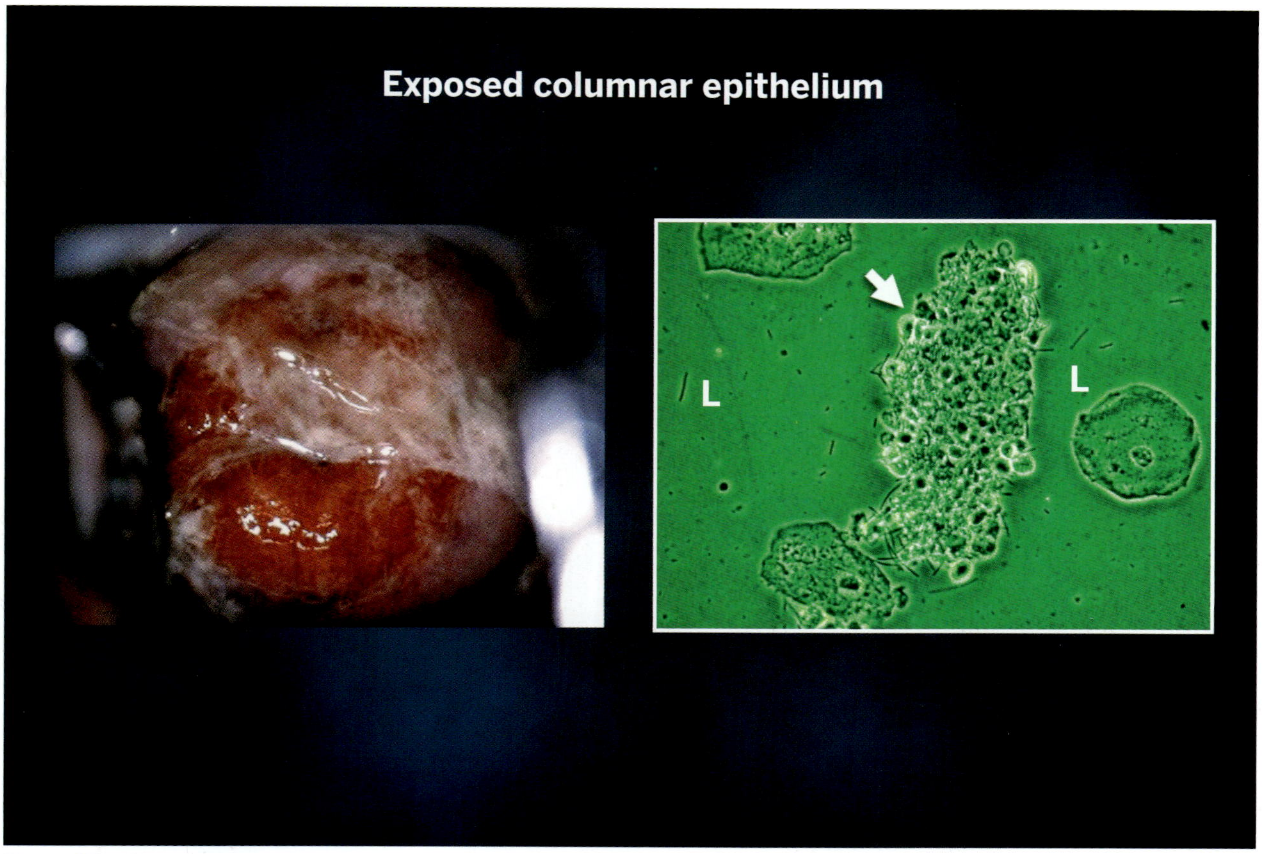

Figure 216 - Cluster of leukocytes (→) associated with Lactobacilli (L) in exposed columnar epithelium.

Localization of occult bleeding and inflammation

When specimens of vaginal discharge and cervical or endometrial secretions are separately collected, the screener is able to distinguish the exact localization of inflammation. Furthermore, it is possible to detect and localize the site of occult bleeding and to establish if it is recent or pre-existing observing the progressive phases of red blood cells degeneration. Fresh erythrocytes appear as roundish biconcave disks (Figure 217) while, as time goes on, red blood cells appear dysmorphic and later spherical and pale. At a late stage of degenerative changes, erythrocytes show a homogeneous content and a sharp edged cytoplasmic membrane.

Post coital spermatozoa morphology and mobility

Phase contrast microscopy enables the observation of spermatozoa left in vagina soon after sexual intercourse in order to evaluate their morphology (Figure 218) and mobility. While still in vagina, spermatozoa lose their tail after a variable amount of time depending on vaginal environmental conditions such as pH or vaginal inflammation. Therefore, it is possible to observe naked heads and free tails. Free tails of spermatozoa (Figure 219) may resemble Lactobacilli but are easily distinguishable because the tail shows a tapered end piece at its tip, following the axial filament.

Bare heads (Figure 220) of spermatozoa may be confused with small spores of Torulopsis glabrata. The distinctive element is represented by a dark pole corresponding to the spermatozoa acrosome (acorn-like aspect), and the frequent budding of blastospores.

Presence of dyskaryotic or atypical cells

Although the colour contrast of the Papanicolaou smear is lacking in unstained specimen, dyskaryotic and atypical cells are detectable for their typical morphology under phase contrast microscope observation.

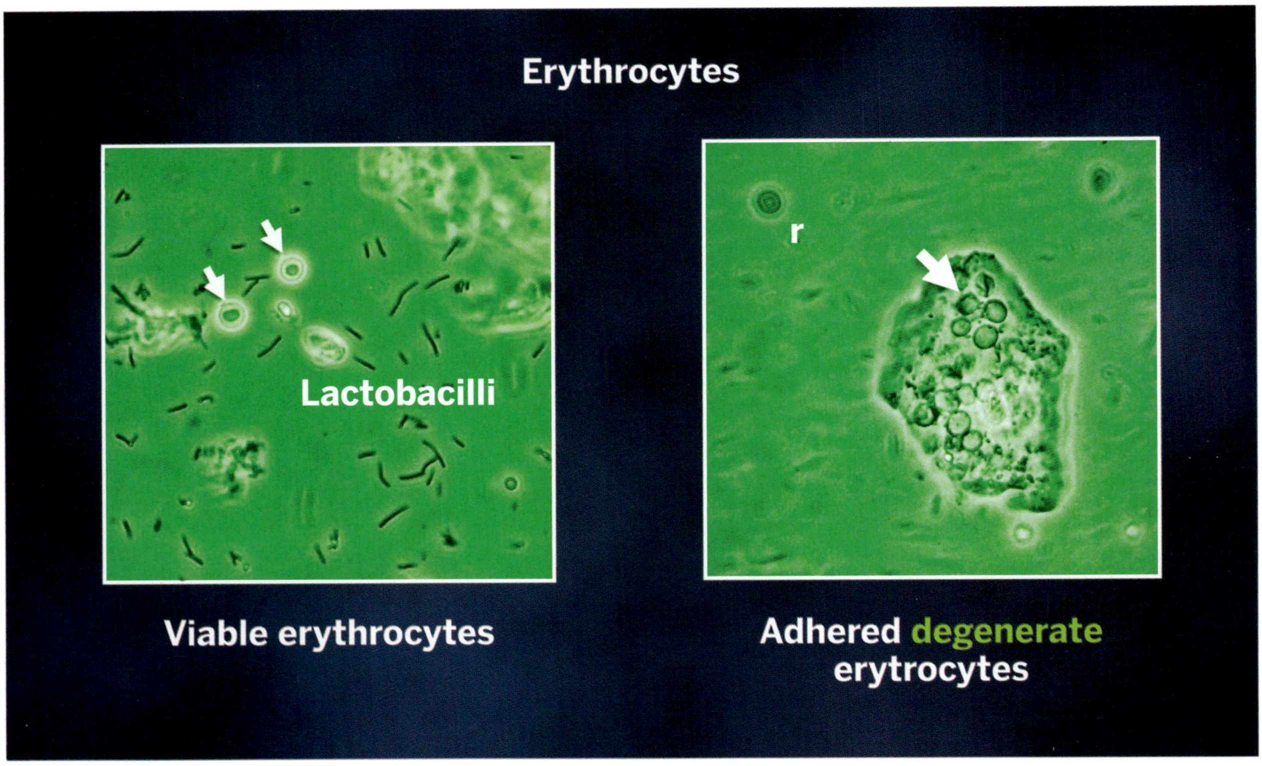

Figure 217 - Viable and degenerate erythrocytes (→). (r) Viable red blood cell.

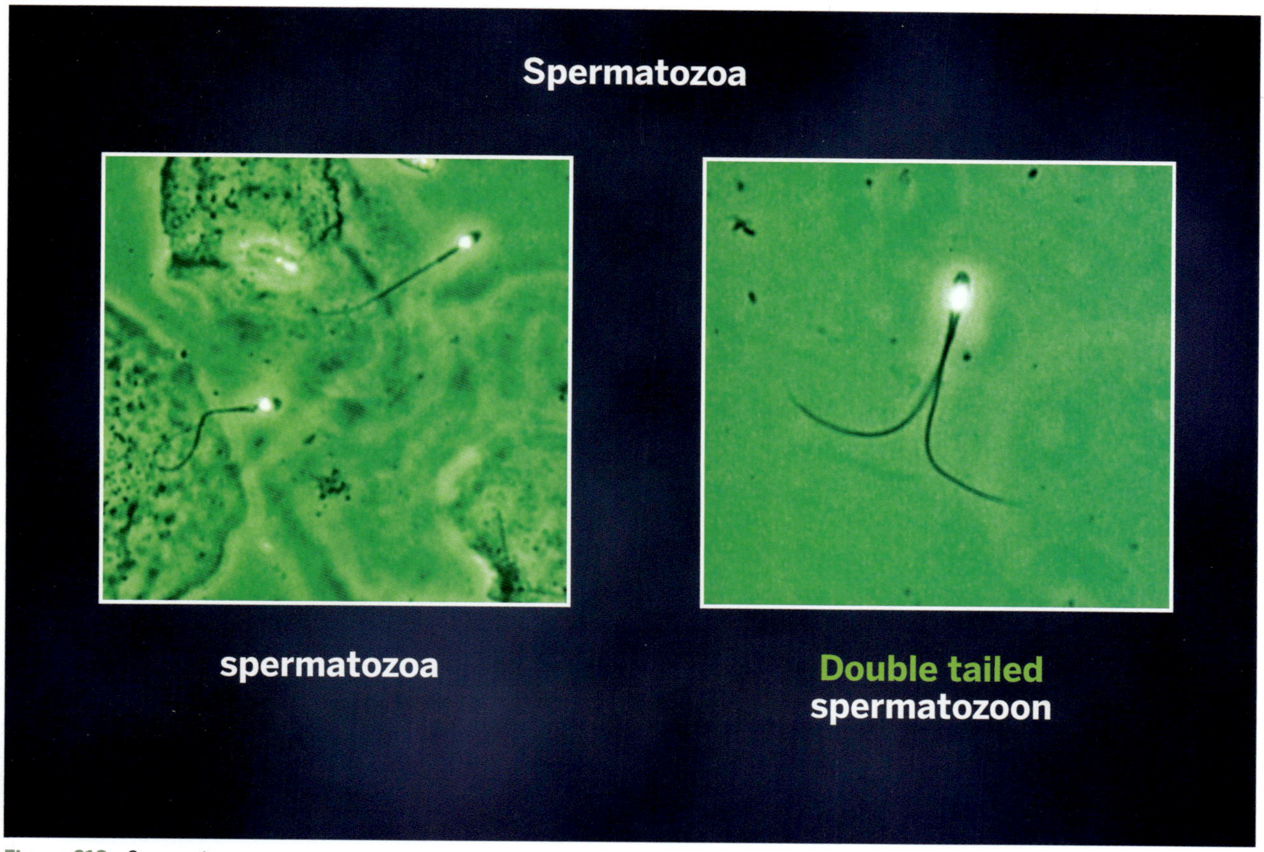

Figure 218 - Spermatozoa.

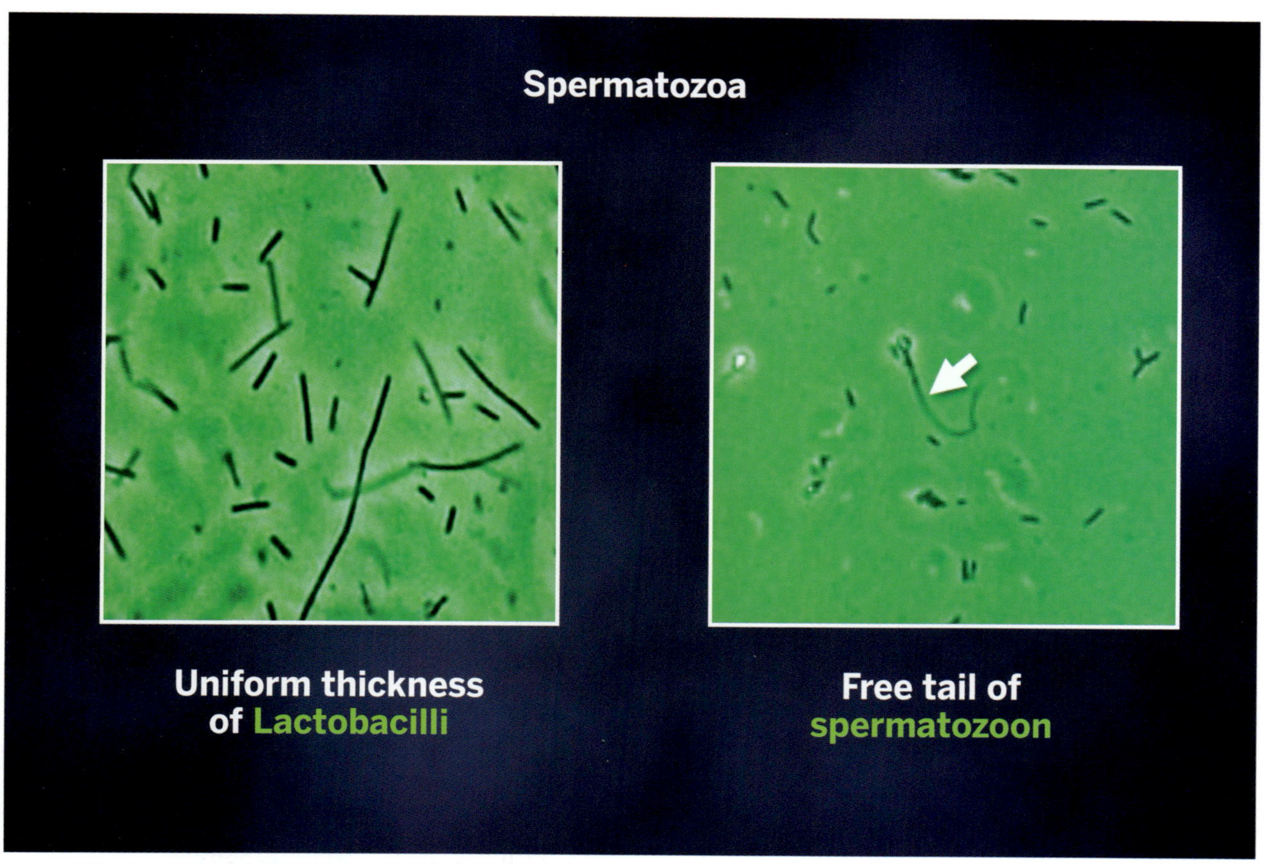

Figure 219 - Comparison between Lactobacilli and tail of spermatozoon.

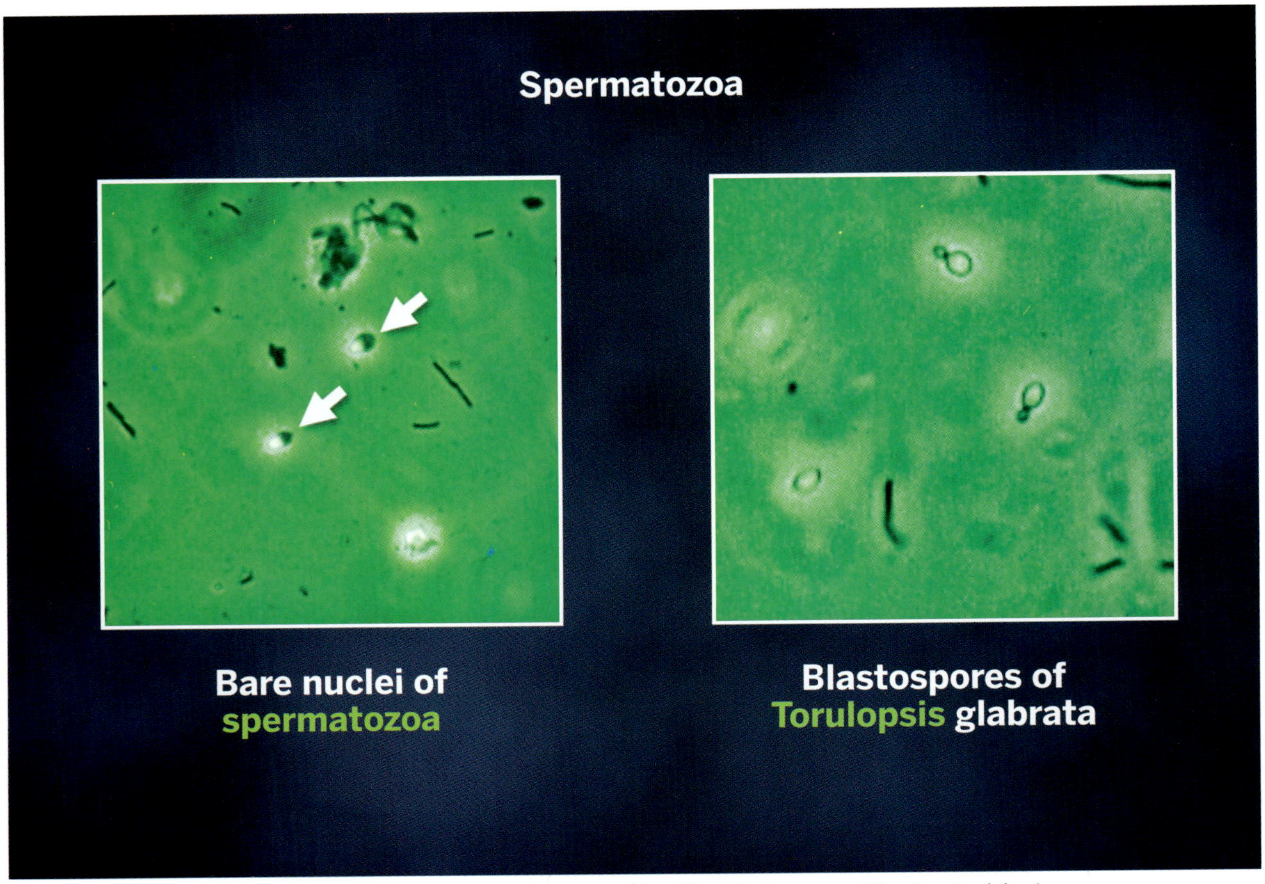

Figure 220 - Comparison between bare heads of spermatozoa and budding blastospores of Torulopsis glabrata.

Cervical cancer (Figures 221, 222) is the second most common cancer affecting women worldwide. Effective methods for early detection of precancerous lesions using cytology (Pap smear and direct microscopy) exist and have been shown to be successful.

A skilful application of direct microscopy enables the observer to detect potentially precancerous changes known as cervical intraepithelial neoplasia (CIN) (Richart CIN grading), cervical dysplasia (Regan WHO) or squamous intraepithelial lesions (SIL) (Bethesda System) (Figure 223).

The screener must follow some criteria for detecting dysplastic or atypical cells in the observation of the cells, the nucleus and the cytoplasm.

Cell

- Different cell sizes and shapes (anisocytosis) (Figures 224, 225)
- Marked fragility of cells with break of the cells and release of bare nuclei (Figure 226).

Nucleus

- Differences in the size and shape of the nucleus (anisokaryosis) (Figure 227)
- Cells with multiple nuclei and anisokaryosis (Figure 228)
- Enlarged (Figure 229) or giant nucleus (Figure 230)
- Ruptured chromatin (Figure 231)
- Variations in the amount of chromatin (Figure 232)
- Clumped chromatin (Figure 233)
- Mitotic figures (Figure 226)
- Eccentric nuclei (Figure 234)
- Multiple (Figures 224, 235) and enlarged nucleoli (Figures 226, 235)
- Differences in the size and number of nucleoli (Figure 235).

Cytoplasm

- Variations in the cytoplasm/nucleus ratio (Figure 227)
- Variable or advanced vacuolization (Figure 236)
- Cell cannibalism (Figure 237).

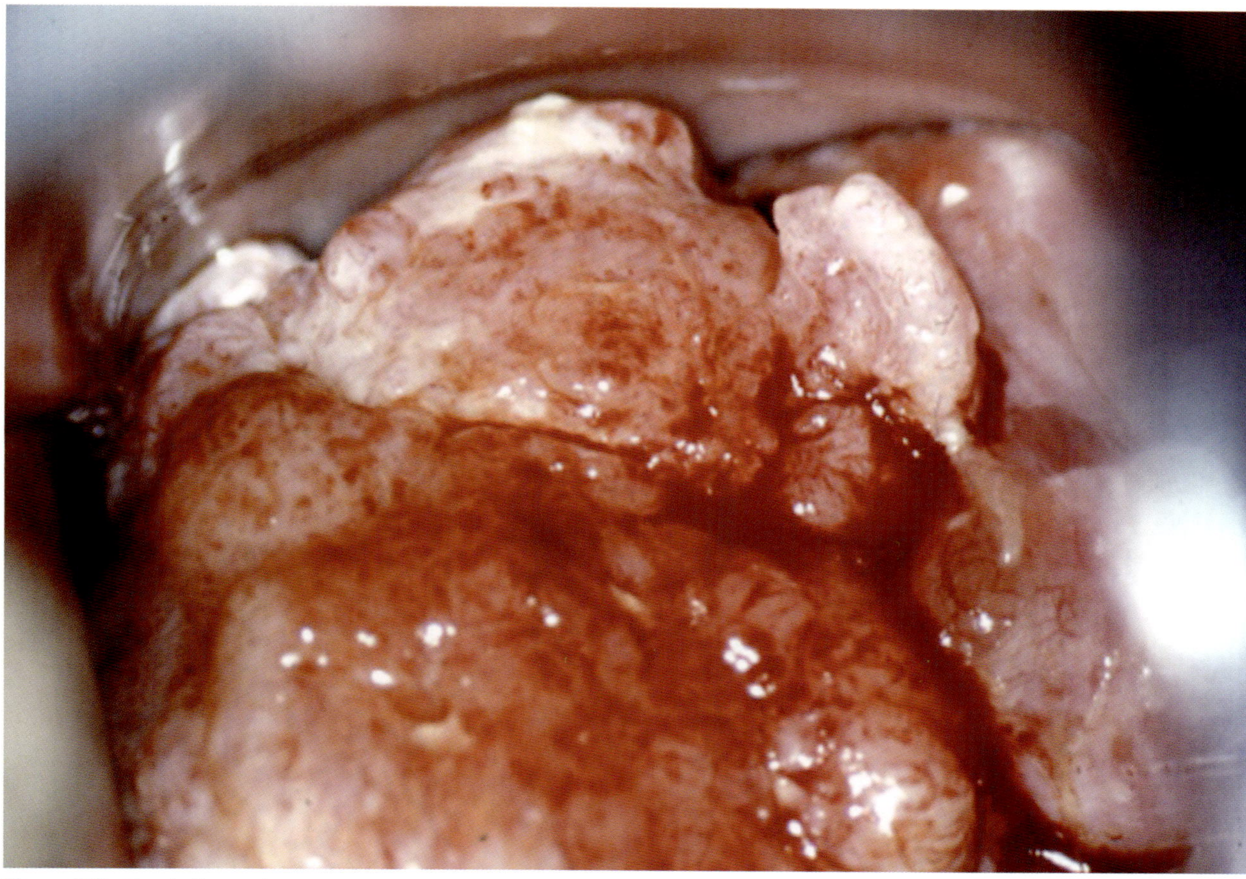

Figure 221 - Exophytic carcinoma.

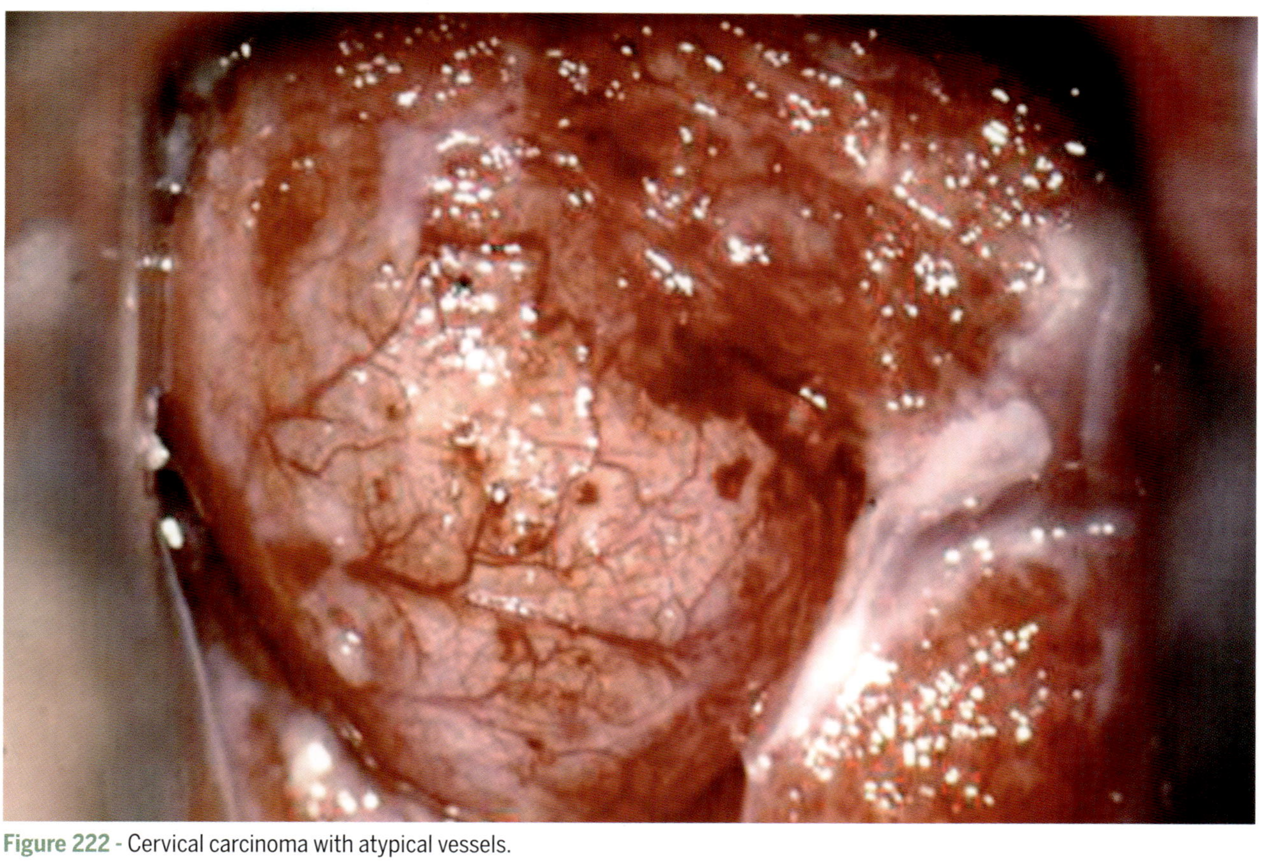

Figure 222 - Cervical carcinoma with atypical vessels.

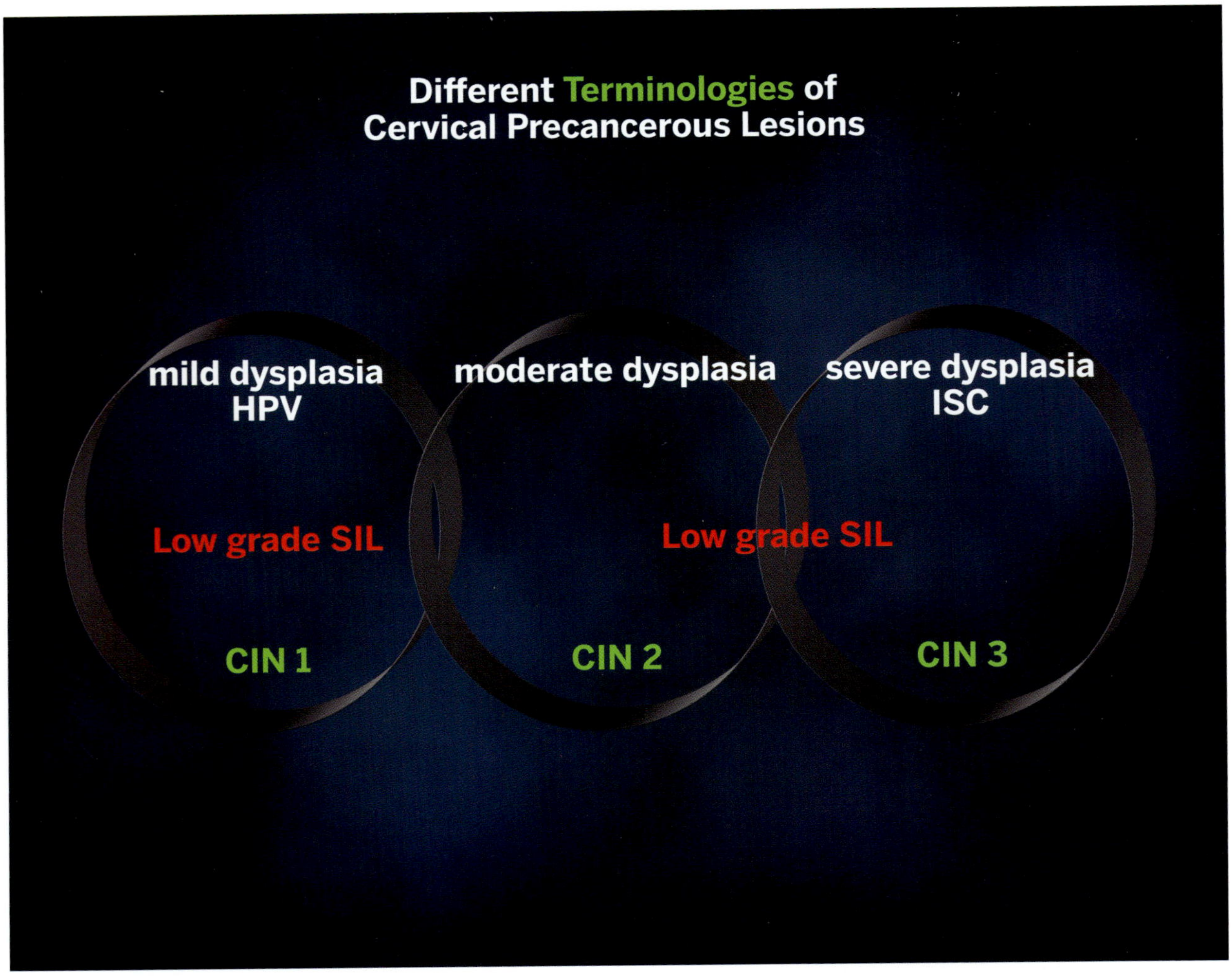

Figure 223 - Different terminologies of cervical precancerous lesions.

Unfortunately wet mount preparations cannot be preserved, therefore it is advisable to document atypical cells photomicrographically, in order to render cytologic assessment more objective and hence free of subjective interpretation.

Sometimes the detection of dysplastic or atypical cells in unstained specimen represents the only warning signal when gynaecological consultation does not include the Pap smear.

Finally, we want to stress that direct cytologic evaluation by phase contrast microscopy does not absolutely exclude the Papanicolaou smear but must be considered as the first step in the diagnostic work-up for cervical cancer screening. This lies on the precious and vital interdisciplinary cooperation between the gynaecologist and histopathologist who must combine their findings to achieve optimum results in the management of female lower genital tract lesions.

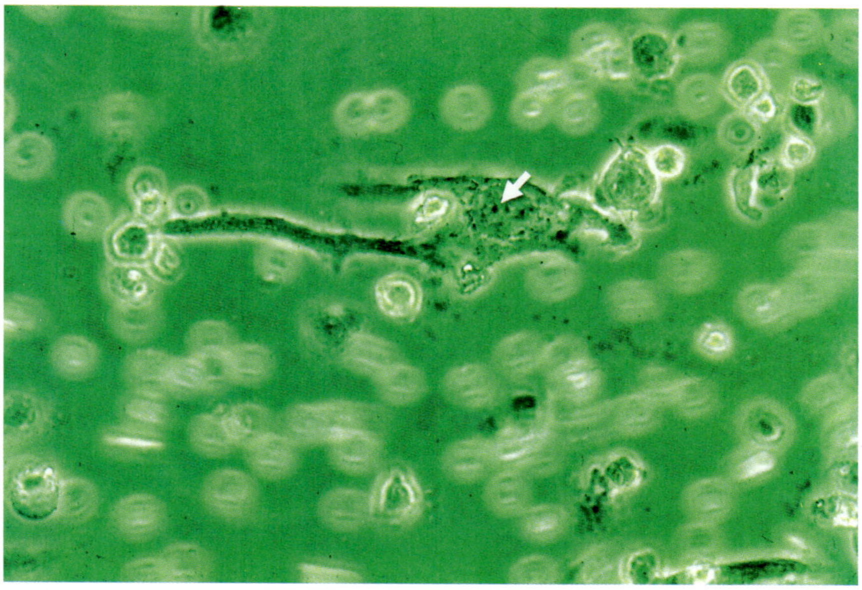

Figure 224 - Different shapes of a malignant cells (anisocytosis). The arrow indicates multiple nucleoli.

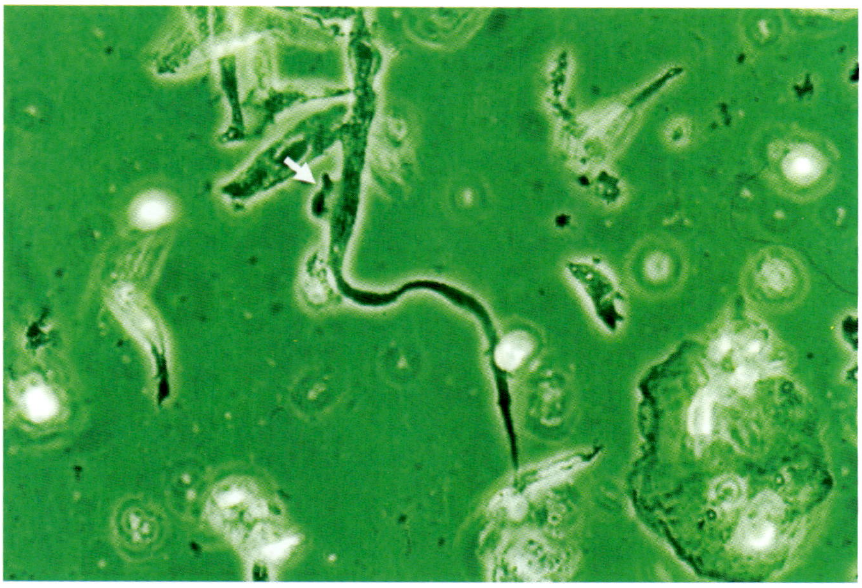

Figure 225 - Malignant fiber cell (→) associated with cells different in shape.

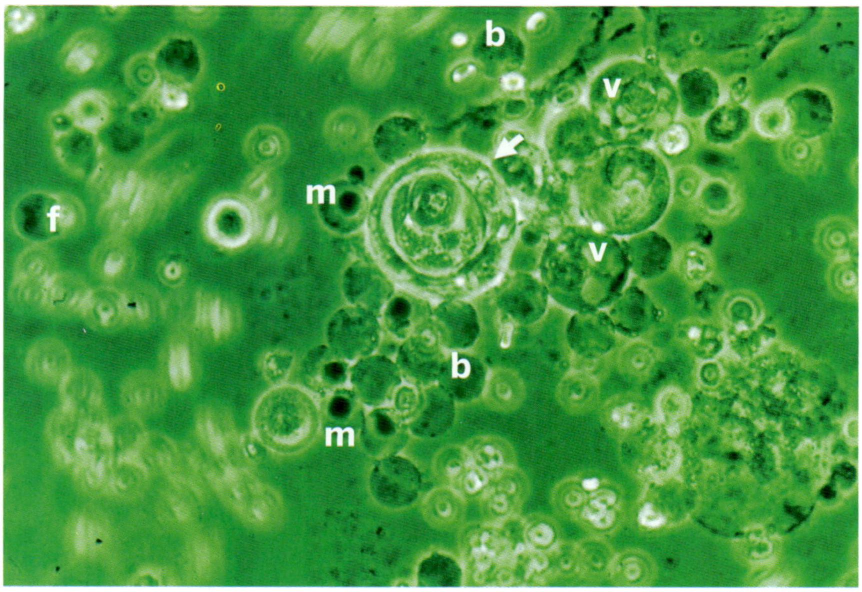

Figure 226 - Marked fragility of cells with break of the cells and release of bare nuclei (b) containing macronucleoli (m). The arrow indicates a malignant epithelial pearl. (v) Cytoplasmic vacuoles, (f) mitotic figure.

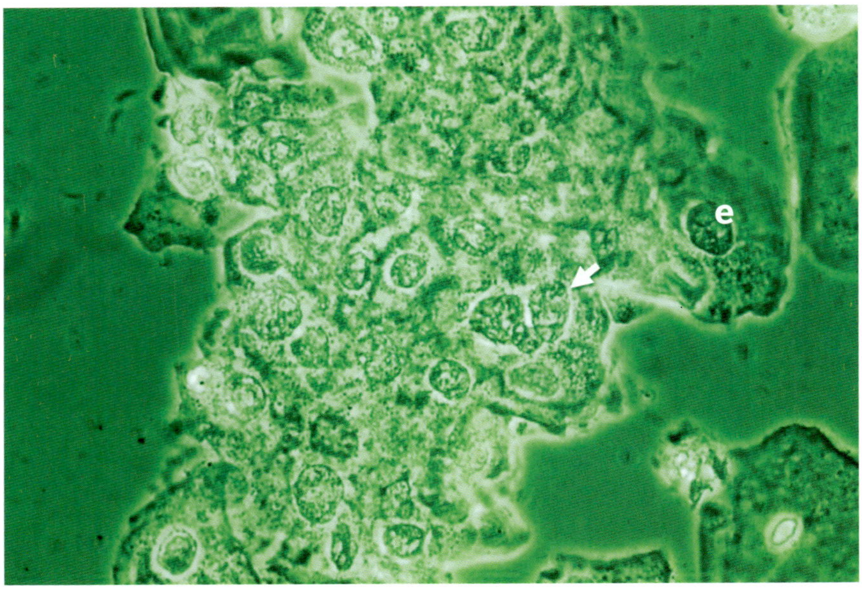

Figure 227 - Multinucleation (→) with nuclei different in shape and size (anisokaryosis). (e) Enlarged and dark nucleus.

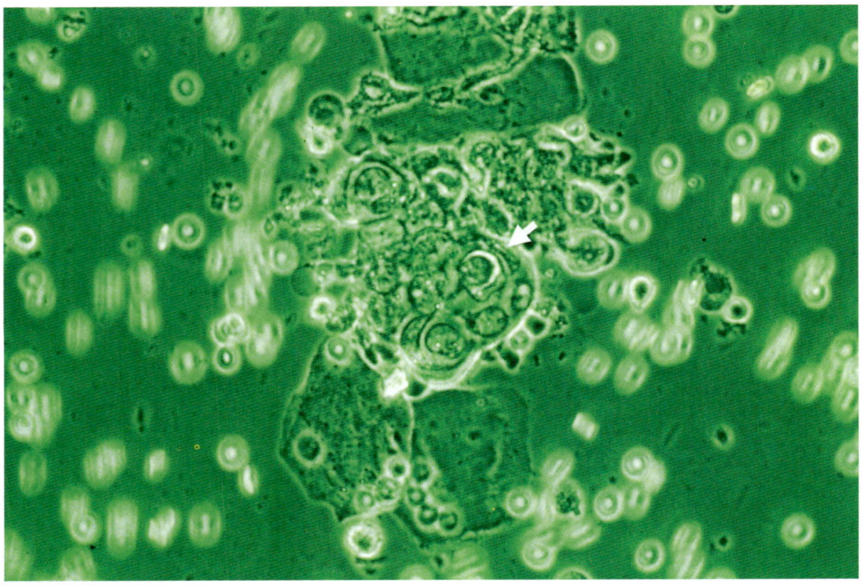

Figure 228 - Multinucleation (→) and anisokaryosis.

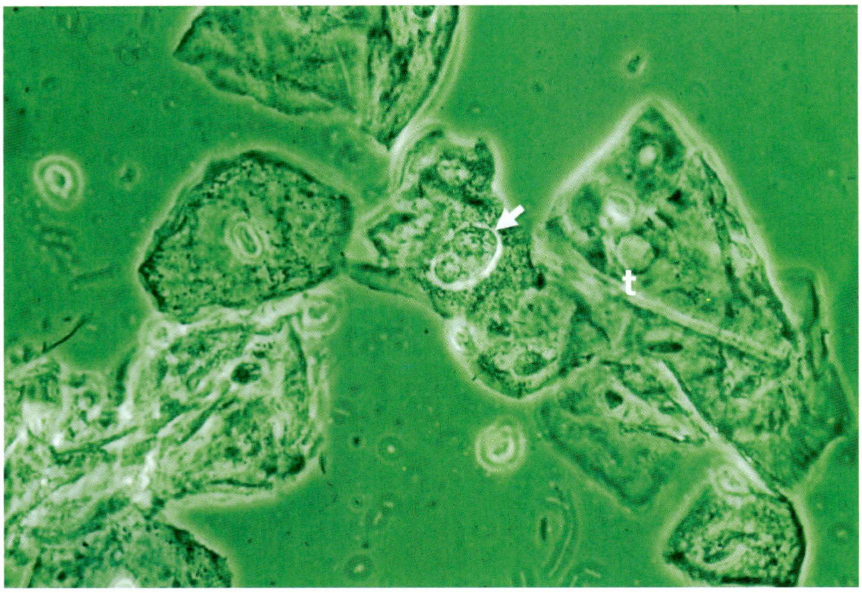

Figure 229 - Multinucleation, anisokaryosis and enlarged nucleus (→). (t) Cytoplasmic tunnel for Candida cytopathy.

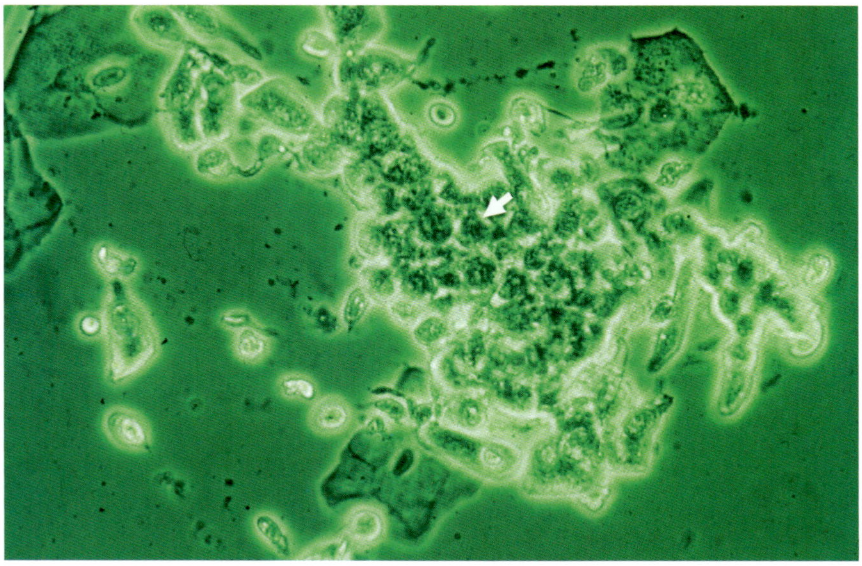

Figure 230 - Giant nucleus.

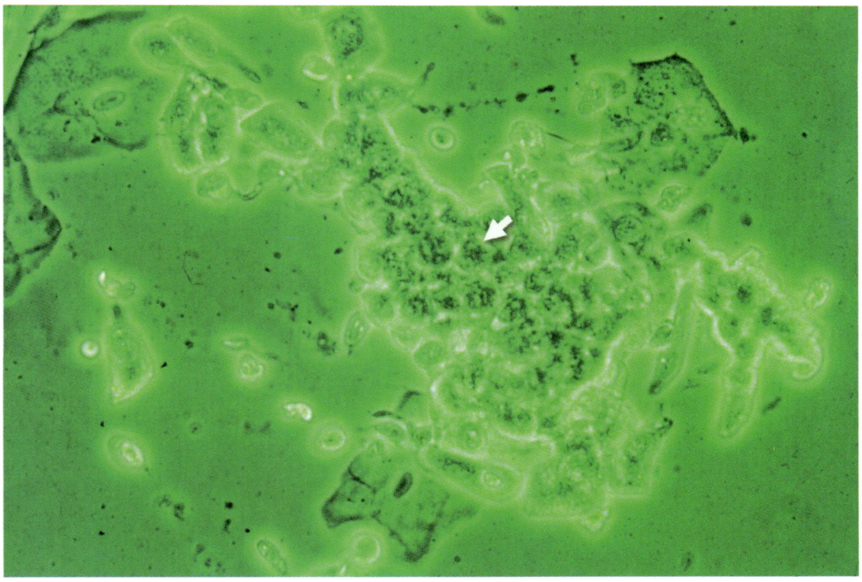

Figure 231 - Ruptured chromatin in a cluster (→) of dyskaryotic glandular cells (adenocarcinoma).

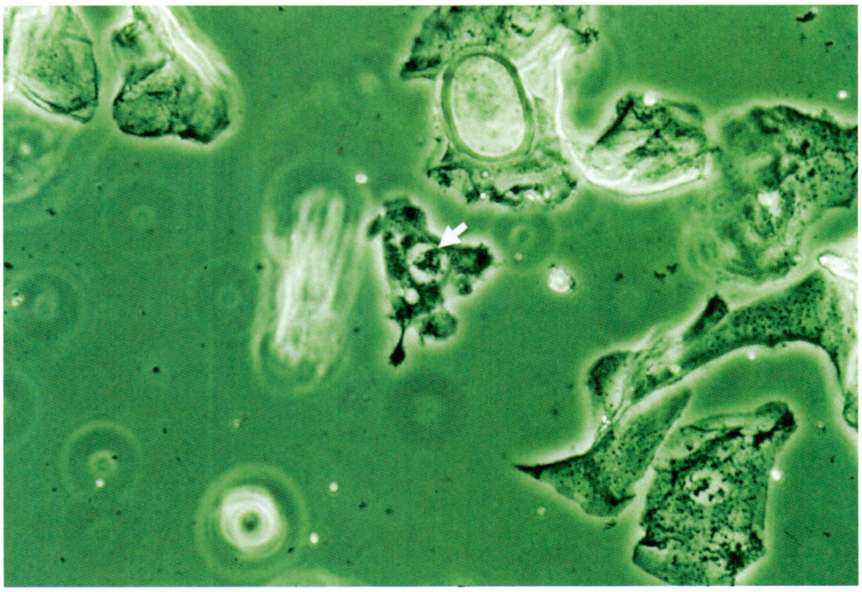

Figure 232 - Clumped chromatin (→) in a dyskaryotic premature metaplastic cell deriving from an immature metaplastic spider cell.

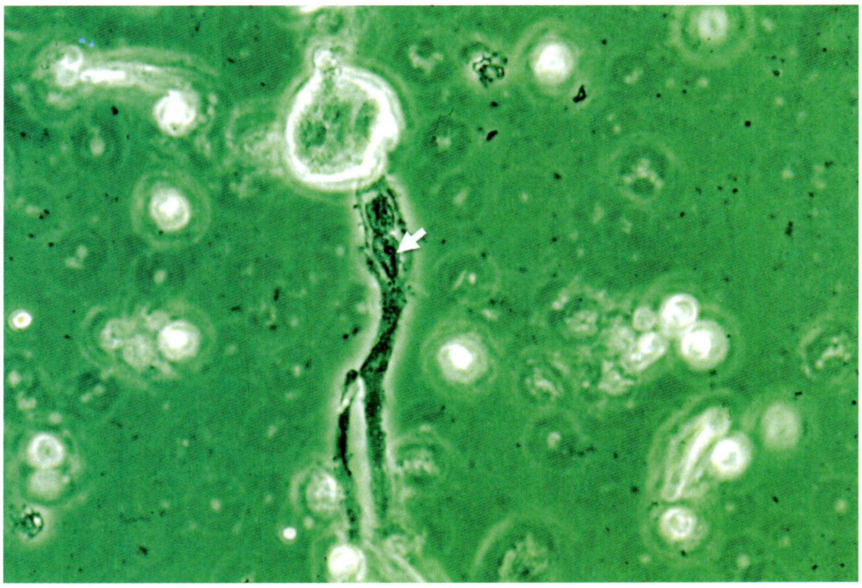

Figure 233 - Equatorial clumped chromatin in a binucleate malignant fiber cell.

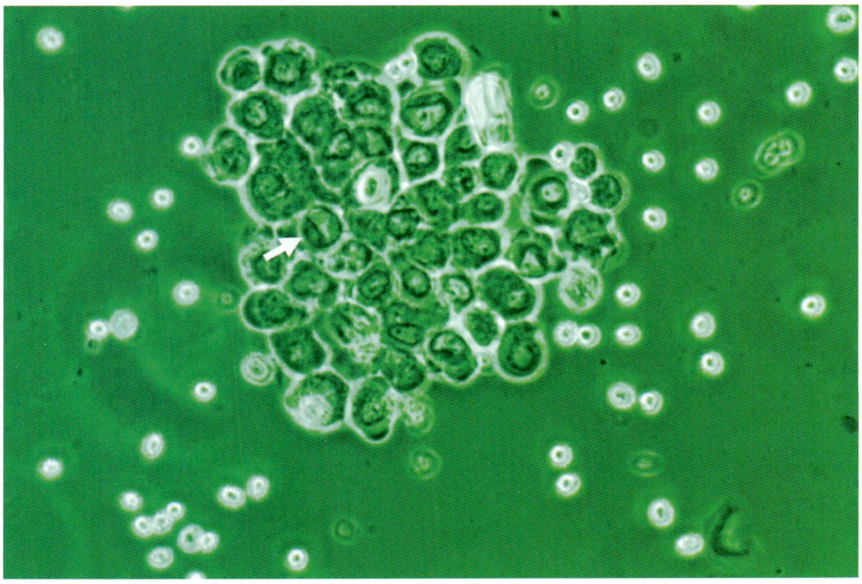

Figure 234 - Eccentric nuclei (→) (adenocarcinoma).

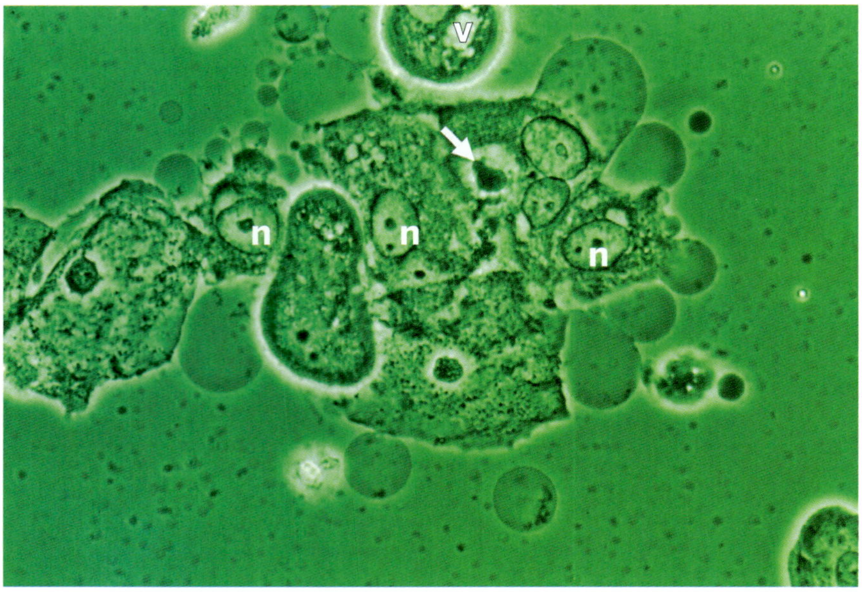

Figure 235 - Nucleoli (n) different in size and number. The arrow indicates a dark nucleus.

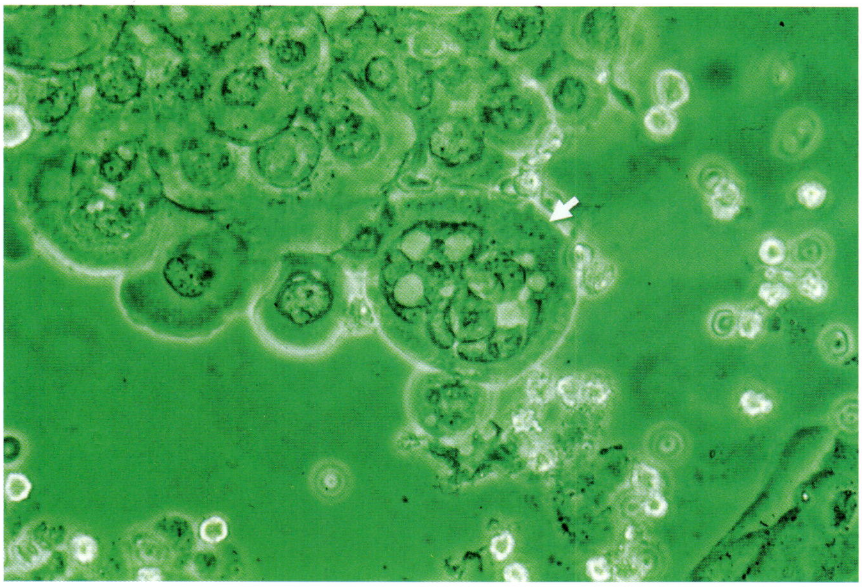

Figure 236 - Multinucleated malignant cell (→) with cytoplasmic vacuoles.

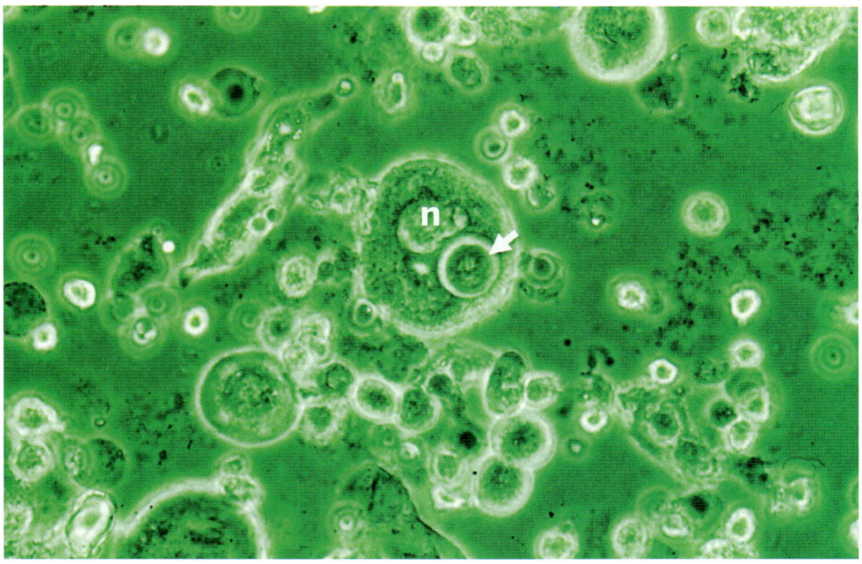

Figure 237 - Cell cannibalism: a malignant cell with irregularly edged nucleus (n) phagocytosing a smaller cell (→).

REFERENCES

- Ault KA. Epidemiology and Natural History of Human Papillomavirus Infections in the Female Genital Tract. Infect Dis Obstet Gynecol. 2006;2006 Suppl:40470.
- Baba AI, Catoi C. Comparative Oncology. The Publishing House of the Romanian Academy. Bucharest, 2007.
- Barakat RR. Oncology Journal, Breast Cancer, Endometrial Cancer, Gynecologic Cancers. Review article, January 31, 1995.
- Cibas ES, Ducatman BS. Cytology. Diagnostic Principles and Clinical Correlates. Elsevier Saunders, 2014.
- Dixit R, Bhavsar C, Marfatia YS. Laboratory diagnosis of human papillomavirus virus infection in female genital tract. Indian J Sex Trasm Dis. 2011;32(1): 50-2.
- Donders G, Bellen G, Rezeberga D. Aerobic vaginitis in pregnancy. BJOG. 2011;118(10):1163-70.
- Eckert LO, Hawes SE, Stevens CE, et al. Vulvovaginal candidiasis: clinical risks factors management algorithm. Obstet Gynecol. 1998;92:757-65.
- Enache-Angoulvant A, Ennequin C. Invasive *Saccharomyces* Infection: a comprehensive review. Clin Infect Dis. 2005;41(11):1559-68.
- EuroCytology Courses. Cervical Cytology (Up to date, 2016).
- Evans DT. Actinomyces israelii in the female genital tract: a review. Article in Genitourin Med.1193;69(1):54-9.
- Gow NA. Germ tube growth of Candida albicans. Curr Top Med Mycol. 1997;8(1-2):43.
- Harp DF, Chowdhury I. Trichomoniasis: evaluation to execution. Eur J Obstet Gynecol Reprod Biol. 2011;157(1):3-9.
- Hillier SL. Diagnostic microbiology of bacterial vaginosis. Am J Obstet Gynecol. 1993;169(2 Pt 2):455-9.
- Usain OAN, Butler EB. A Colour Atlas of Gynaecological Cytology. Wolfe Medical Publications Ltd, 1989.
- Ahic M, Mulavdic M, Nurkic J, Jahic E, Nurkic M. Clinical Characteristics of Aerobic Vaginitis and Its Association to Vaginal Candidiasis, Trichomonas Vaginitis and Bacterial Vaginosis. Med Arch. 2013;67(6):428.
- Kavikcioglu F, Akif Akgul M, Haberal A, Faruk Demir O. Actinomyces infection in female genital tract. Eur J Obstet Gynecol Reprod Biol. 2005;118(1):77-80.
- Koneman EW, Allen SD, Dowel VR-J, Janda WM, Sommers HM, Winn WC-J. Color atlas and textbook of diagnostic microbiology; JB Lippincott Company, 1988.
- Majeroni BA. Bacterial vaginosis: an update. Am Fam Physician. 1998 Mar 15;57(6):1285-9.

- Malarewicz A, Florczak K. Cytologia fazowo-kontrastowa w diagnostyce ginekologicznej. Digital Medicine in the Future, 2006.
- Marinho-Dias J, Ribeiro J, Monteiro P, Loureiro J, Baldaque I, Medeiros R, Sousa H. Characterization of cytomegalovirus and epstein-barr virus infection in cervical lesions in Portugal. J Med Virol. 2013;85(8):1409-13.
- Miniello G. Citogramma Vaginale - Vaginal Cytogram. CIC Edizioni Internazionali, 1994.
- Miniello G. Sindrome uretrale e urocitogramma a fresco. CIC Edizioni Internazionali, 1996.
- Miniello G. Colposcopia e microscopia a fresco – Colposcopy and Phase Contrast Microscopy. CIC Edizioni Internazionali, 1998.
- Miniello G. Le micosi vaginali in microscopia a fresco. Vaginal Fungal Infections by phase contrast microscopy. CIC Edizioni Internazionali, 2001-2012.
- Miniello G, Saraiya U. Color Atlas of Cytology and Colposcopy. CBS Publishers, New Delhi, 1999.
- Miniello G. Gynecological Urology, Wet Mount Urocytogram in Recurrent Urinary Tract Infections. Orient Longman Eds, p.52, 2001.
- Miniello G. Microscopia a fresco nella diagnostica delle MST. Da: Trattato di Patologia Vulvare. Malattie Infettive del distretto vulvo-vestibolo-vaginale. Cap. 5, 2009.
- Miniello G. Micosi. Da: Frega A, Moscarini M, Caserta D, Biamonti A, French D, Scirpa P. Infezioni in Ginecologia. Manuale Pratico di diagnosi e terapia, p.179, Momento Medico, 2011.
- Miniello G. Role of Phase Contrast or Direct Microscopy in Daily Gynecologic Practice. From: AA Khan. Cytohormonal Profile of a Female from Birth to Postmenopausal Phase. A Review. CBS Publishers Distributors Pvt Ltd, 2017.
- Paavonen J, Vesterinen E, Meyer B, Saksela E. Colposcopic and histologic findings in cervical chlamydial infection. Obstet Gynecol. 1982;59(6):712-5.
- Redgrove KA, McLaughlin EA. The role of the immune response in Chlamydia trachomatis infection of the male genital tract: a double-edged sword. Review Article Front. Immunol., 27 October 2014.
- Roan NR, Starnbach MN. Immune-mediated control of Chlamydia infection. Cell Microbiol. 2008;10(1):9-19.
- Saraiya UB, Miniello G. HPV Infections and its Role in Cervical Cancer. From: Principles & Practice of Obstetrics and Gynecology for Postgraduates. Ch. 111, p. 1006, Jaypee Brothers Medical Publishers LTD, 2008.
- Saraiya UB, Miniello G. Atlas of Cytology and Colposcopy. Jaypee Brothers Medical Publishers, 2009.
- Singer A, Monaghan JM. Lower Genital Tract Precancer. Colposcopy, Pathology and Treatment. Blackwell Science, Inc, 2nd edition, april 2008.
- Sobel JD, Faro S, Force RW, Foxman B, Ledger WJ, Nyirjesy PR, Reed BD, Summers PR. Vulvovaginal candidiasis: epidemiologic, diagnostic, and therapeutic considerations. Am J Obstet Gynecol. 178(2):203-11.
- Sobel JD. Bacterial Vaginosis, Uptodate website, August 28, 2015.
- Stoll P, Dallenbach-Hellweg G. Cytology in Gynecological Practice. An Atlas of Phase Contrast Microscopy - Gynäkologische Vitalzytologie in der Praxis. Atlas der Phasenkontrastmikroskopie. Springer-Verlag, 1993.
- Suresh A, Rajesh A, Bhat RM, Rai Y. Cytolytyc vaginosis. Indian J Sex Transm Dis. 2009;30(1):48-50.
- Tempera G, Furneri PM. Management of aerobic vaginitis. Gynecol Obstet Invest. 2010;70(4):244-9.
- Szalay L. Cytolology of the uterine cervix. Wilhelm Maudrich-Medical Publishers, 1990.
- Yazdanparast SA, Barton RC. Arthroconidia production in Trichophyton rubrum and a new ex vivo model of onychomycosis. J Med Microbiol. 2006;55(Pt 11);1577-81.
- Wojciech R. The diagnostic value of cytology and colposcopy in women with cervical intraepithelial neoplasia. Ginekol Pol. 2011;82(8):607-11.

DIRECT MICROSCOPY IMMERSION

The pictures contained in this chapter do not follow any etiological order or plan, but are occasionally presented, as they may be observed in daily microscopical practice.

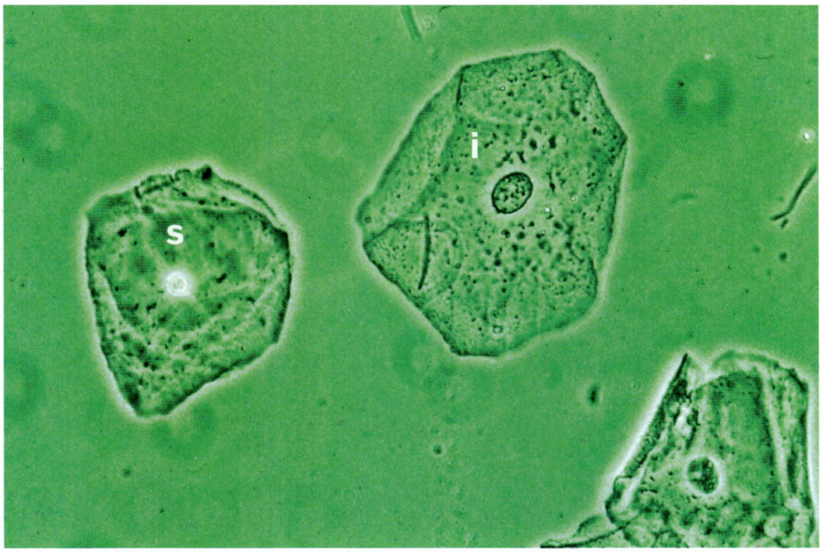

Figure 238 - Intermediate (i) and superficial cells (s).

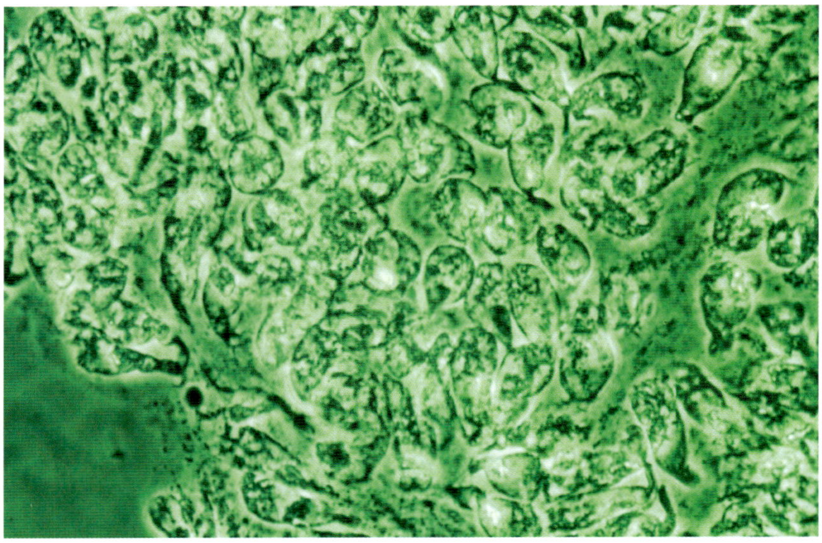

Figure 239 - Secretory endocervical cells.

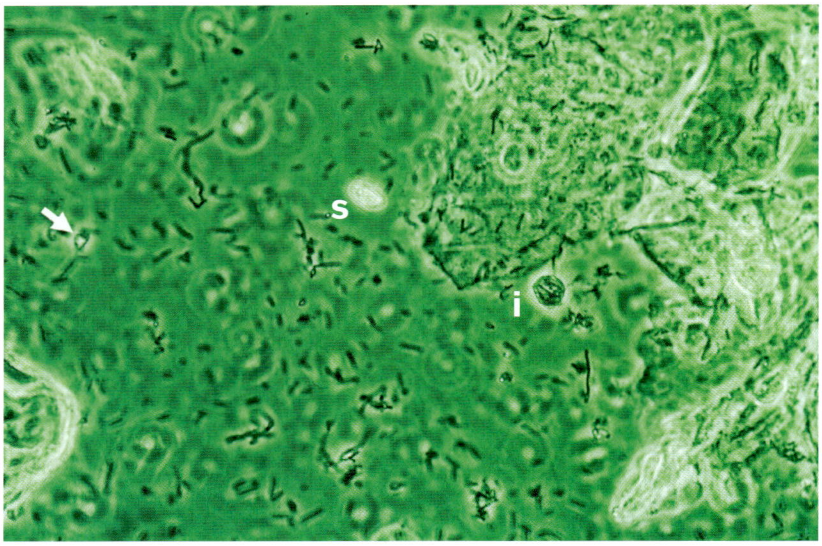

Figure 240 - Cytolytic smear showing naked nuclei of a superficial (s) and an intermediate cell (i). The arrow indicates the released top of a ciliated endocervical cell.

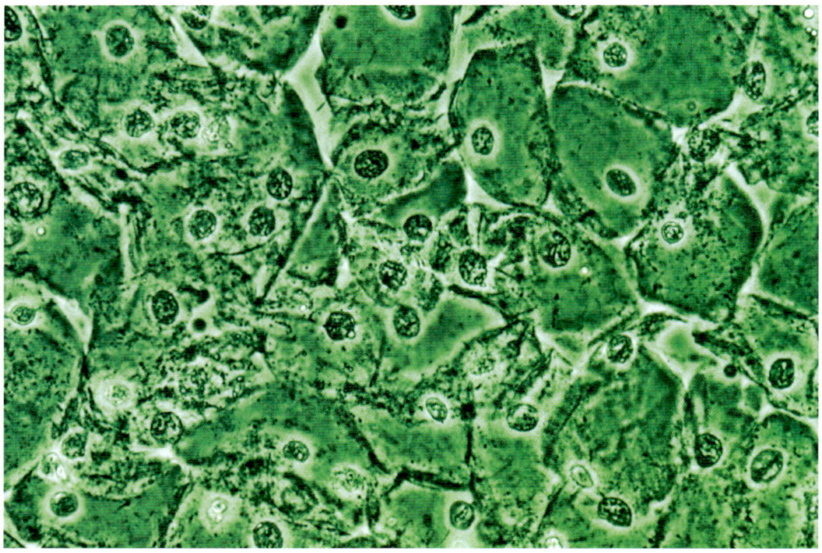

Figure 241 - Intermediate cells (intermediate pattern).

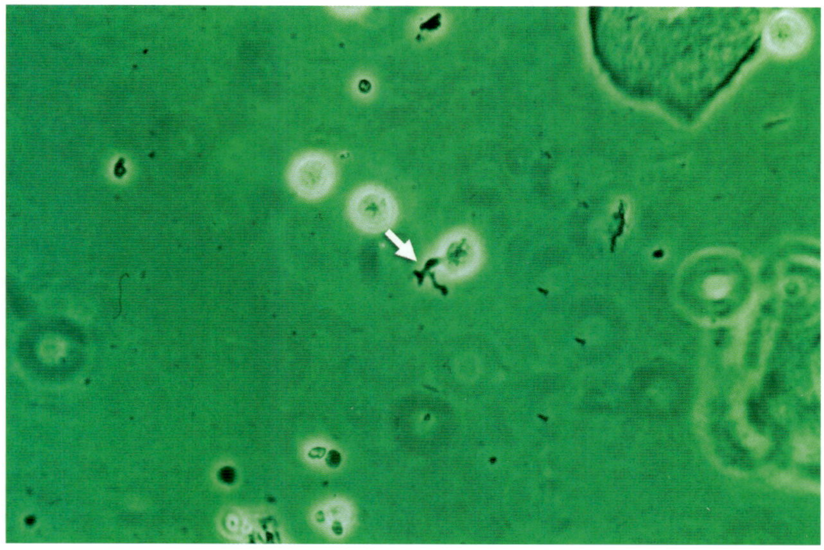

Figure 242 - Granulocyte provided with two pseudopodia (→).

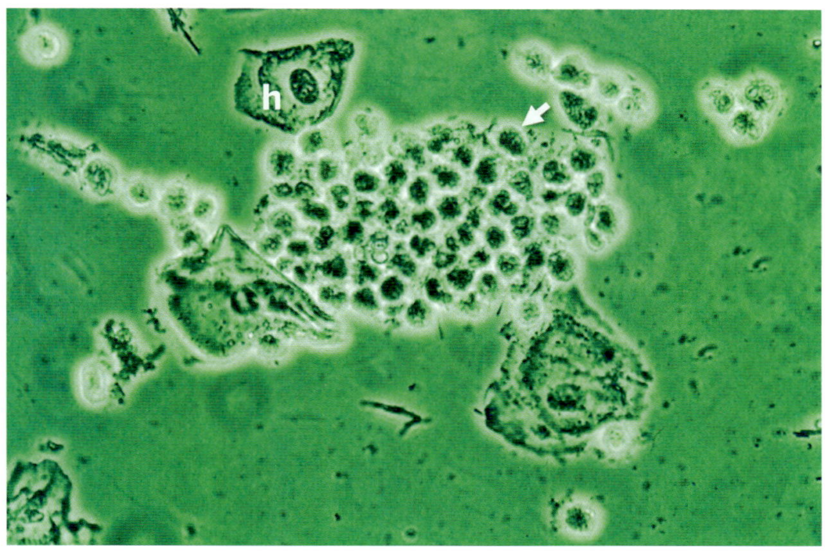

Figure 243 - Cluster of activated granulocytes (→). Wide perinuclear halo (h) without a sharply condensed edge (false koilocyte), surrounding a dark nucleus.

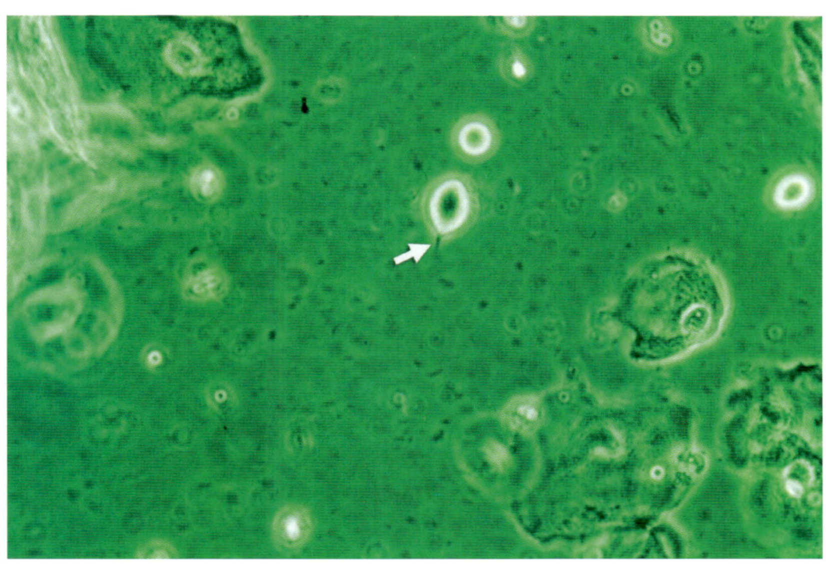

Figure 244 - Trichomonas vaginalis. The arrow indicates the axostyle.

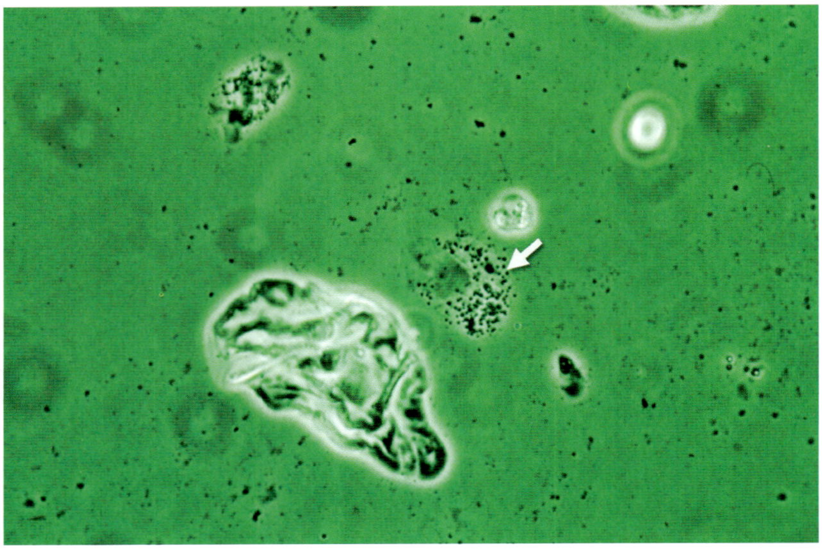

Figure 245 - Lysis of a macrophage and release (→) of digested material.

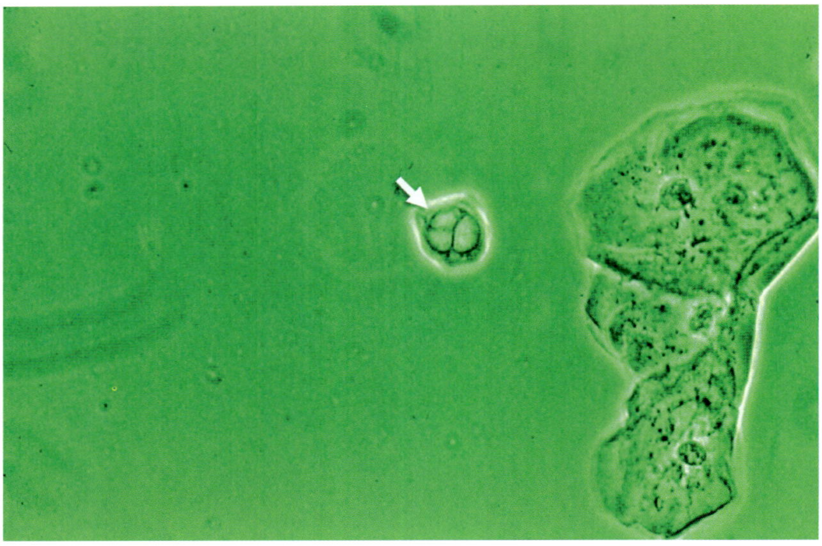

Figure 246 - Polykaryocyte (→) by HSV.

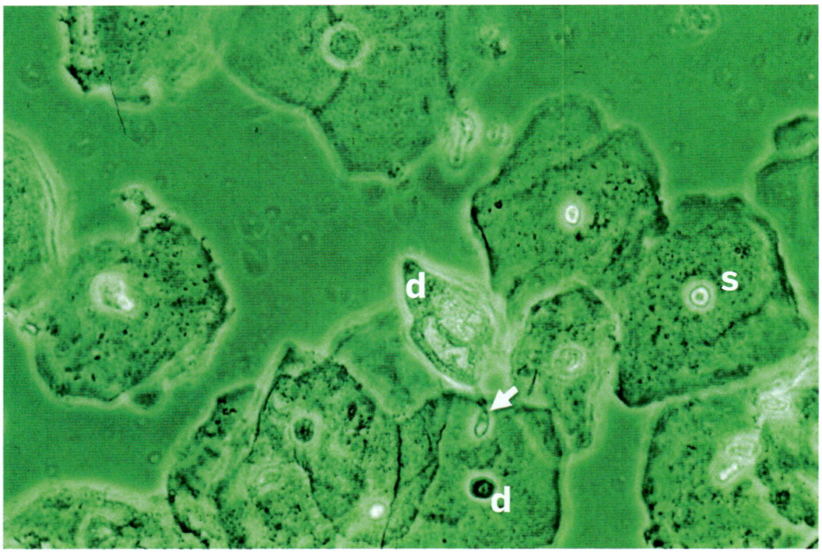

Figure 247 - The arrow indicates the short cytoplasmic process of a dysplastic premature metaplastic cell deriving from an immature metaplastic tadpole cell, containing two differently shaped nuclei (anisokaryosis) which alter the C/N ratio. (s) Superficial cell, (d) dark nucleus.

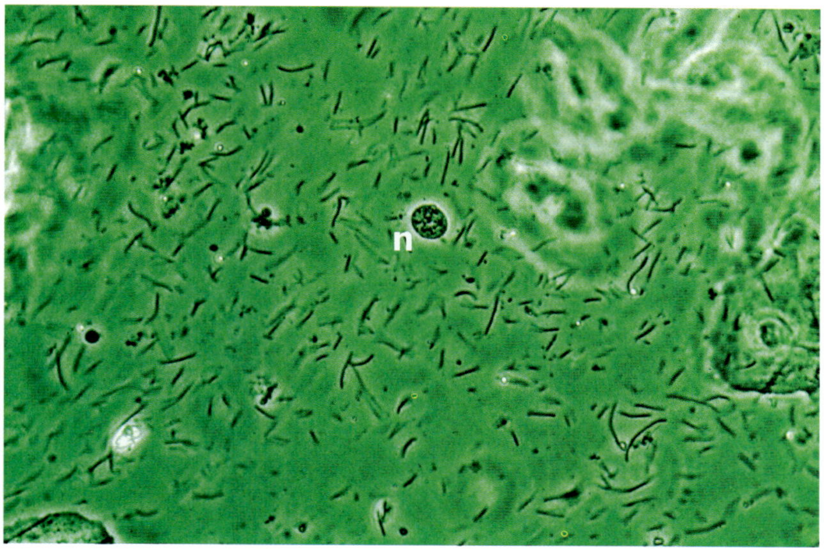

Figure 248 - Cytolytic smear.
(n) Naked nucleus of an intermediate cell.
Background of Lactobacilli.

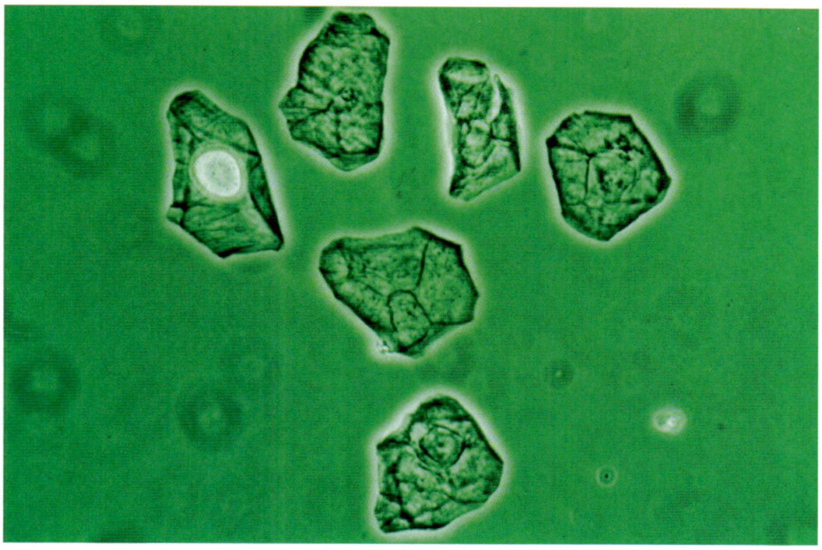

Figure 249 - Horny cells.

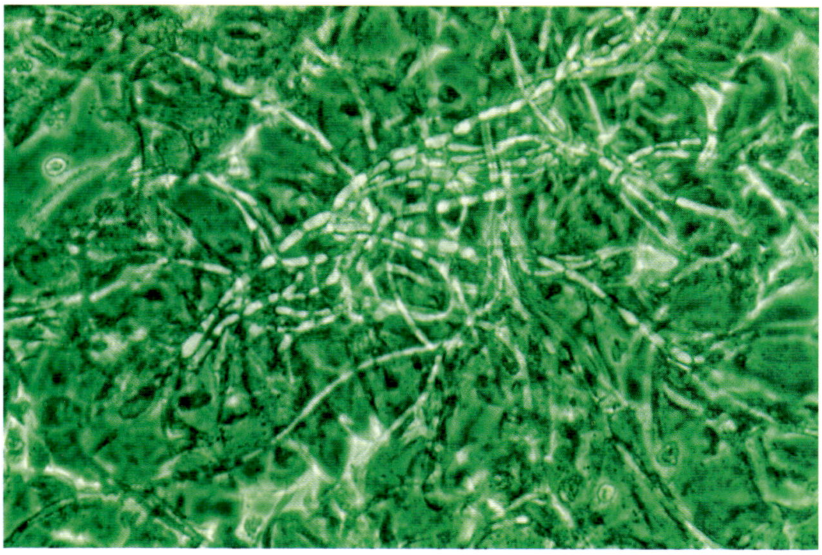

Figure 250 - Diaphanous aspect
of intraepithelial hyphae.

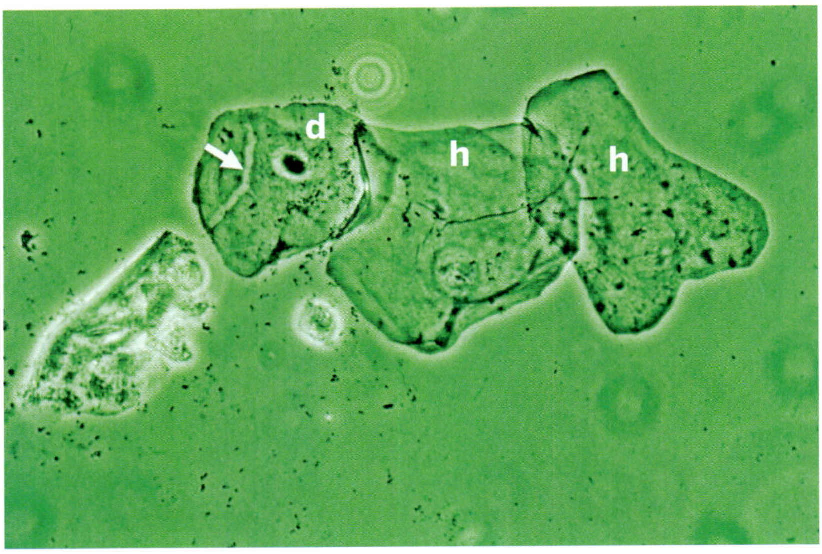

Figure 251 - Candida cytopathy: cytoplasmic groove (→) in a cell containing a dark nucleus (d). (h) Horny cells.

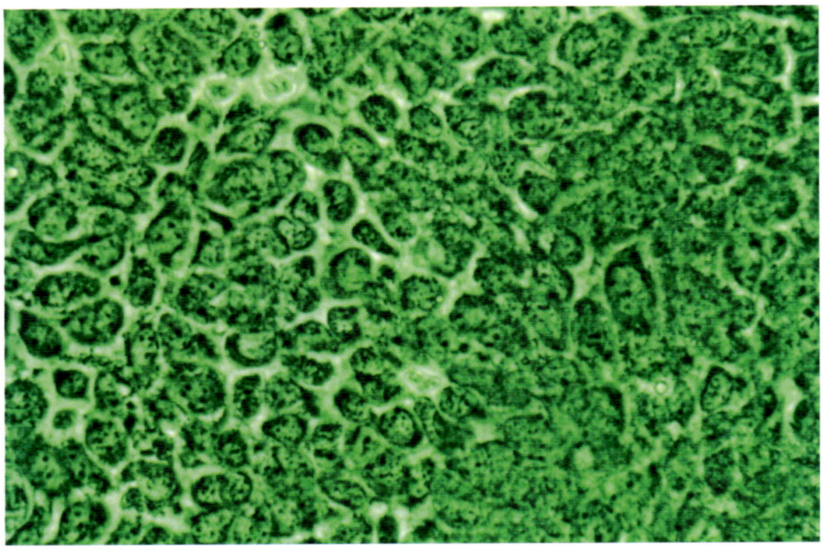

Figure 252 - Highly dyskaryotic glandular cells (adenocarcinoma).

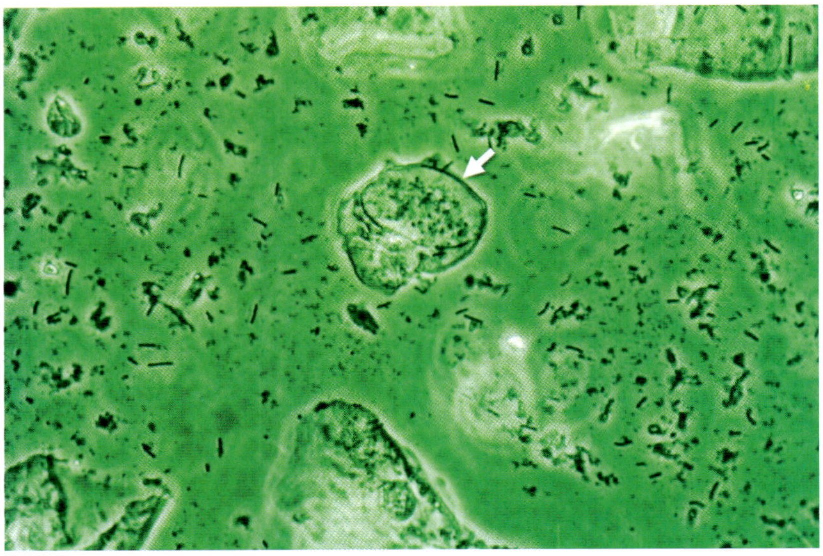

Figure 253 - Giant nucleus (→).

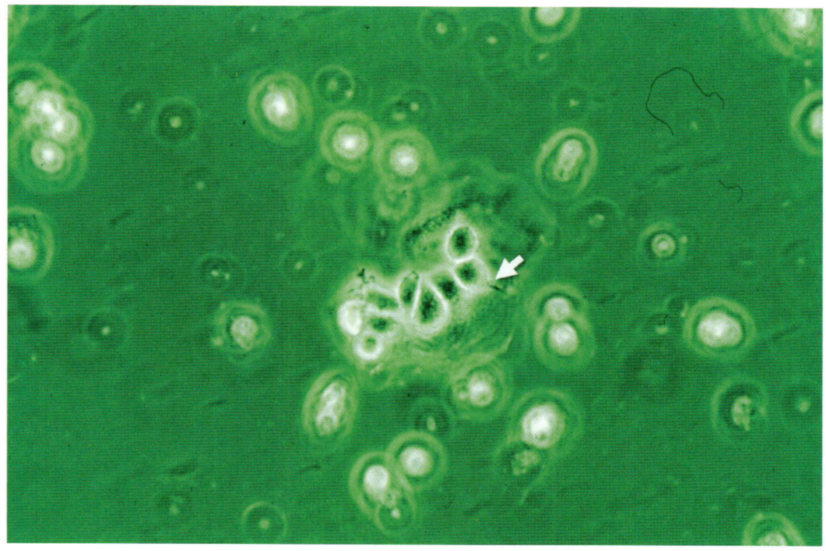

Figure 254 - Cluster of trichomonads. The arrow indicates an axostyle.

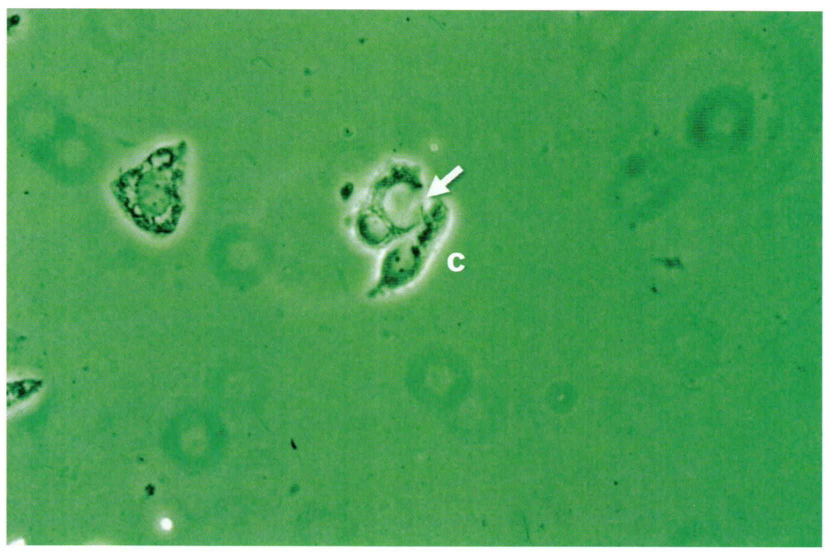

Figure 255 - Rupture (→) of an inclusion of Chlamydia trachomatis. (c) Columnar cell.

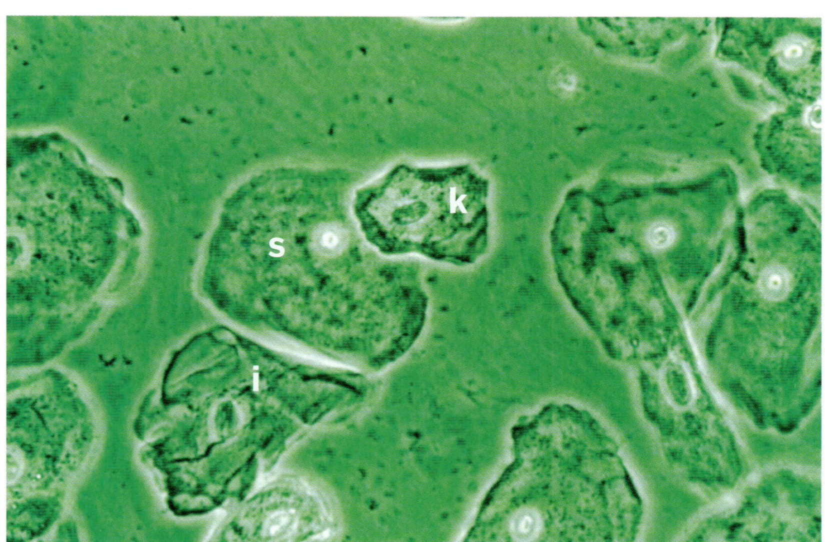

Figure 256 - Koilocyte (k). (i) Intermediate cell, (s) superficial cell.

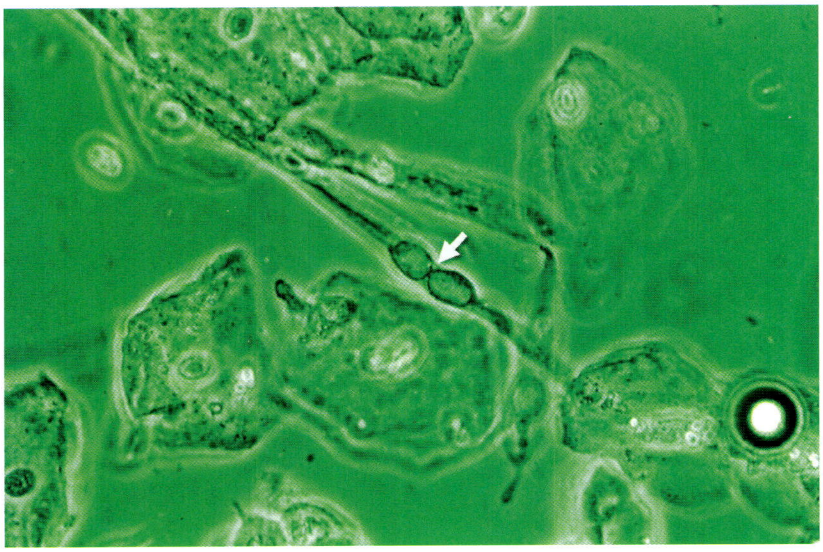

Figure 257 - Binucleate benign fiber cell (→) (HPV infection).

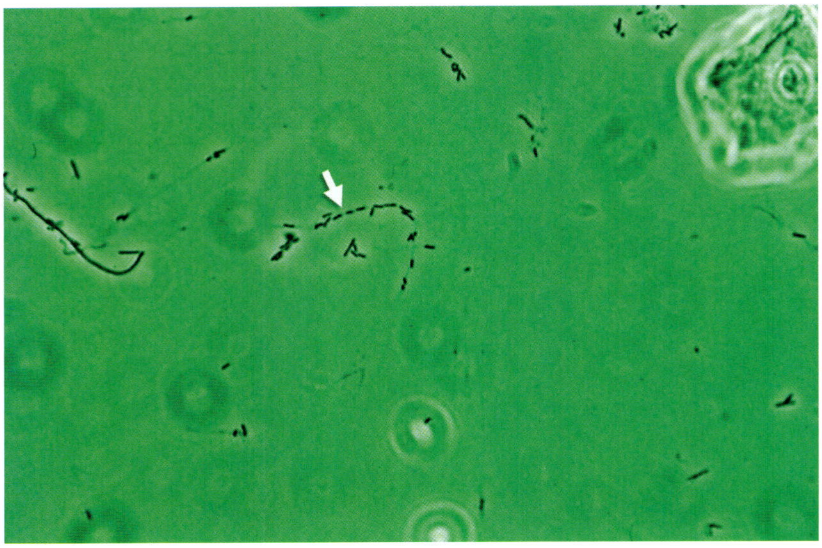

Figura 258 - Short and plump bacilli (→) (Escherichia coli).

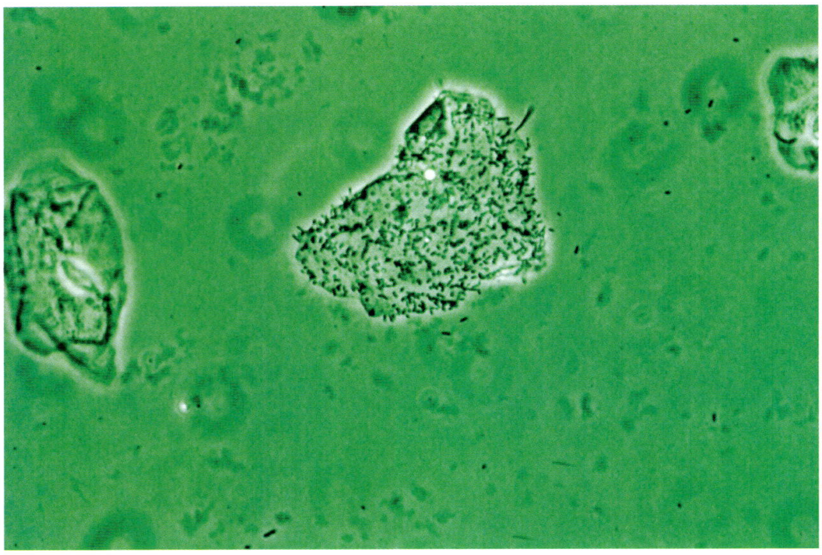

Figure 259 - Clue cell (Bacterial vaginosis).

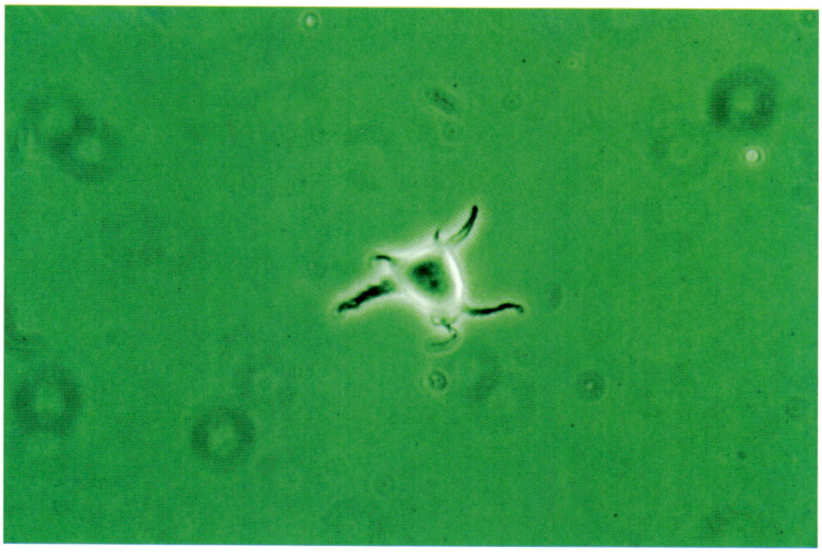

Figure 260 - Immature metaplastic spider cell.

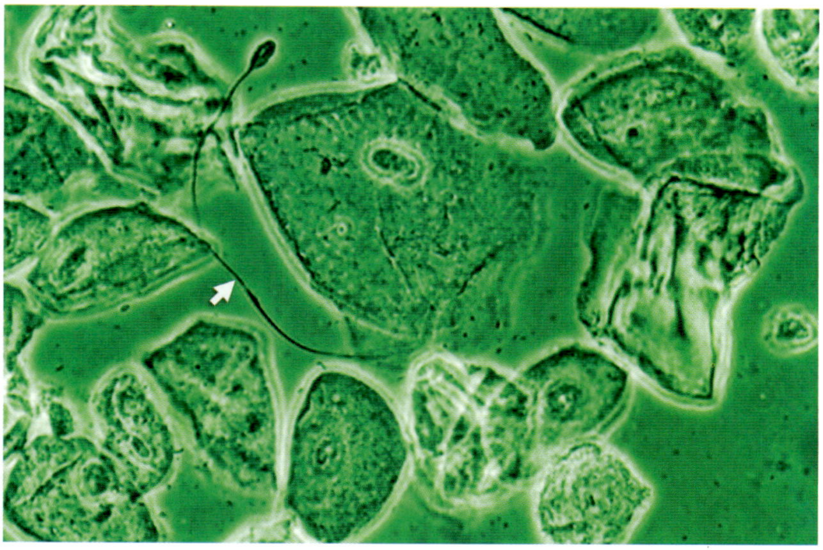

Figure 261 - Premature metaplastic cell deriving from an immature metaplastic tadpole cell. The arrow indicates the long cytoplasmic process.

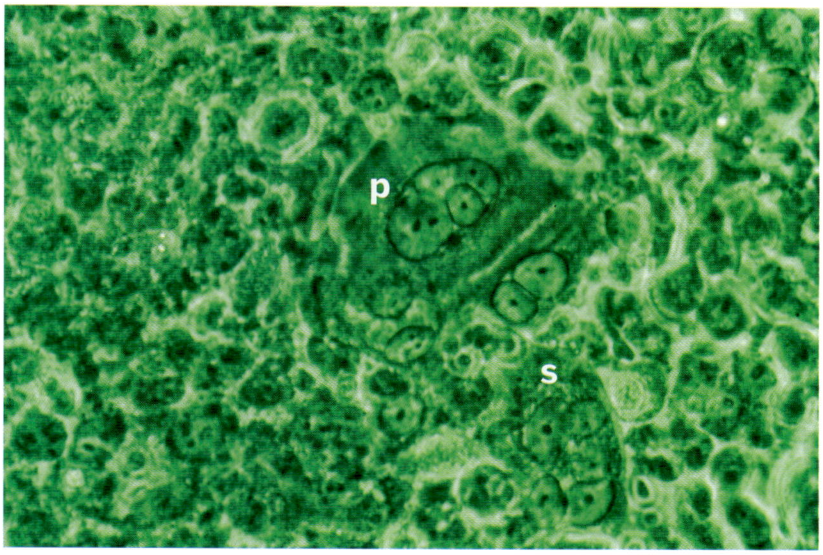

Figure 262 - Polykaryocyte (p) by HSV. (s) Cell syncytium.

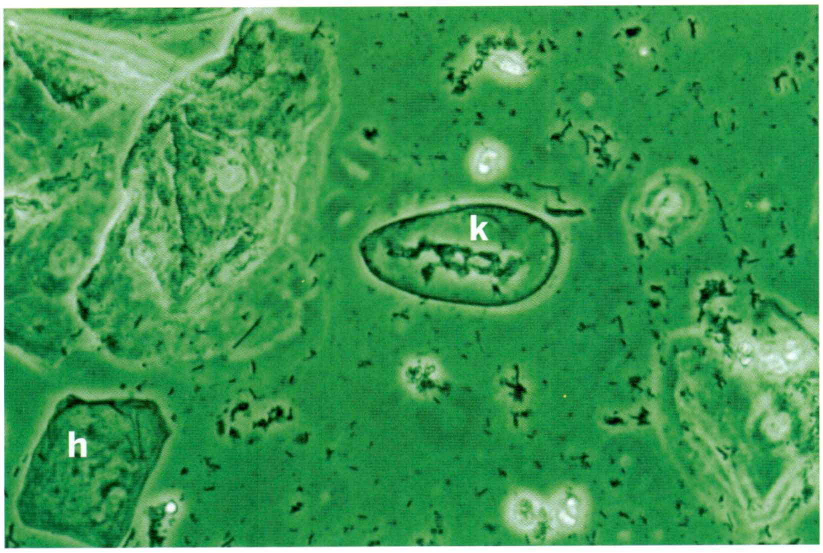

Figure 263 - Horny cell (h) and horny cell with a highly keratinized edge (k).

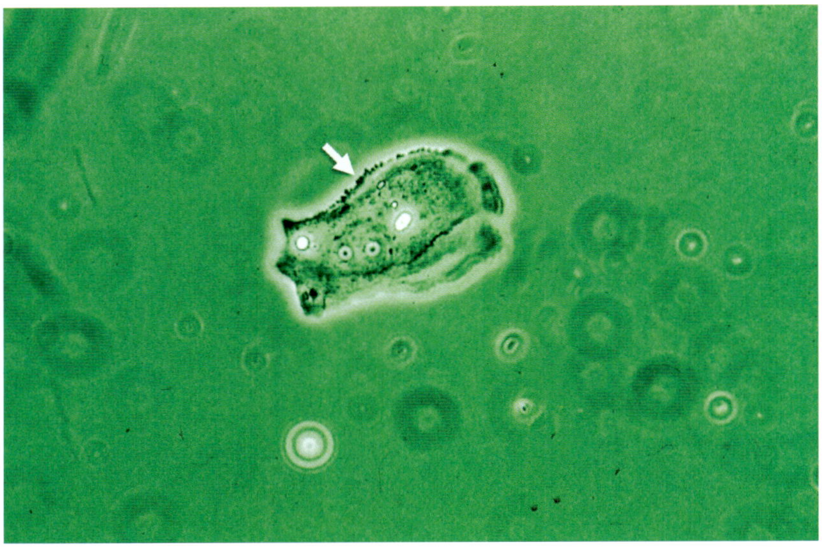

Figure 264 - Superficial cell. The arrow indicates the small cytoplasmic indentations for the connection with the neighbourig cells.

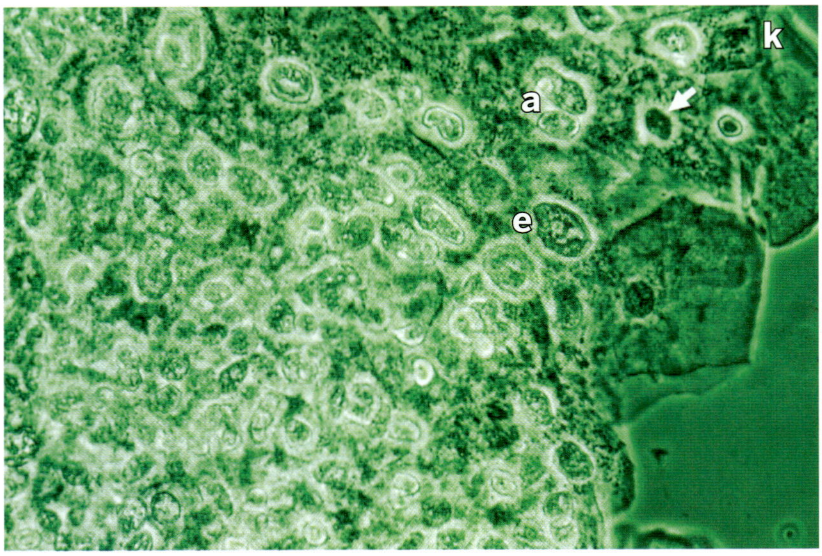

Figure 265 - Sheet of dysplastic cells: (e) enlarged and dysmorphic nucleus, (a) anisokaryosis of a binucleate cell, (k) koilocyte. The arrow indicates a dark nucleus.

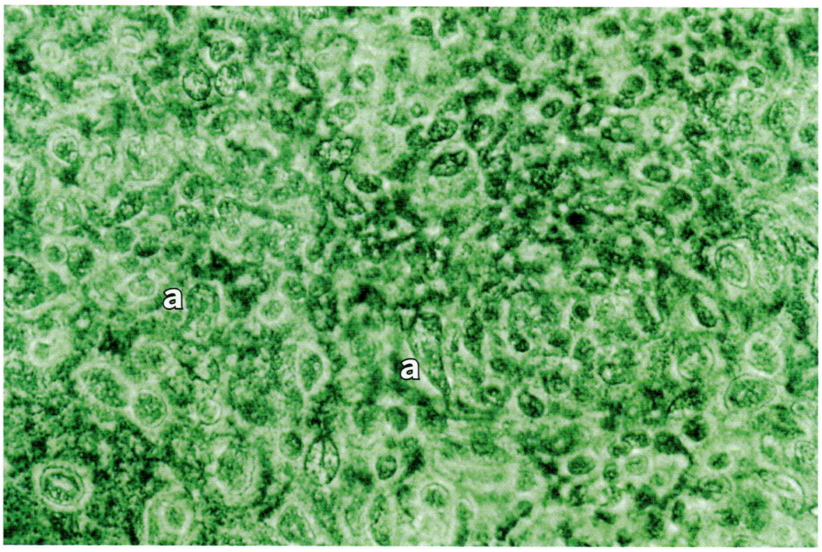

Figure 266 - Sheet of dyskaryotic cells with abnormal nuclei (a).

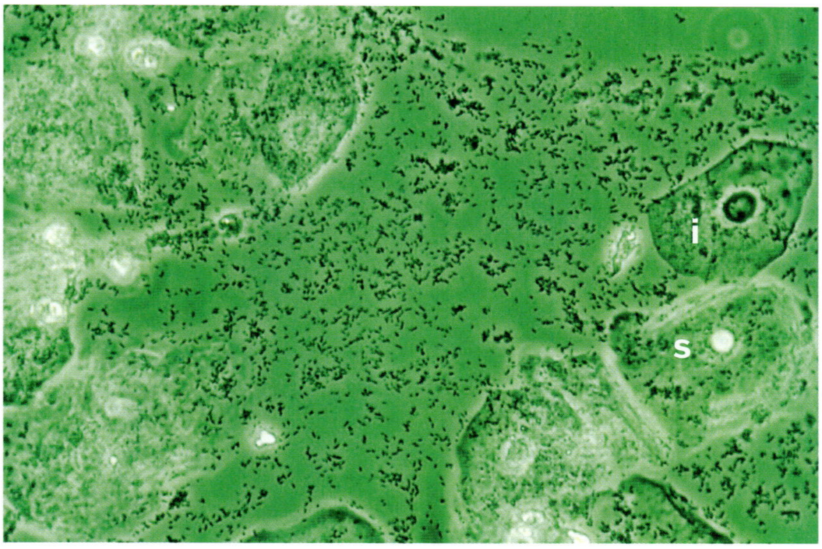

Figure 267 - Pleomorphic bacteria in Bacterial vaginosis. (i) Intermediate cell, (s) superficial cell.

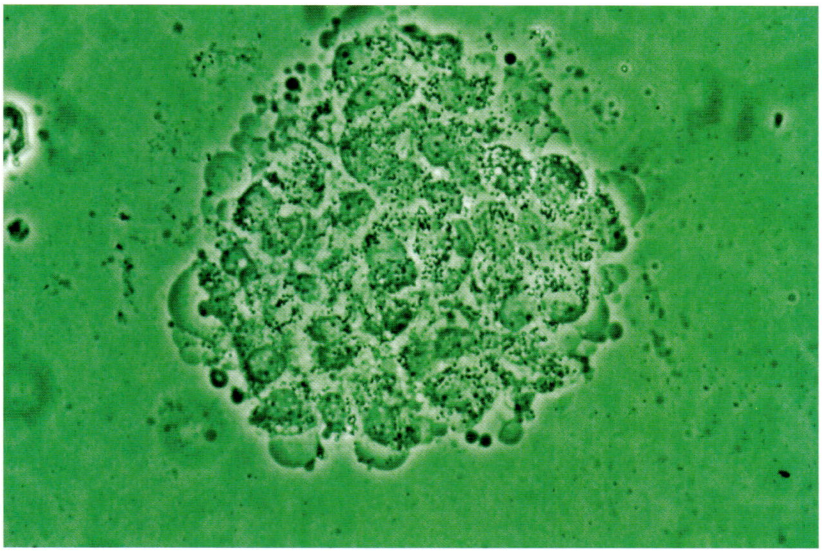

Figure 268 - Cocci adhered to a cluster of columnar cells.

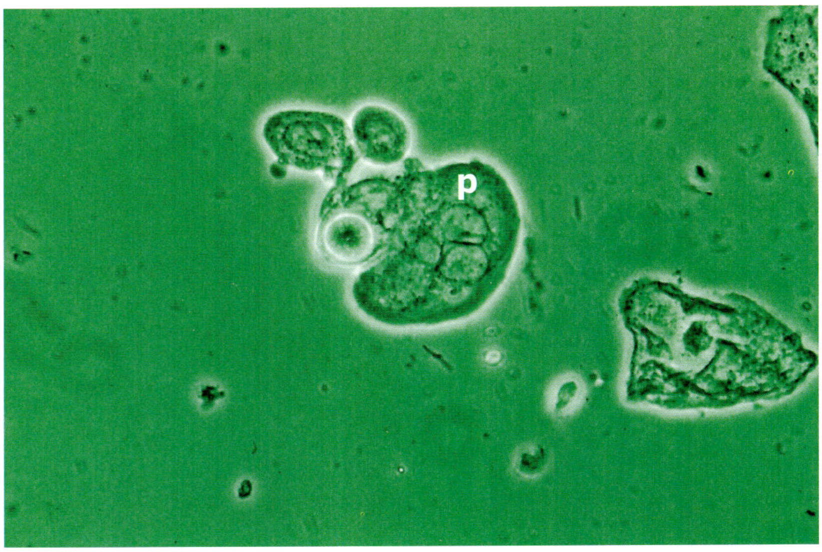

Figure 269 - Polykaryocyte (p) by HSV.

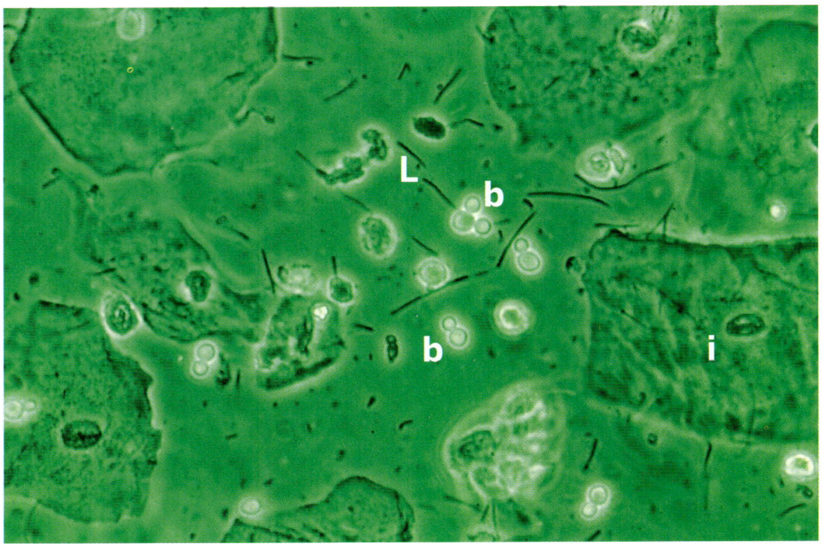

Figure 270 - Lactobacilli (L) and budding blastospores (b). (i) Intermediate cell.

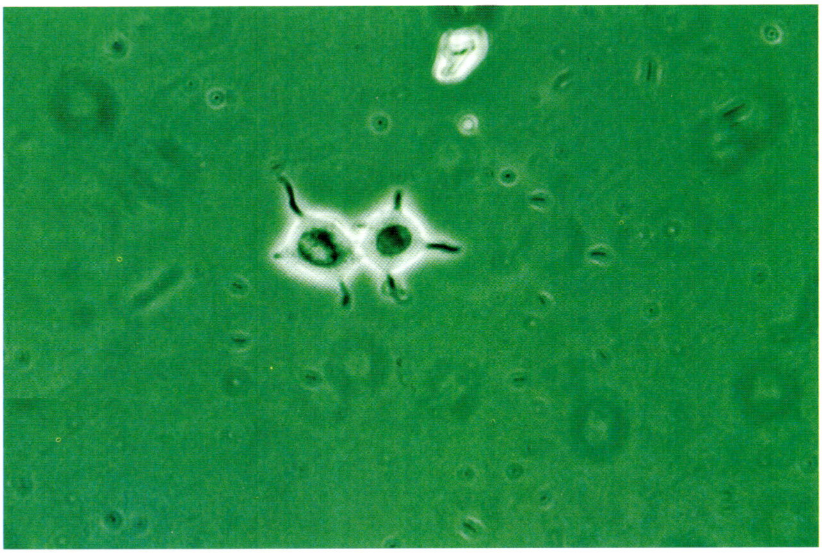

Figure 271 - Connecting immature metaplastic spider cells.

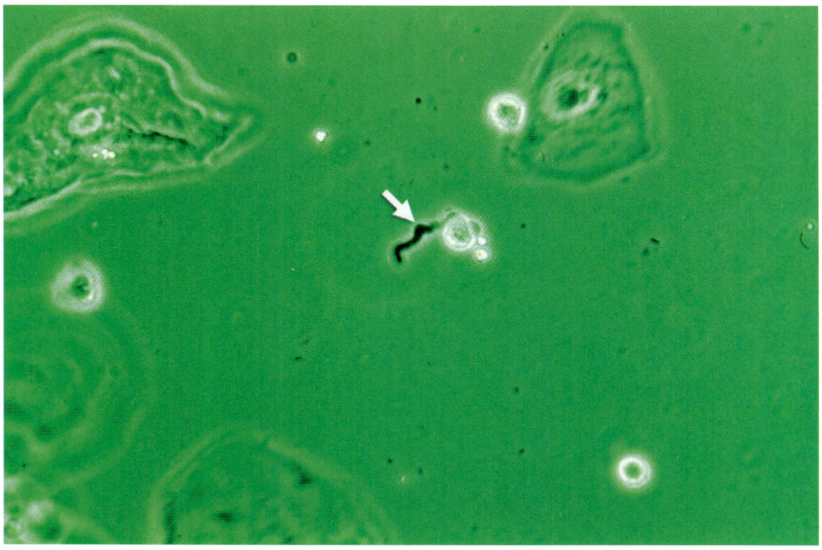

Figure 272 - Lymphocyte provided with a pseudopod (→).

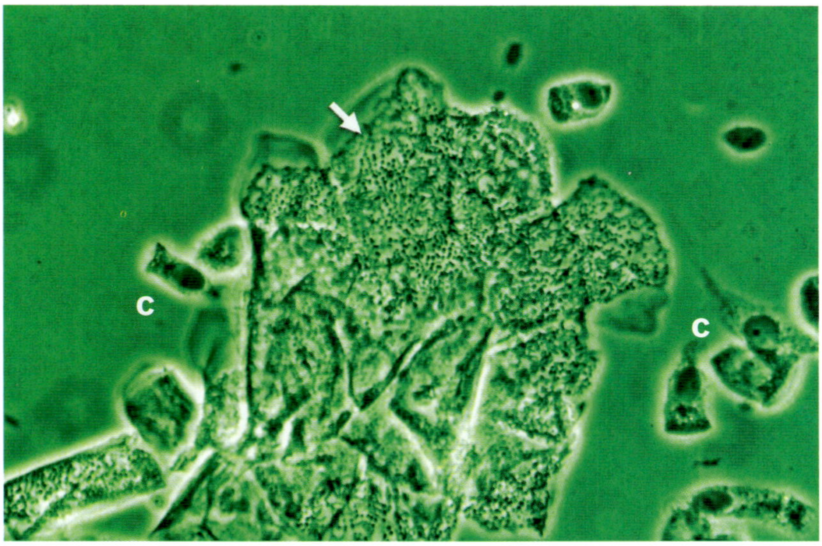

Figure 273 - Adhesion of cocci (→). (c) columnar cells.

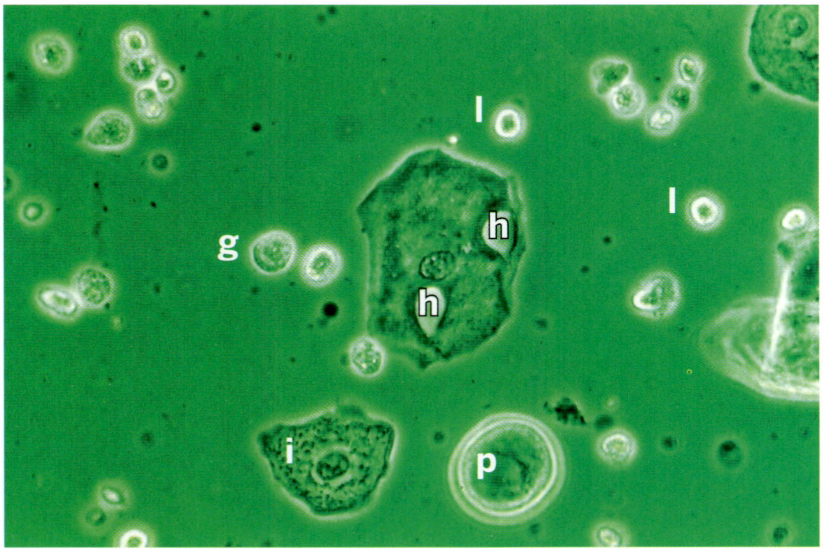

Figure 274 - Candida cytopathy: cytoplasmic holes (h). (i) Small intermediate cell, (p) parabasal cell, (l) lymphocytes, (g) granulocyte.

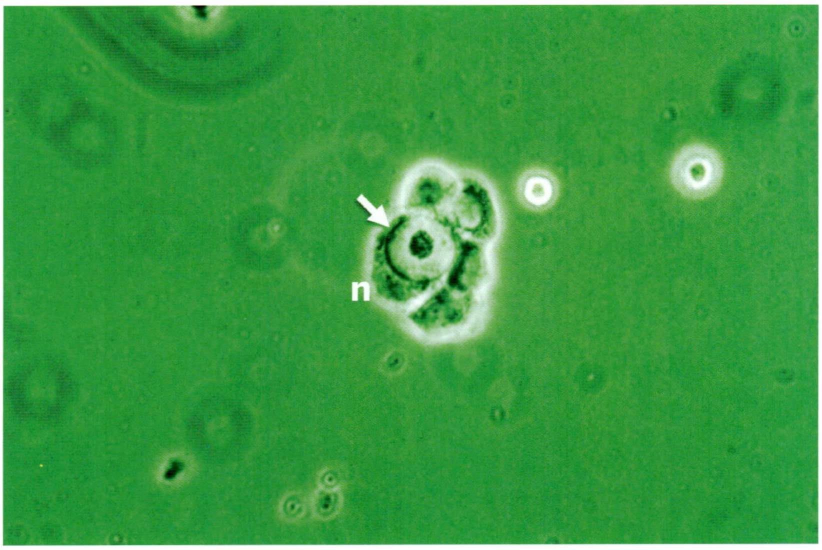

Figure 275 - Inclusion (→) of Chlamydia trachomatis containing a condensed body. (n) Nucleus.

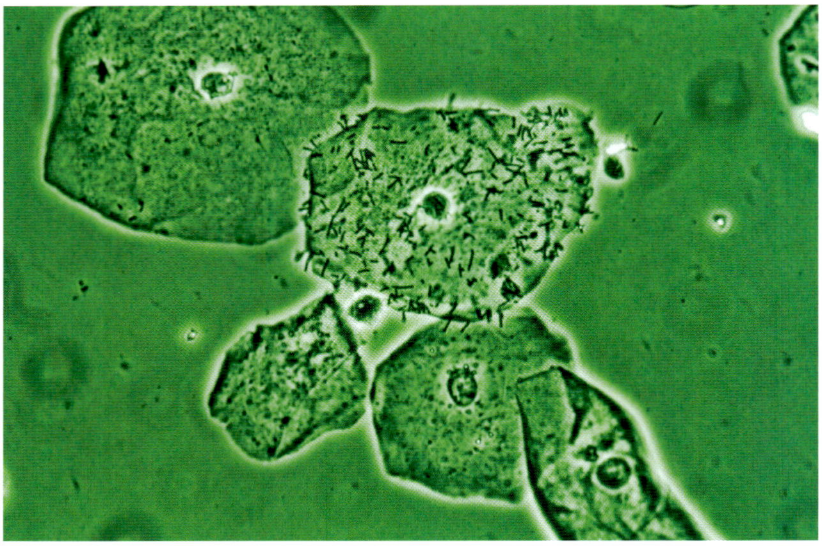

Figure 276 - Selective adhesion of Lactobacilli.

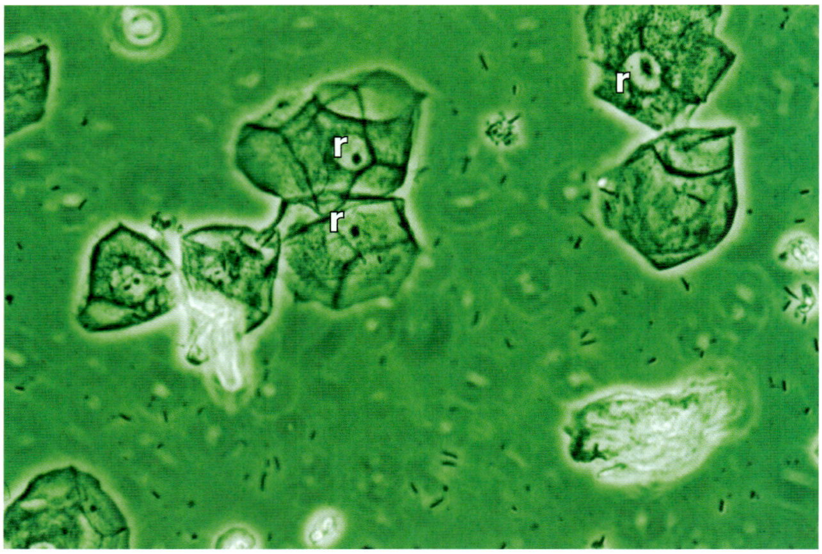

Figure 277 - Horny cells with residual chromatin (r).

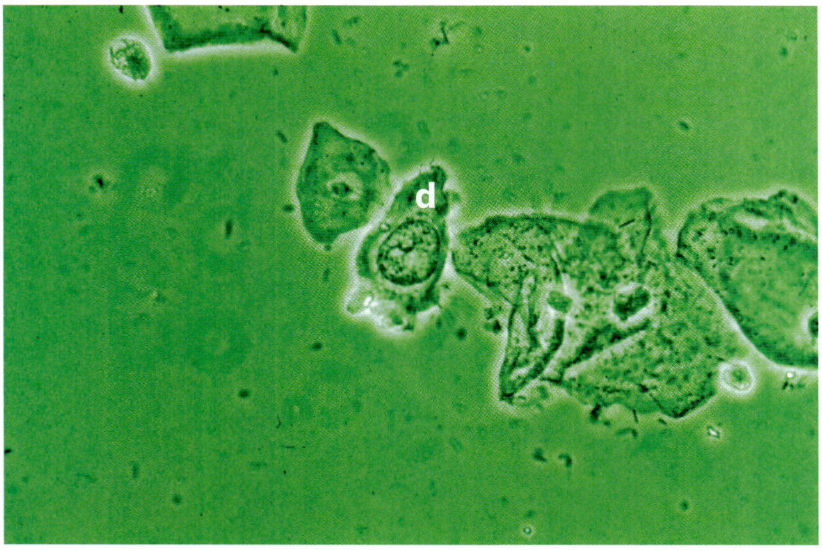

Figure 278 - Dyskaryotic cell (d) with an enlarged nucleus.

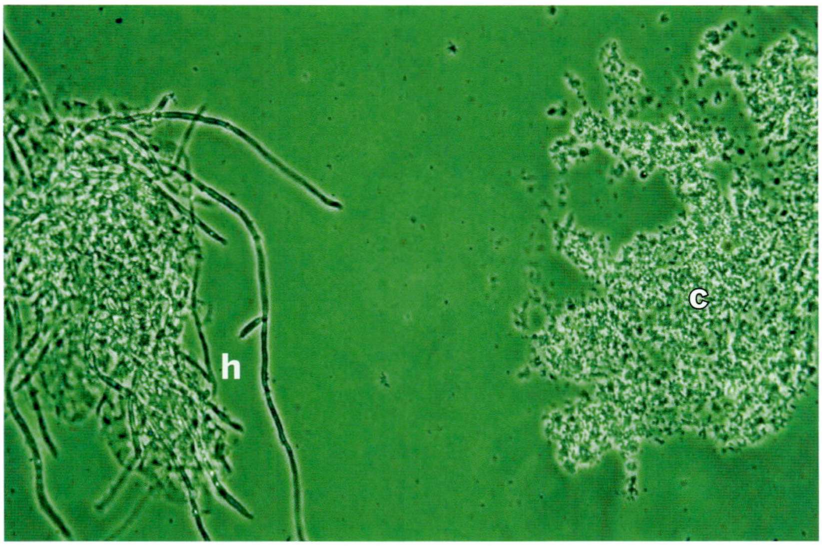

Figure 279 - Candida hyphae (h) and clue cells (c).

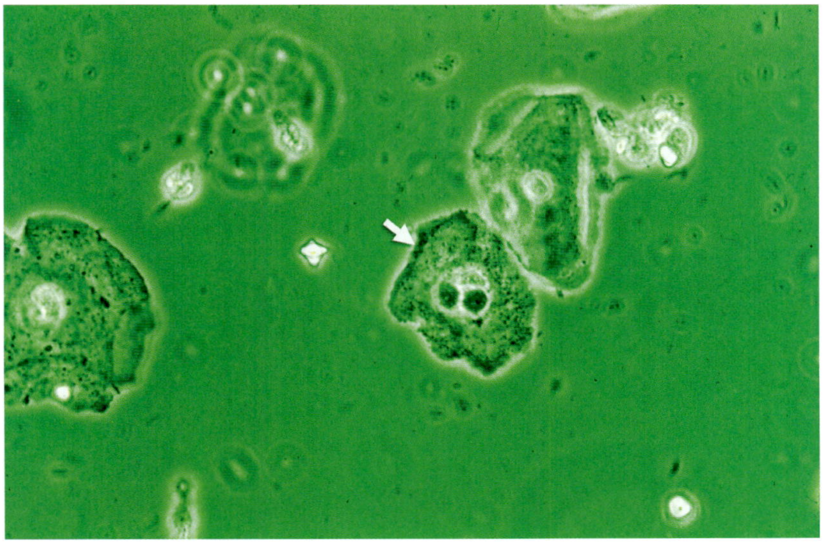

Figure 280 - The arrowed cell contains two dark nuclei and a third normal nucleus.

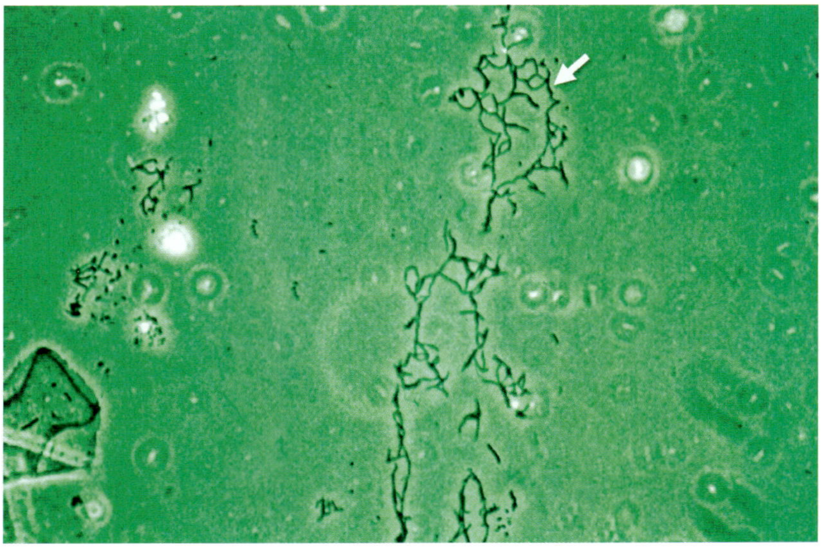

Figure 281 - Connecting Lactobacilli (social behavior).

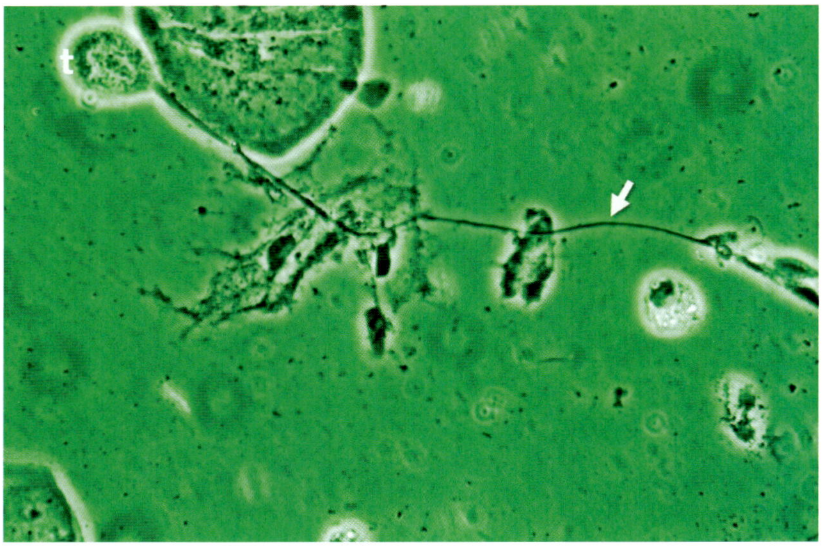

Figure 282 - Immature metaplastic tadpole cell (t) with a very long cytoplasmic process (→).

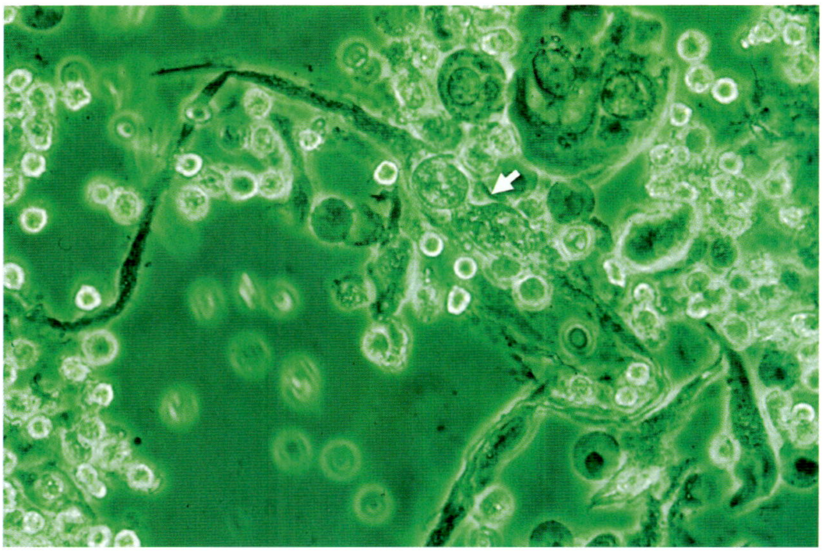

Figure 283 - Malignant fiber cell (→) with abnormal nuclei.

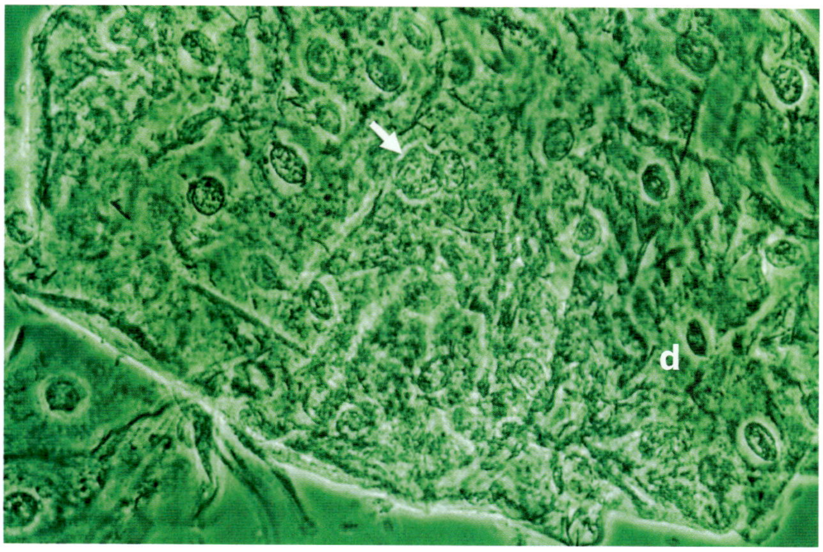

Figure 284 - Dyskaryotic cell (→) with overlapping nuclei. (d) Dark nucleus.

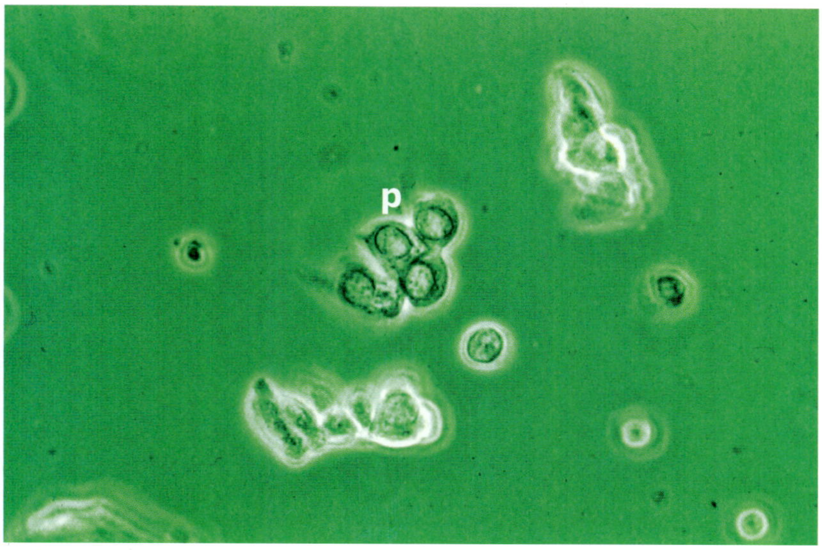

Figure 285 - Atrophic smear with parabasal cells (p).

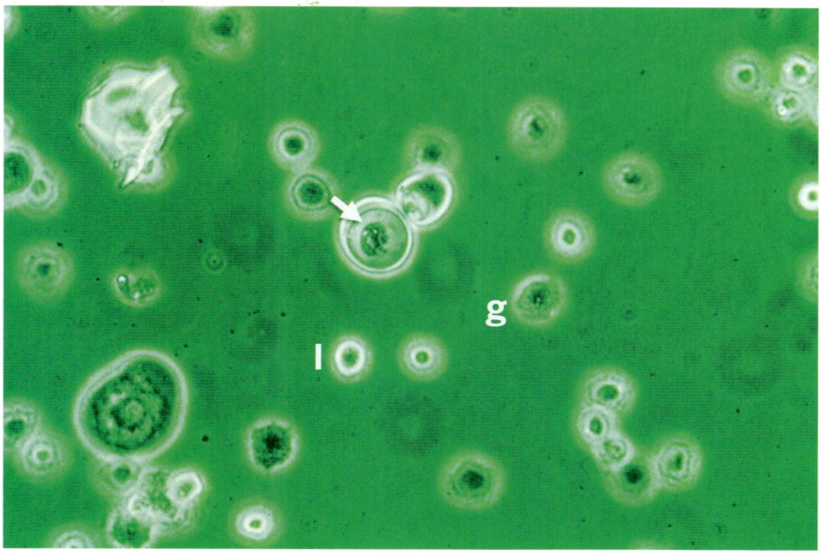

Figure 286 - Reserve cell changing into an immature parabasal-like cell. The arrow indicates ruptured chromatin. (l) Lymphocyte, (g) granulocyte.

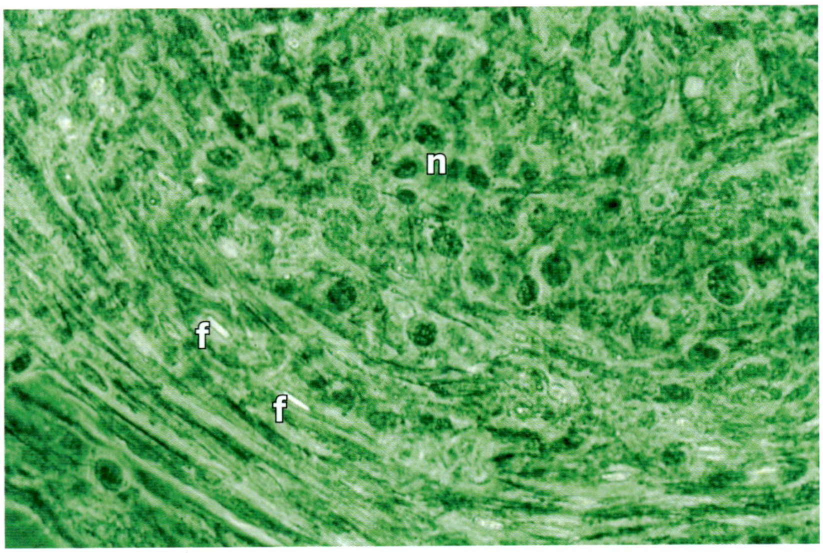

Figure 287 - Fiber superficial cells (f) and crowded nuclei (n) of intermediate cells (acanthosis).

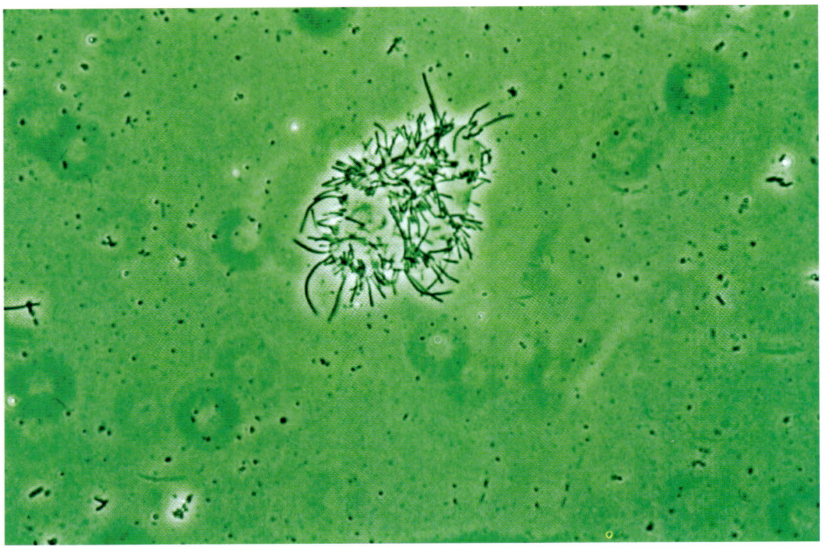

Figure 288 - Lactobacilli adhered to a horny cell. Background of cocci.

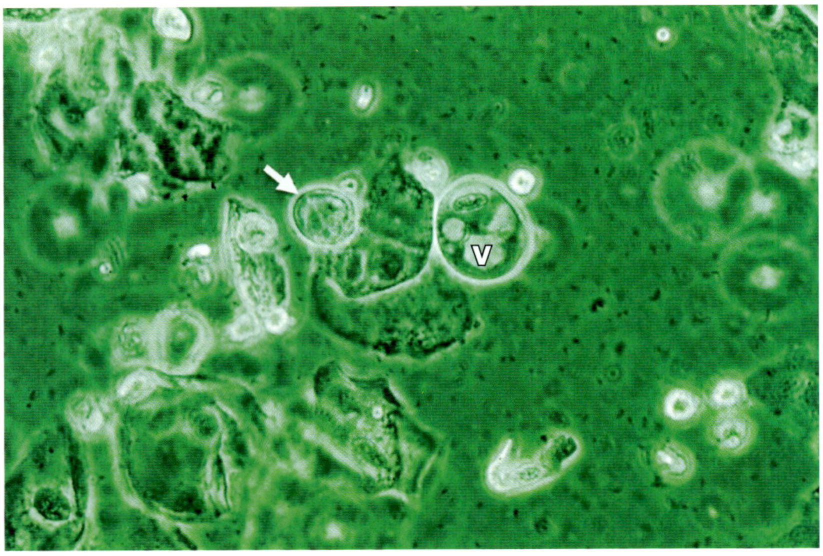

Figure 289 - Dyskaryotic cell (→) with an enlarged nucleus. Cytoplasmic vacuoles (v).

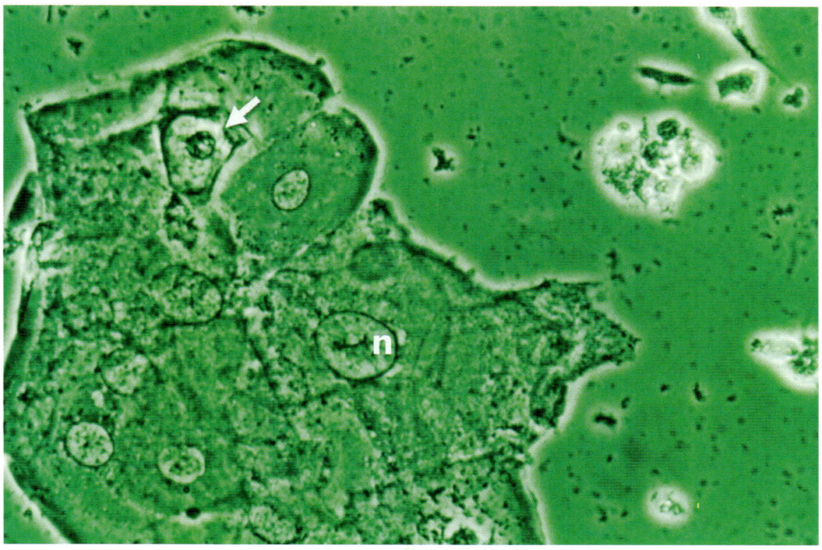

Figure 290 - Koilocyte (→) and enlarged nucleus (n).

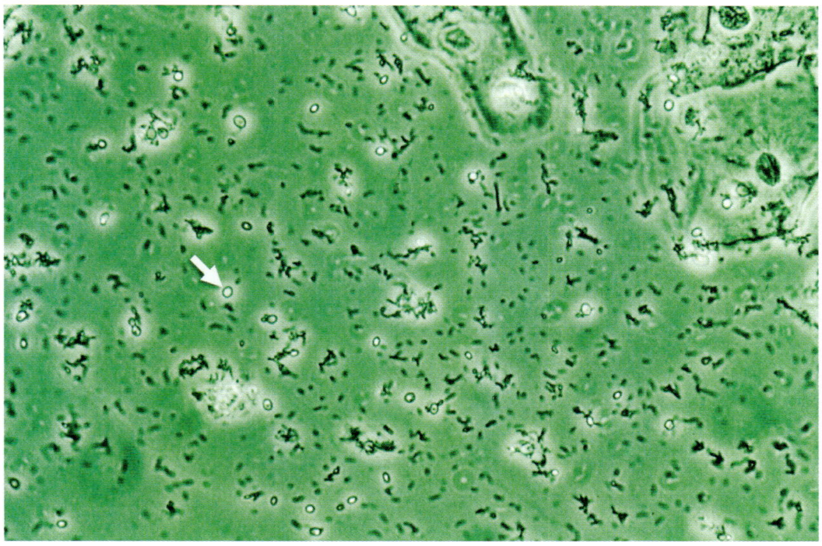

Figure 291 - Small spores of Torulopsis glabrata (→) associated with pleomorphic bacteria (Bacterial vaginosis).

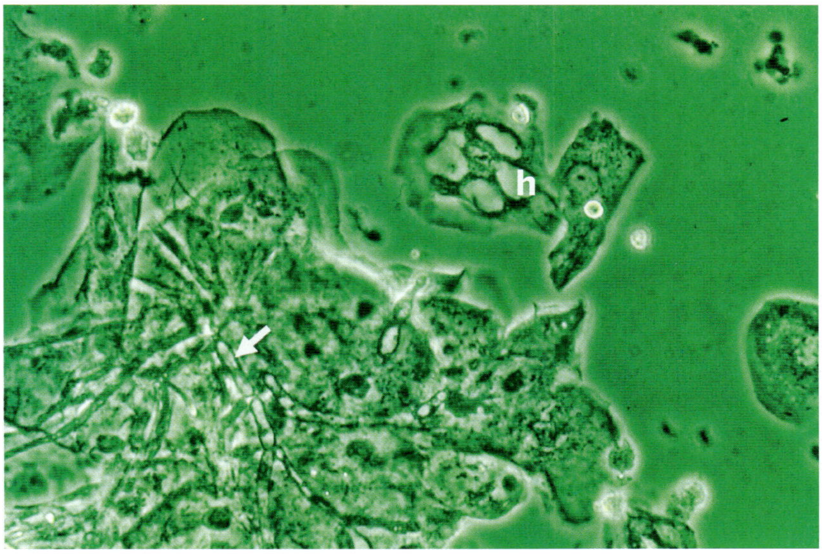

Figure 292 - Diaphanous aspect of intraepithelial hyphae (→) and cytoplasmic holes (h) (Candida cytopathy).

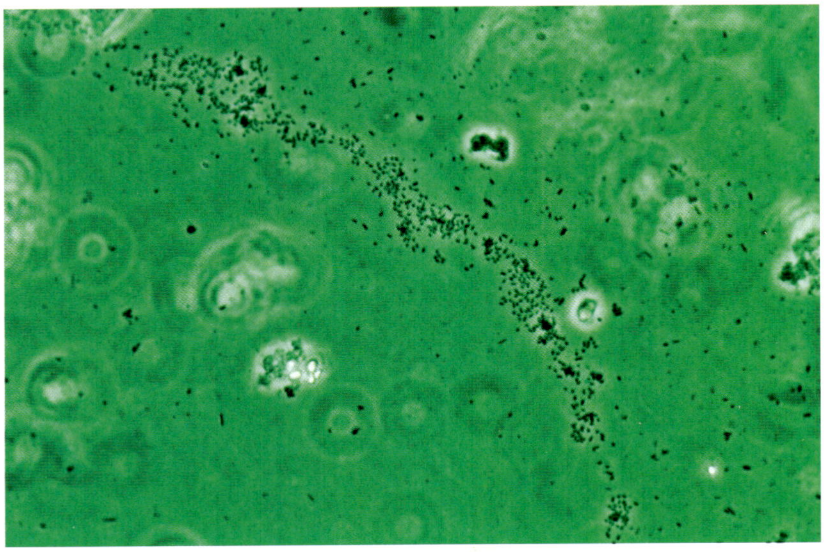

Figure 293 - Pleomorphic bacteria (Bacterial vaginosis).

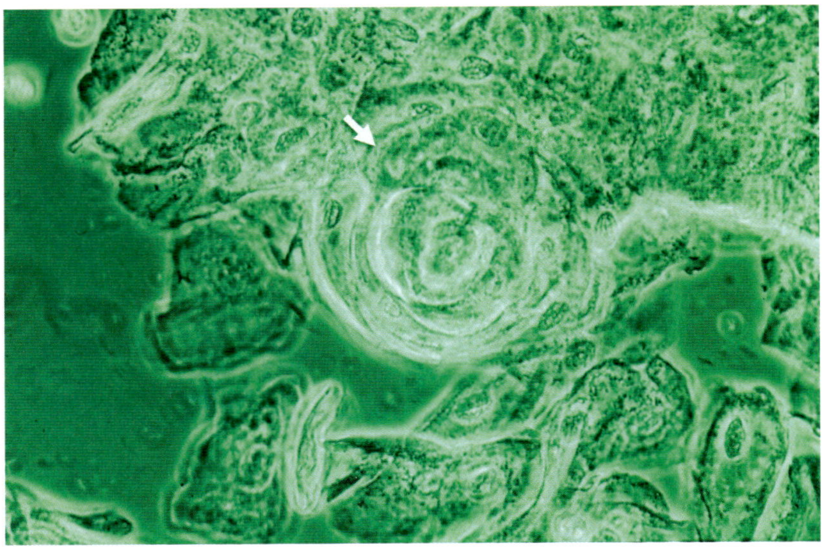

Figure 294 - Benign epithelial pearl (→).

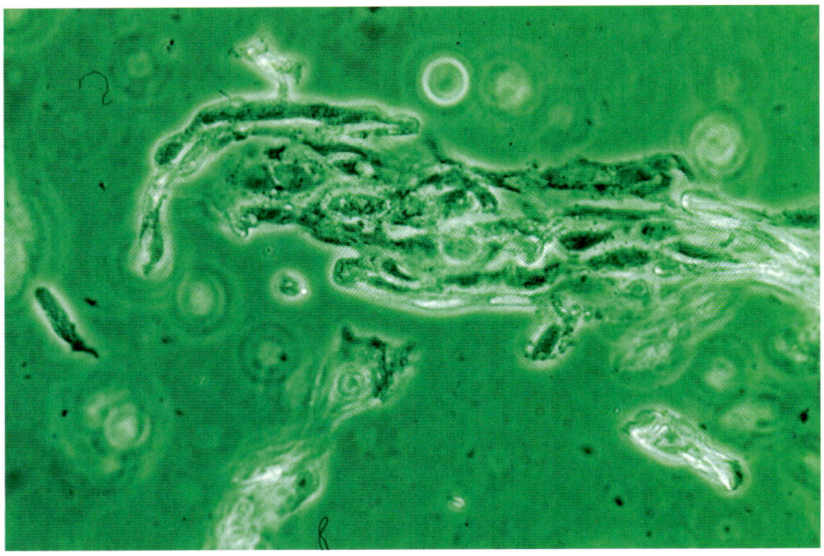

Figure 295 - Malignant cells.

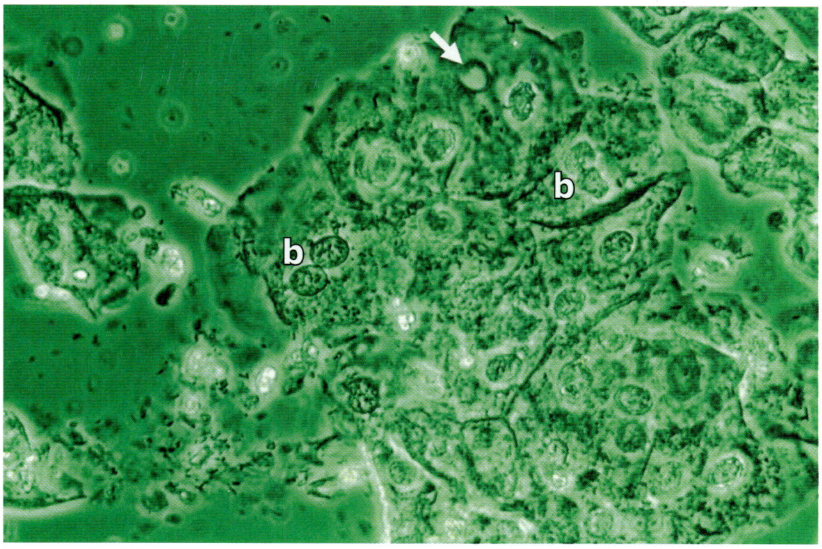

Figure 296 - Binucleate cells (b) and cytoplasmic hole (→) (Candida cytopathy).

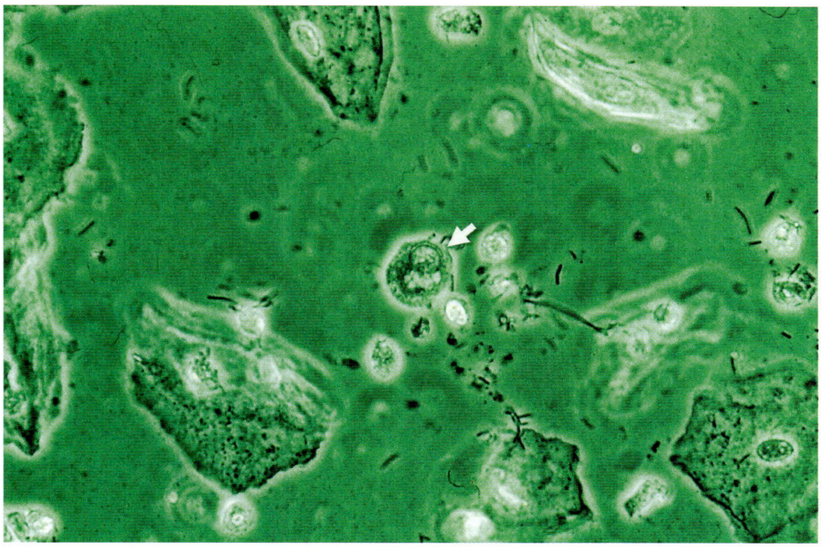

Figure 297 - Binucleate dyskaryotic cell (→) with anisokaryosis.

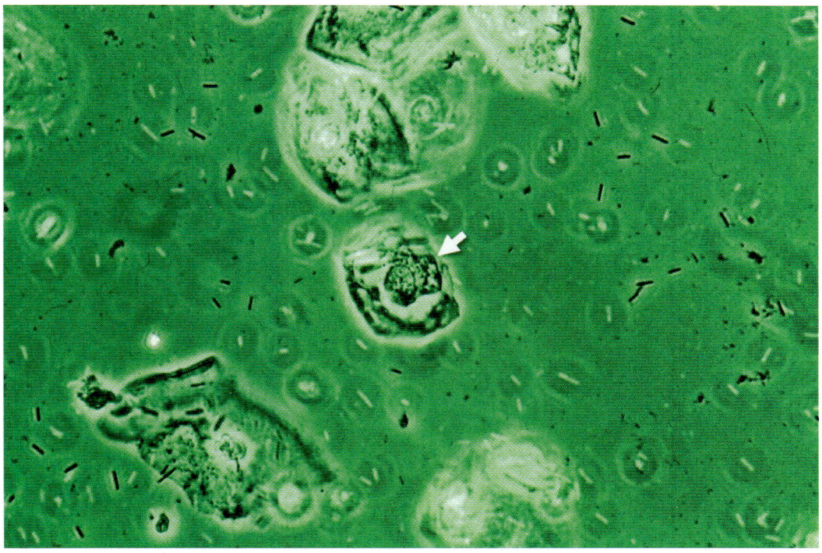

Figure 298 - Koilocyte (→) containing three overlapping nuclei.

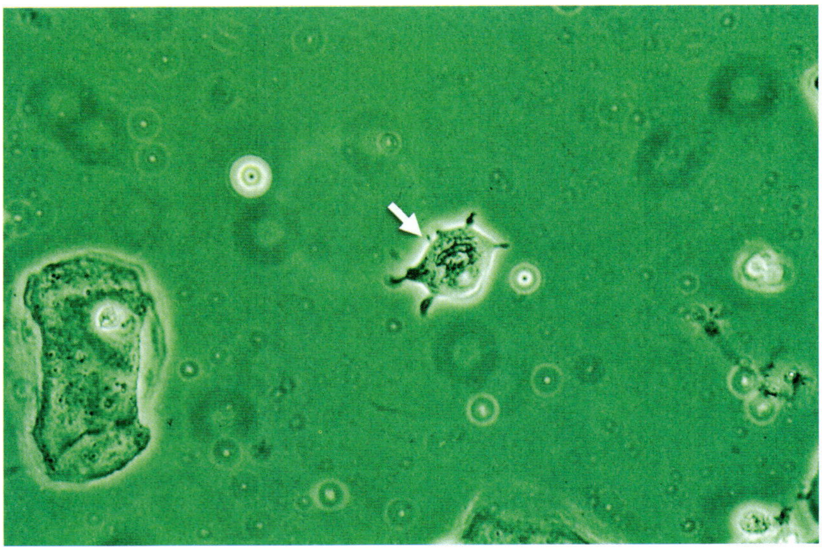

Figure 299 - Dyskaryotic binucleate immature metaplastic spider cell with anisokaryosis.

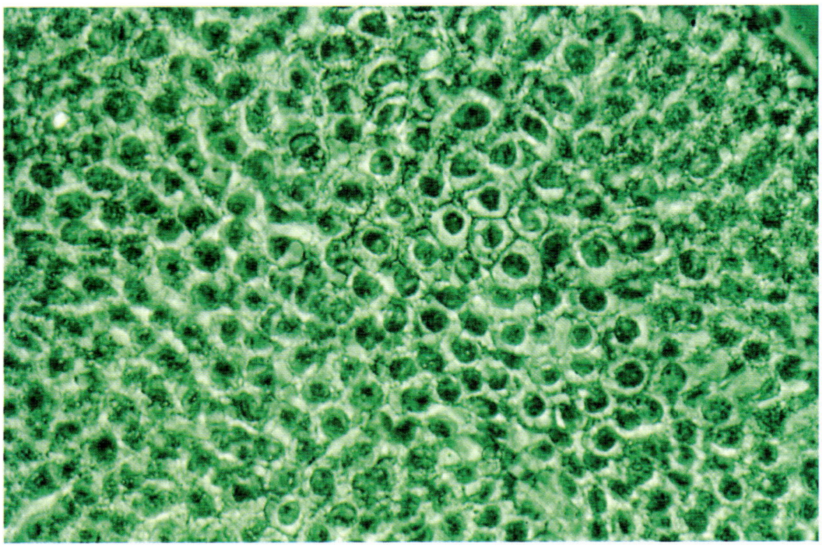

Figure 300 - Sheet of endometrial cells with clumped chromatin.

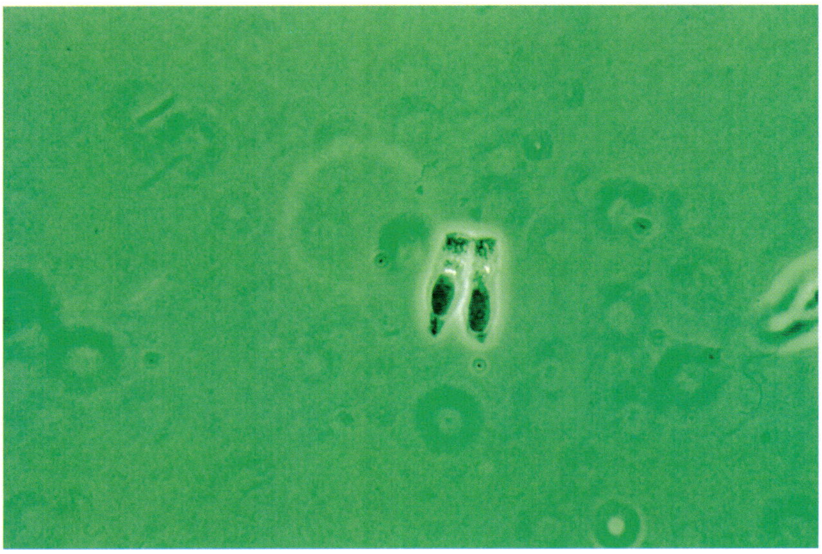

Figure 301 - Endocervical columnar cells with dark nuclei (HPV infection).

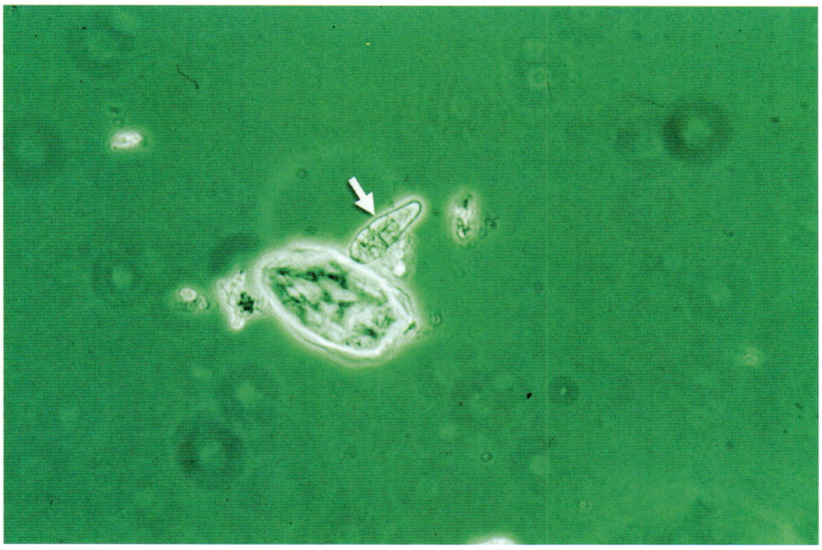

Figure 302 - Blastoconidium of Alternaria (→).

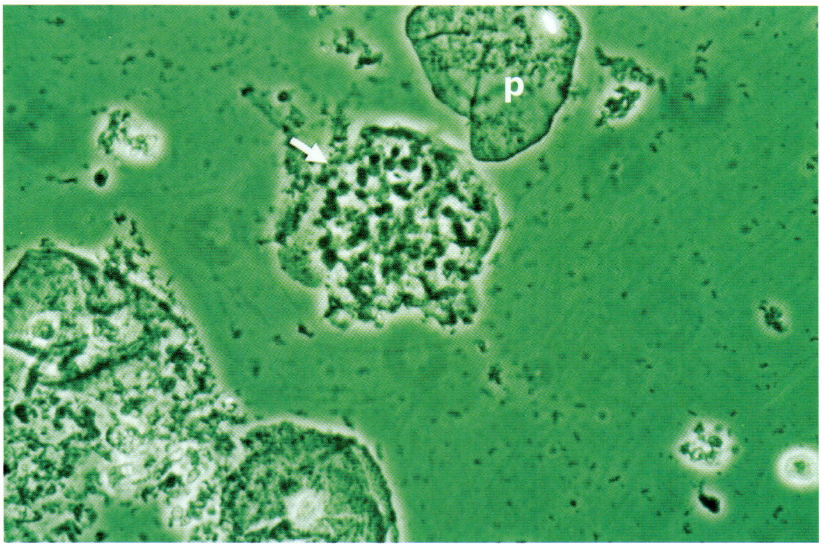

Figure 303 - Adhered degenerate fungal spores (→). (p) Parakeratotic cell.

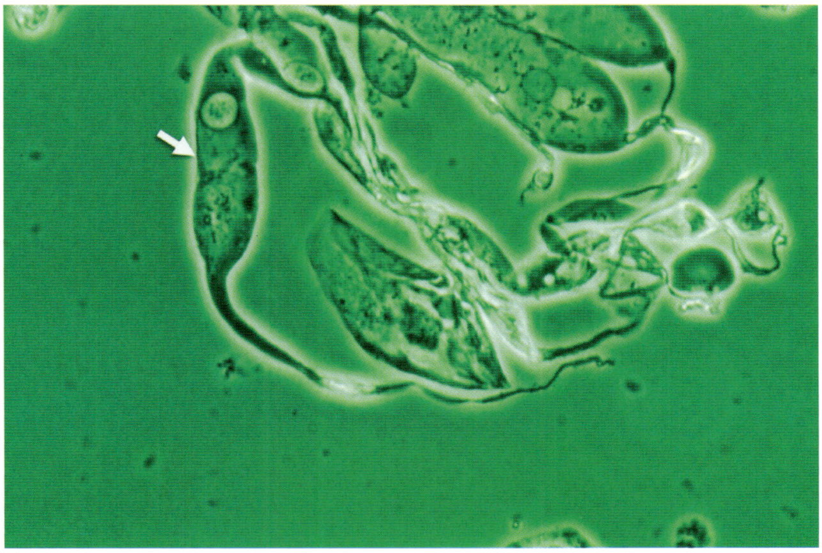

Figure 304 - Immature metaplastic tadpole cell (→).

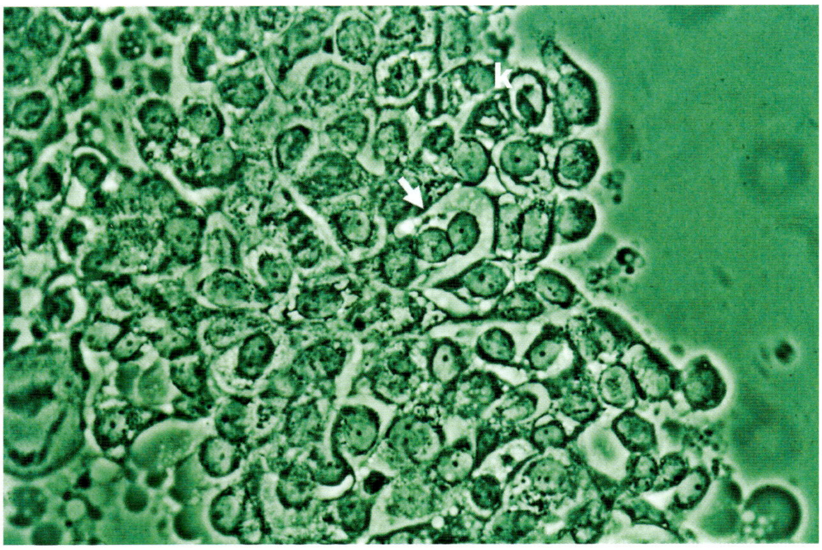

Figure 305 - Sheet of endocervical cells. The arrow indicates a binucleate koilocyte. (k) Koilocyte with dark nucleus.

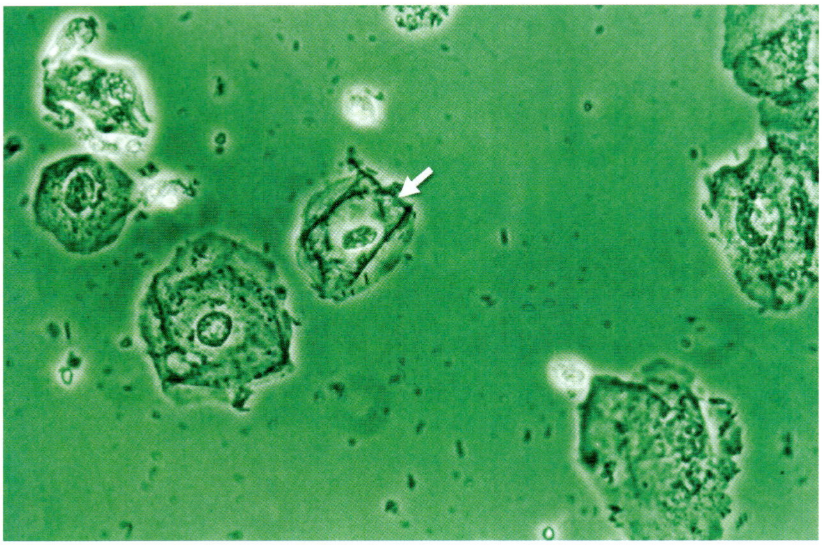

Figure 306 - Koilocyte (→).

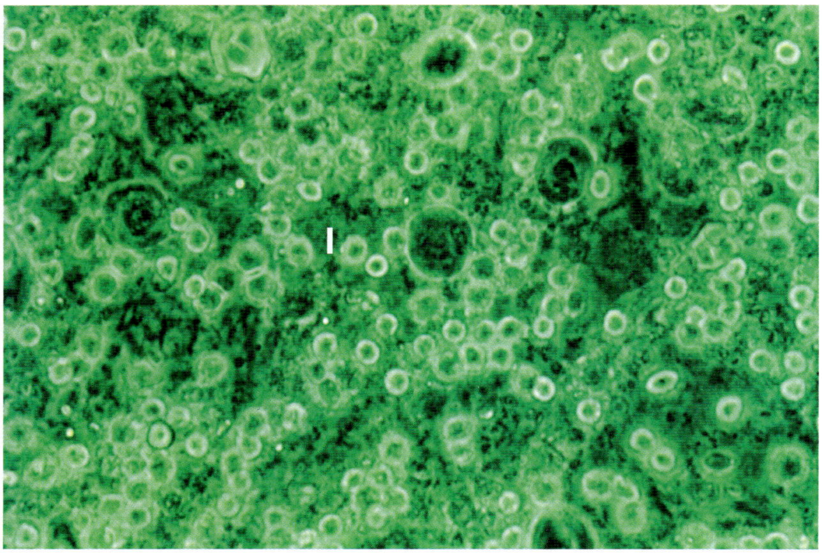

Figure 307 - Background of lymphocytes (l) in HSV infection.

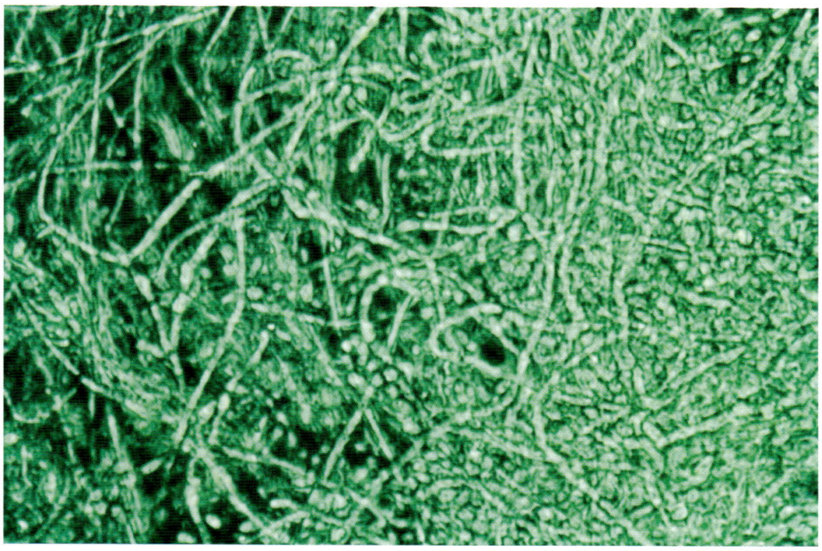

Figure 308 - Diaphanous aspect of intraepithelial Candida hyphae.

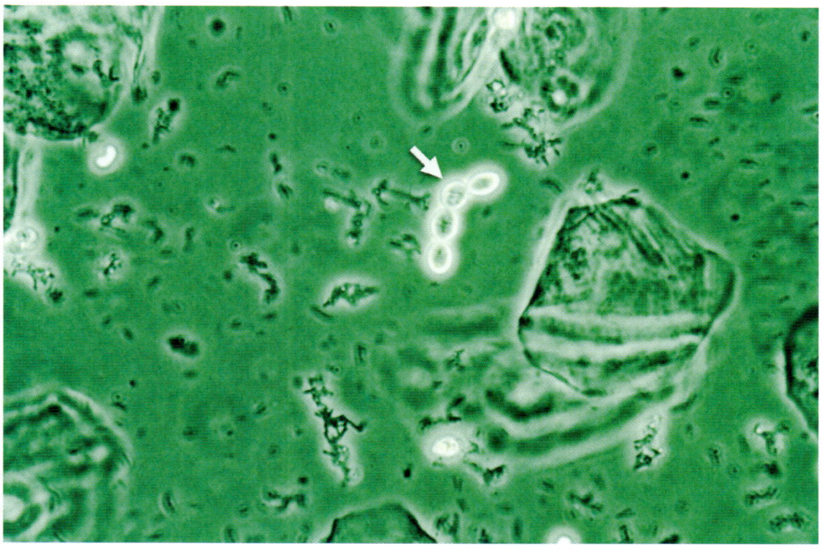

Figure 309 - Budding blastospores of Saccharomyces (→).

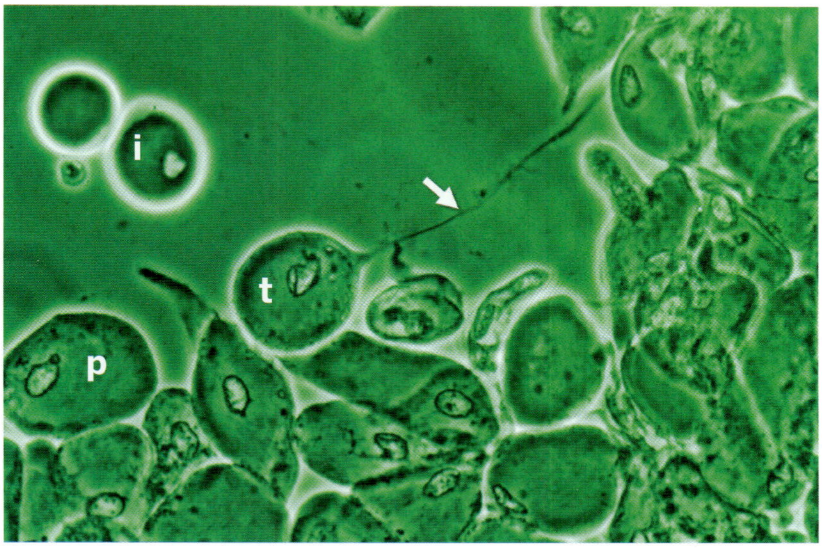

Figure 310 - Metaplastic immature tadpole cell (t) with a long cytoplasmic process (→). The partial dark esoplasmic ring indicates that the cell is turning into a metaplastic maturing cell. (i) Metaplastic immature parabasal-like cell, (p) metaplastic premature cell deriving from a metaplastic immature parabasal-like cell.

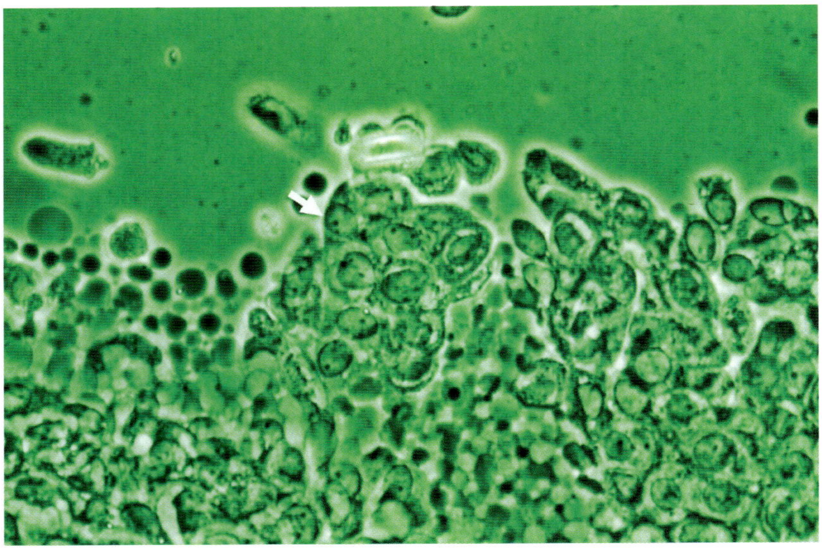

Figure 311 - Cell syncytium (→) by HSV.

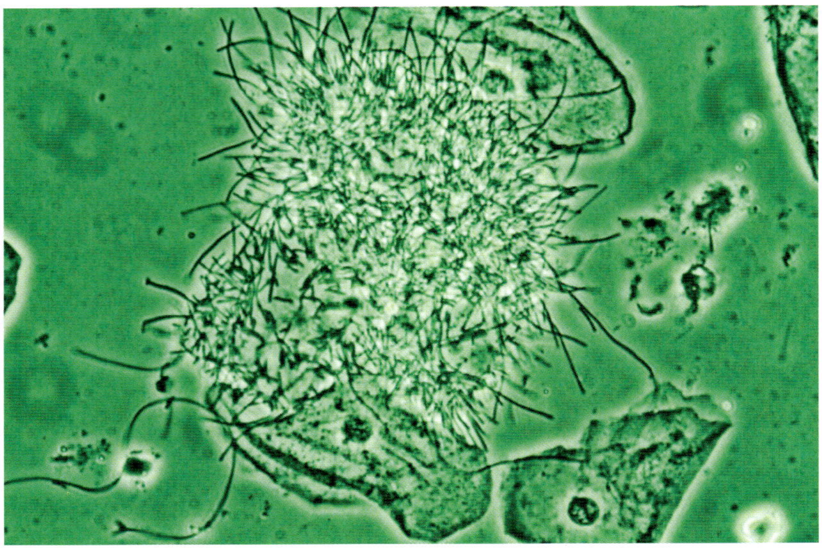

Figure 312 - Tip adhesion of long filamentous Lactobacilli.

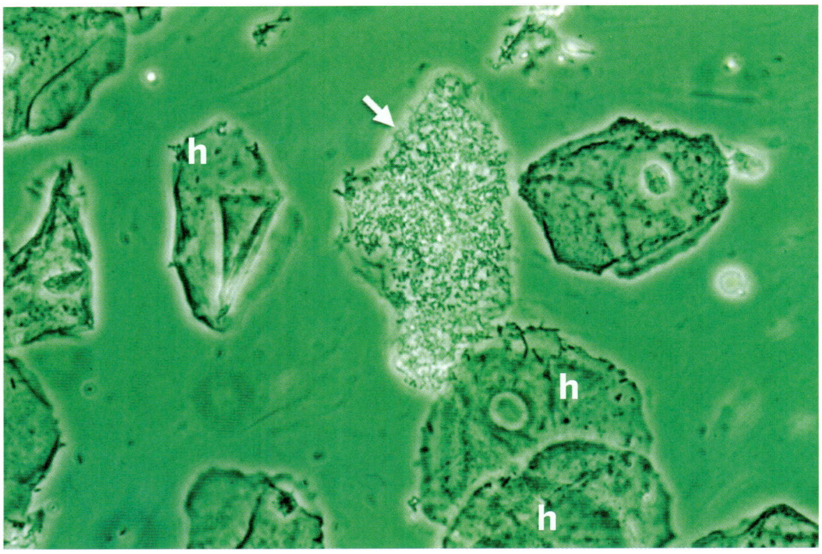

Figure 313 - Clue cell (→) (Bacterial vaginosis). (h) Horny cells.

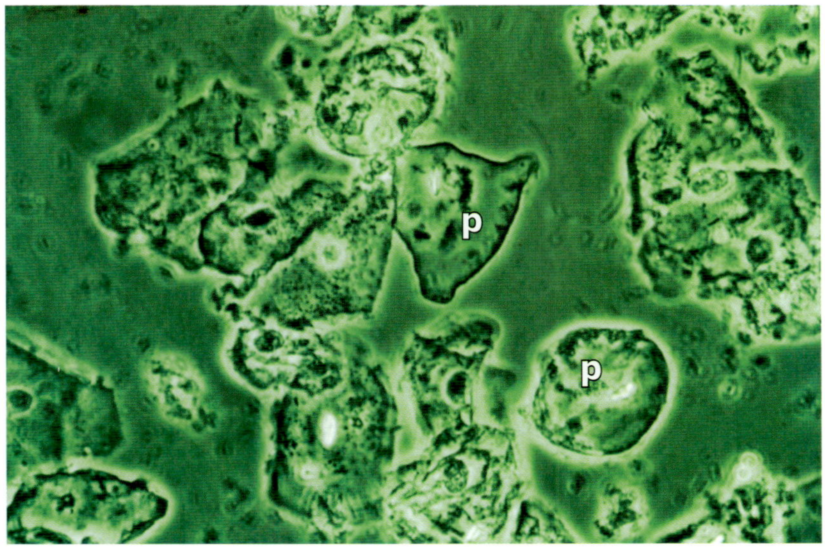

Figure 314 - Parakeratotic cells (p).

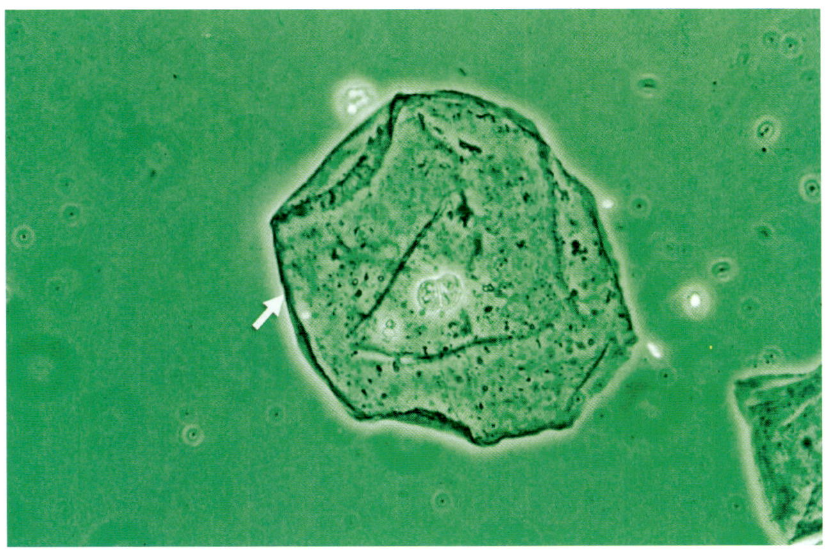

Figure 315 - Binucleate superficial cell with marginal keratinization (→).

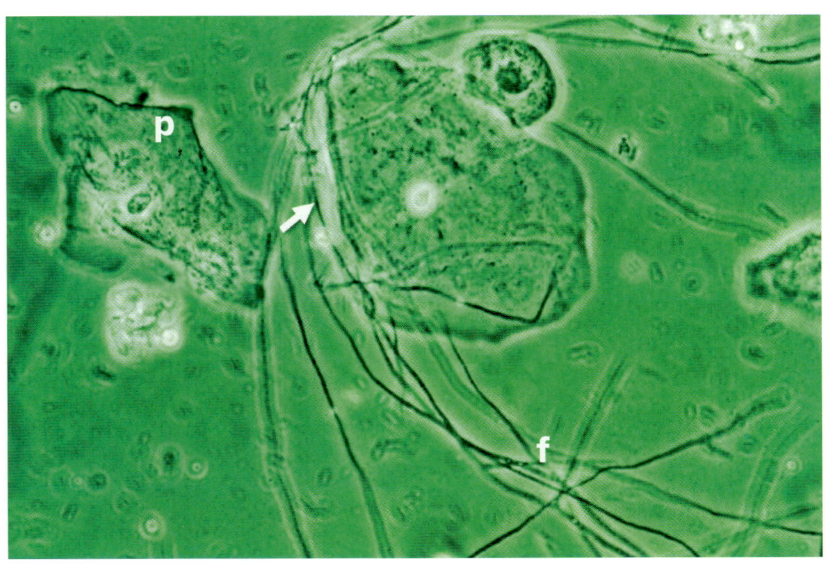

Figure 316 - Thin filaments (f) of Nocardia asteroides. The arrow indicates a cytoplasmic groove (Candida cytopathy). (p) Parakeratotic cell.

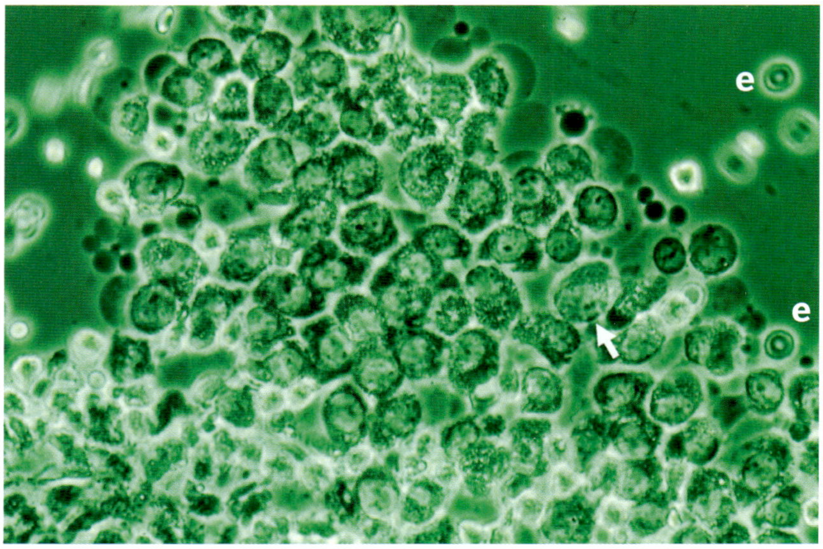

Figure 317 - Endocervical cells with a flocculent cytoplasm, pale nuclei and evident nucleoli. The arrow indicates sex chromatin (Barr body). (e) Erythrocytes.

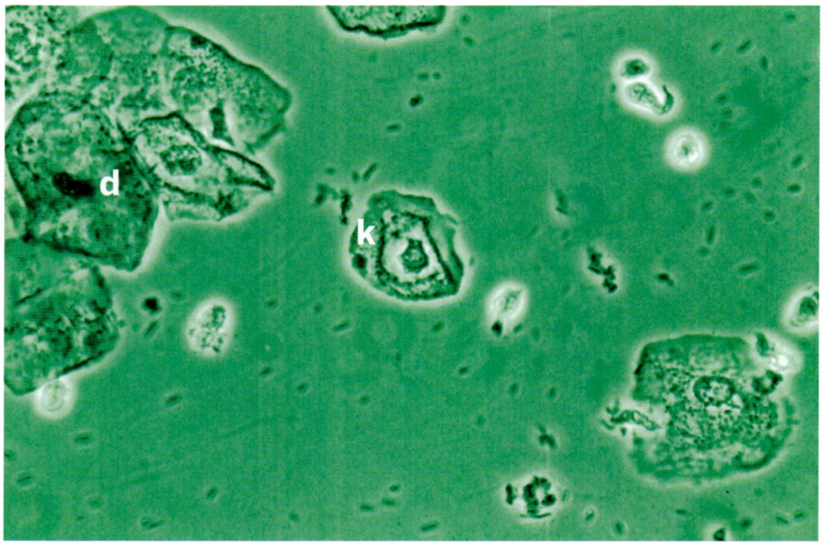

Figure 318 - Koilocyte (k) and dark nucleus (d) by HPV.

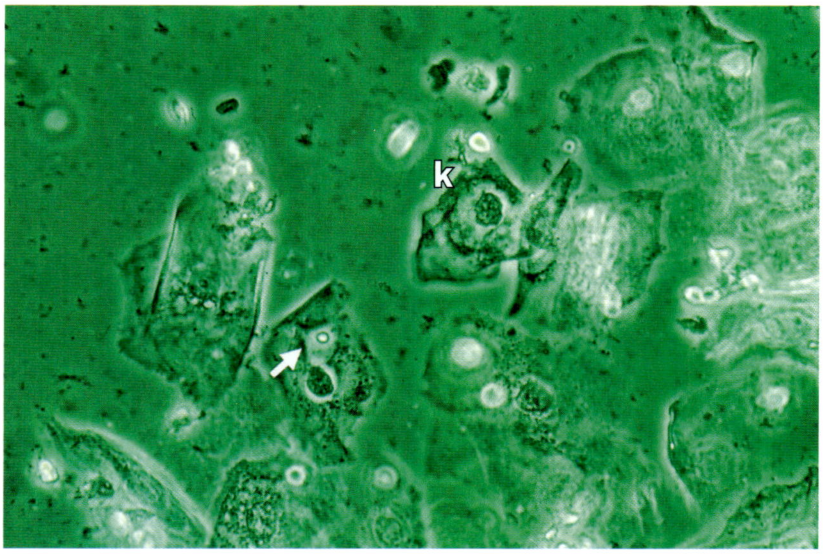

Figure 319 - The arrow indicates a cytoplasmic hole (Candida cytopathy) containing a fungal spore. (k) Koilocyte.

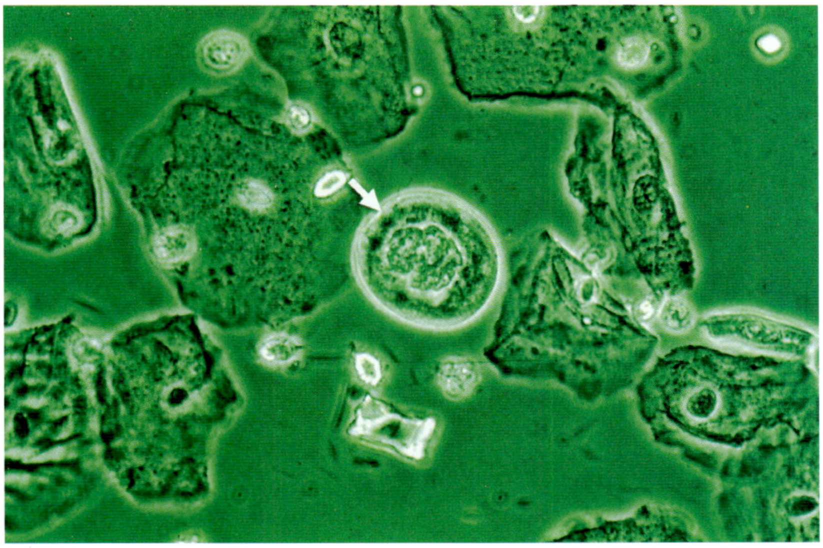

Figure 320 - Dyskaryotic cell (→) with multiple overlapping nuclei (HPV infection).

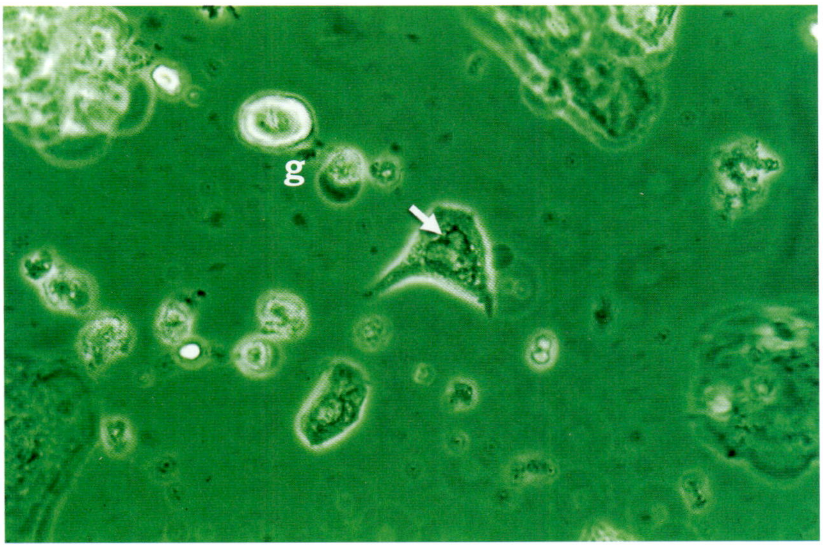

Figure 321 - Dyskaryotic immature metaplastic spider cell with a clear-cut indentation into the nucleoplasm (→). (g) Granulocyte expelling a vescicle of exocytosis.

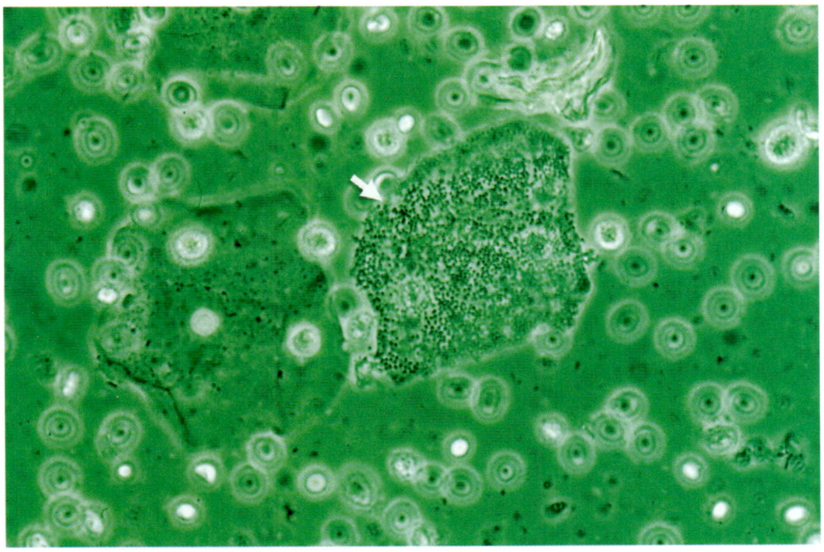

Figure 322 - Adhesion of cocci (→) and background of erythrocytes during menstruation.

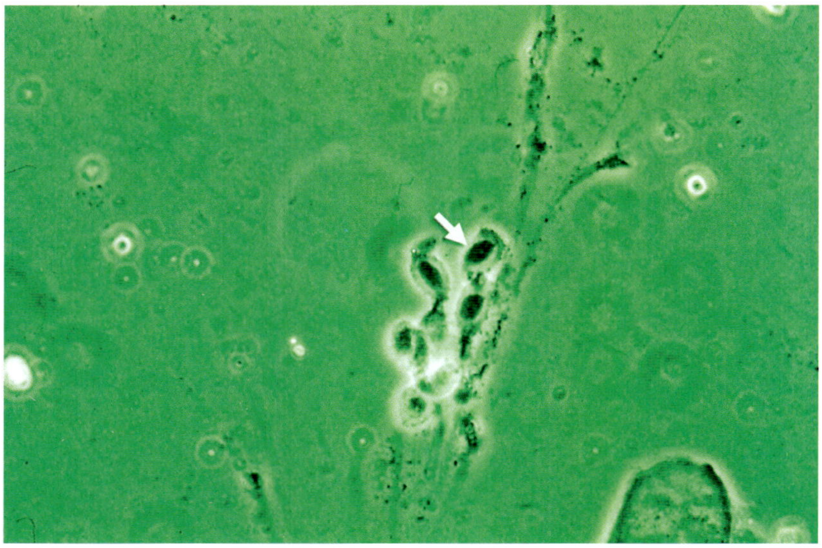

Figure 323 - Endocervical columnar cells with dark nucleus (→) (HPV infection).

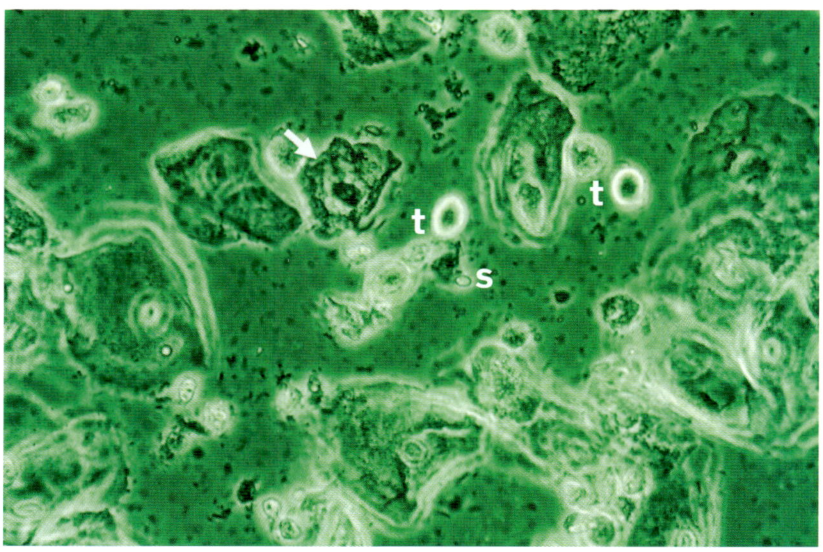

Figure 324 - The arrow indicates a koilocyte. (t) trichomonads, (s) fungal spore.

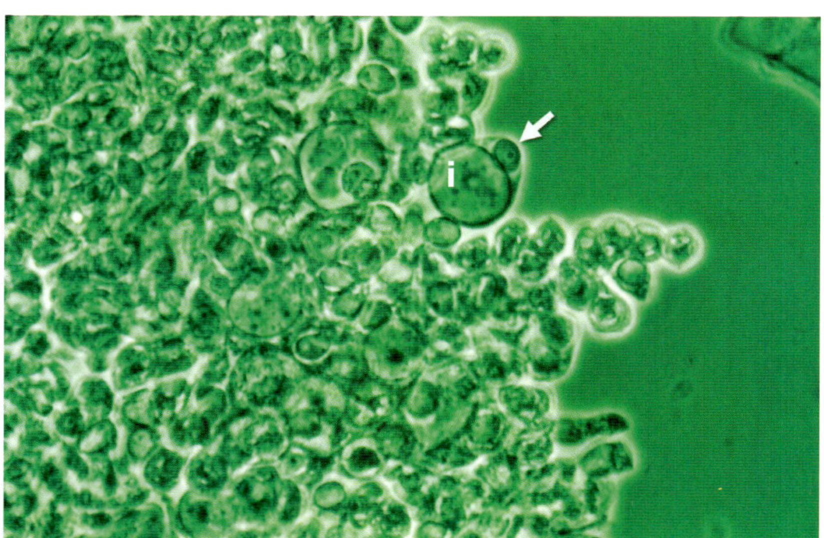

Figure 325 - Cell (→) containig a large inclusion (i) of Chlamydia trachomatis. The nucleus is pushed against one pole of the cell.

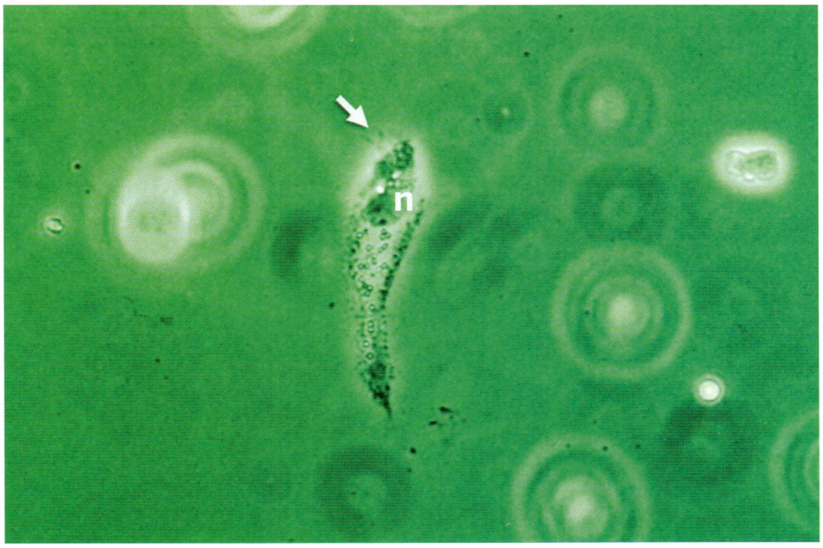

Figure 326 - Ciliated (→) and secretory endocervical cell. The nucleus (n) is displaced by the vacuoles of mucus and pushed toward the upper portion of the cell.

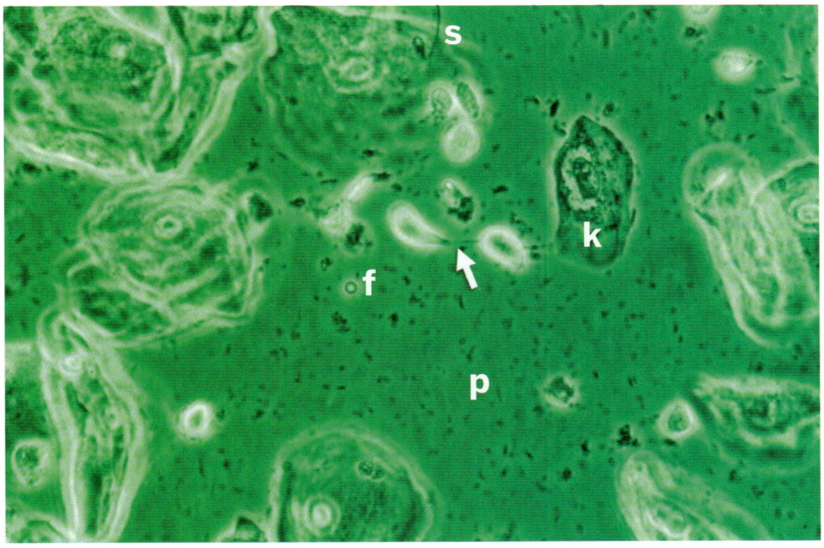

Figure 327 - Mixed vaginal infection: (k) koilocyte by HPV, (f) fungal spore, (p) pleomorphic bacteria of Bacterial vaginosis, two trichomonads connected by their axostyle (→). (s) Spermatozoon.

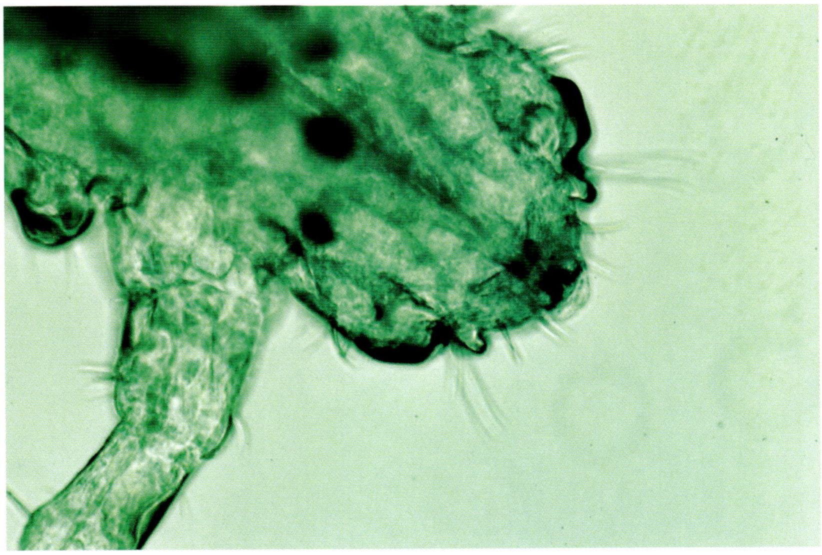

Figure 328 - Head of pubic louse (contaminant).